CLINICS IN CHEST MEDICINE

Pulmonary Considerations in Organ and Hematopoietic Stem Cell Transplantation

GUEST EDITORS
Robert M. Kotloff, MD, and
Vivek N. Ahya, MD

December 2005 • Volume 26 • Number 4

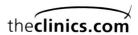

SAUNDERS

An Imprint of Elsevier, Inc.
PHILADELPHIA   LONDON   TORONTO   MONTREAL   SYDNEY   TOKYO

W.B. SAUNDERS COMPANY
A Division of Elsevier Inc.

Elsevier, Inc. • 1600 John F. Kennedy Boulevard • Suite 1800 • Philadelphia, Pennsylvania 19103-2899

http://www.chestmed.theclinics.com

CLINICS IN CHEST MEDICINE   **Volume 26, Number 4**
December 2005   **ISSN 0272-5231**
Editor: Sarah E. Barth   **ISBN 1-4160-2813-7**

Reprints: For copies of 100 or more, of articles in this publication, please contact the Commercial Reprints Department, Elsevier Inc., 360 Park Avenue South, New York, New York 10010-1710. Tel. (212) 633-3813 Fax: (212) 462-1935 e-mail: reprints@elsevier.com.

The ideas and opinions expressed in *Clinics in Chest Medicine* do not necessarily reflect those of the Publisher. The Publisher does not assume any responsibility for any injury and/or damage to persons or property arising out of or related to any use of the material contained in this periodical. The reader is advised to check the appropriate medical literature and the product information currently provided by the manufacturer of each drug to be administered to verify the dosage, the method and duration of administration, or contraindications. It is the responsibility of the treating physician or other health care professional, relying on independent experience and knowledge of the patient, to determine drug dosages and the best treatment for the patient. Mention of any product in this issue should not be construed as endorsement by the contributors, editors, or the Publisher of the product or manufacturers' claims.

Clinics in Chest Medicine (ISSN 0272-5231) is published quarterly by W.B. Saunders Company. Corporate and editorial offices: Elsevier, Inc., 1600 John F. Kennedy Boulevard, Suite 1800, Philadelphia, PA 19103-2899. Accounting and circulation offices: 6277 Sea Harbor Drive, Orlando, FL 32887-4800. Periodicals postage paid at Orlando, FL 32887, and additional mailing offices. Subscription price is $195.00 per year (US individuals), $300.00 per year (US institutions), $215.00 per year (Canadian individuals), $360.00 per year (Canadian institutions), $250.00 per year (international individuals), and $360.00 per year (international institutions). International air speed delivery is included in all *Clinics* subscription prices. All prices are subject to change without notice. POSTMASTER: Send address changes to *Clinics in Chest Medicine* (ISSN 0272-5231), W.B. Saunders Company, Periodicals Fulfillment, Orlando, FL 32887-4800. **Customer Service: 1-800-654-2452 (US). From outside of the US, call 1-407-345-4000.**

Clinics in Chest Medicine is covered in *Index Medicus, Current Contents/Clinical Medicine, EMBASE/Excerpta Medica, Science Citation Index,* and *ISI/BIOMED.*

Printed in the United States of America.

GUEST EDITORS

VIVEK N. AHYA, MD, Medical Director, Lung Transplantation Program; and Assistant Professor of Medicine, Pulmonary, Allergy, and Critical Care Division, University of Pennsylvania School of Medicine, Philadelphia, Pennsylvania

ROBERT M. KOTLOFF, MD, Chief, Section of Advanced Lung Disease and Lung Transplantation, Pulmonary, Allergy, and Critical Care Division, University of Pennsylvania Medical Center, Philadelphia, Pennsylvania

CONTRIBUTORS

BEKELE AFESSA, MD, Associate Professor of Medicine, Division of Pulmonary and Critical Care Medicine, Mayo Clinic College of Medicine, Rochester, Minnesota

VIVEK N. AHYA, MD, Medical Director, Lung Transplantation Program; and Assistant Professor of Medicine, Pulmonary, Allergy, and Critical Care Division, University of Pennsylvania School of Medicine, Philadelphia, Pennsylvania

BARBARA D. ALEXANDER, MD, Assistant Professor of Medicine; Director of Transplant Infectious Diseases Service; and Head of Clinical Mycology Laboratory, Division of Infectious Diseases and International Health, Department of Medicine, Duke University Medical Center, Durham, North Carolina

JOSEPH H. ANTIN, MD, Professor of Medicine, Harvard Medical School; Director of Stem Cell Transplantation, Division of Medical Oncology, Dana-Farber Cancer Institute; and Brigham and Women's Hospital, Boston, Massachusetts

TODD D. BARTON, MD, Assistant Professor of Medicine, Division of Infectious Diseases; and Associate Program Director, Internal Medicine Residency Program, Hospital of the University of Pennsylvania, Philadelphia, Pennsylvania

ROY D. BLOOM, MD, Associate Professor of Medicine, Renal, Electrolyte, and Hypertension Division, University of Pennsylvania Medical Center, Philadelphia, Pennsylvania

EMILY A. BLUMBERG, MD, Associate Professor of Medicine, Division of Infectious Diseases, Hospital of the University of Pennsylvania, Philadelphia, Pennsylvania

SYLVIA F. COSTA, MD, Associate in Medicine, Division of Pulmonary, Allergy and Critical Care, Department of Medicine, Duke University Medical Center, Durham, North Carolina

COREY CUTLER, MD, MPH, FRCP(C), Instructor in Medicine, Harvard Medical School; Division of Medical Oncology, Dana-Farber Cancer Institute; and Brigham and Women's Hospital, Boston, Massachusetts

THOMAS W. FAUST, MD, Assistant Professor of Medicine, Gastroenterology Division, University of Pennsylvania Medical Center, Philadelphia, Pennsylvania

JAY A. FISHMAN, MD, Associate Professor of Medicine, Harvard Medical School; and Director, Transplant Infectious Disease and Compromised Host Program, Infectious Disease Division, Massachusetts General Hospital, Boston, Massachusetts

LEANNE B. GASINK, MD, Division of Infectious Diseases, Department of Medicine, University of Pennsylvania, Philadelphia, Pennsylvania

LEE R. GOLDBERG, MD, MPH, Assistant Professor of Medicine, Heart Failure/Transplant Program, Cardiovascular Disease Division, University of Pennsylvania Medical Center, Philadelphia, Pennsylvania

MARSHALL I. HERTZ, MD, Professor of Medicine, Division of Pulmonary, Allergy, and Critical Care Medicine, University of Minnesota, Minneapolis, Minnesota

MICHAEL G. ISON, MD, MS, Transplant Infectious Disease and Compromised Host Program, Infectious Disease Division, Massachusetts General Hospital, Boston, Massachusetts

STEVEN M. KAWUT, MD, MS, Assistant Professor of Clinical Medicine and Epidemiology, Division of Pulmonary, Allergy, and Critical Care Medicine and Department of Epidemiology, Columbia University College of Physicians and Surgeons, New York, New York

ROBERT M. KOTLOFF, MD, Chief, Section of Advanced Lung Disease and Lung Transplantation, Pulmonary, Allergy, and Critical Care Division, University of Pennsylvania Medical Center, Philadelphia, Pennsylvania

MICHAEL J. KROWKA, MD, Professor of Medicine, Division of Gastroenterology and Hepatology; and Vice-Chair, Division of Pulmonary & Critical Care, Mayo Clinic College of Medicine, Rochester, Minnesota

ALISON W. LOREN, MD, MS, Instructor of Medicine, Division of Hematology/Oncology; and Faculty Fellow, Center for Clinical Epidemiology and Biostatistics, University of Pennsylvania School of Medicine, Philadelphia, Pennsylvania

WALLACE MILLER, Jr, MD, Associate Professor in Radiology, Division of Thoracic Radiology, Hospital of the University of Pennsylvania, Philadelphia, Pennsylvania

STEVE G. PETERS, MD, Professor of Medicine, Division of Pulmonary and Critical Care Medicine, Mayo Clinic College of Medicine, Rochester, Minnesota

ROSITA M. SHAH, MD, Clinical Associate Professor in Radiology, Division of Thoracic Radiology, Hospital of the University of Pennsylvania, Philadelphia, Pennsylvania

DONALD E. TSAI, MD, PhD, Assistant Professor of Medicine, Division of Hematology/Oncology, University of Pennsylvania School of Medicine, Philadelphia, Pennsylvania

ANDREW Y. WANG, MD, Fellow, Gastroenterology Division, University of Pennsylvania Medical Center, Philadelphia, Pennsylvania

TIMOTHY P.M. WHELAN, MD, Assistant Professor of Medicine, Division of Pulmonary, Allergy, and Critical Care Medicine, University of Minnesota, Minneapolis, Minnesota

DOROTHY A. WHITE, MD, Attending Physician, Department of Medicine, Memorial Sloan Kettering Cancer Center; and Professor of Medicine, Department of Medicine, Weill Medical College of Cornell University, New York, New York

CONTENTS

> This article is a broad overview of hematopoietic stem cell transplantation, covering topics such as indications for transplantation, types of transplantation procedures, HLA matching of donors and recipients, procurement of stem cells from donors, and outcomes of transplantation. The major complications of transplantation, such as graft-versus-host disease, and the mechanisms of tissue injury after transplantation are discussed, as are the nature of immunologic impairment and reconstitution after transplantation. Finally future directions in stem cell transplantation are discussed.

> Once a medical curiosity, solid organ transplantation is now a common place occurrence, with more than 27,000 procedures performed in the United States in 2004 alone. This article offers an overview of the various solid organ transplant procedures to provide a context within which subsequent articles on pulmonary complications can be viewed.

> The aim of this article is to clarify radiographic definitions associated with common parenchymal patterns encountered in the transplant population and to discuss the most common pathologic causes responsible for each pattern. The article also touches on radiographic findings signifying complications of other intrathoracic structures, including the airways, pleural space, and mediastinum.

FORTHCOMING ISSUES

RECENT ISSUES

THE CLINICS ARE NOW AVAILABLE ONLINE!

Access your subscription at:
http://www.theclinics.com

Clin Chest Med 26 (2005) xi

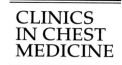

Dedication

To my parents, Leon and Jean, for leading me to the path.

To my mentors and patients, for guiding me down it.

To my wife, Debbie, and sons, Eric, Brian, and Ethan, for making sure that I step off of it once in a while.

—Robert M. Kotloff

To my father, Narendra, whose strength and courage during his struggle with multiple myeloma inspires me to strive to become a better physician and whose constant support and encouragement helped me to become the person I am today.

—Vivek N. Ahya

doi:10.1016/j.ccm.2005.08.005

CLINICS
IN CHEST
MEDICINE

Clin Chest Med 26 (2005) xiii – xiv

Preface

Pulmonary Considerations in Organ and Hematopoietic Stem Cell Transplantation

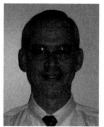 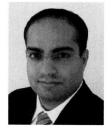

Robert M. Kotloff, MD   Vivek N. Ahya, MD
Guest Editors

On December 23, 1954, Dr. Joseph Murray and his surgical colleagues at the Peter Bent Brigham Hospital performed the first successful human organ transplantation, removing a kidney from a healthy donor and implanting it into the body of an identical twin suffering from advanced renal disease. At approximately the same time that Murray was conducting his work in solid organ transplantation, Dr. Donnall Thomas and associates at the Mary Imogene Basset Hospital in Cooperstown, New York, began a series of attempts to treat patients with terminal leukemias by ablating their bone marrow with total body irradiation and subsequently infusing bone marrow derived from healthy donors. Clinical organ transplantation and bone marrow transplantation, landmark achievements of twentieth century medicine, were thus inaugurated. Over the ensuing decades, organ transplantation expanded to include liver, heart, lung, and pancreas transplantation, and introduction of novel immunosuppressive agents resulted in markedly improved allograft survival rates. Use of peripheral blood and umbilical cord blood as alternative sources of hematopoietic stem cells extended the boundaries of "bone marrow transplantation" and resulted in adoption of new nomenclature (i.e., hematopoietic stem cell transplantation) to more accurately

describe the field. Drs. Murray and Thomas, the two early pioneers of transplantation, went on to share the Nobel Prize for Medicine in 1990.

Solid organ transplantation is now widely applied in the treatment of vital organ failure and hematopoietic stem cell transplantation in the treatment of a variety of malignant, hematologic, autoimmune, and genetic diseases. While these procedures offer the potential for extended survival to many patients with otherwise lethal conditions, they are associated with substantial risks. Prominent among these are pulmonary complications, both infectious and noninfectious, that contribute significantly to the morbidity and mortality associated with transplantation. As transplantation has become more commonplace, there has been a progressive shift in the care of recipients from the university hospitals to the community setting. Thus, it is now imperative that all practicing pulmonologists be familiar with the potential complications affecting these complex patient populations.

This issue of the *Clinics in Chest Medicine* was assembled with the goal of providing the general pulmonologist with information essential to addressing pulmonary complications in organ and hematopoietic stem cell transplant recipients. The issue begins with two articles offering broad overviews of these respective fields of transplantation. The next section is comprised of articles detailing non-infectious pulmonary complications that arise from a variety of insults, including underlying disease, transplantation surgery, chemoradiation regimens used to prepare for hematopoietic stem cell transplantation, and alloimmune mechanisms that trigger graft-versus-host and host-versus-graft reactions. The issue concludes with a series of articles detailing the broad spectrum of pulmonary infectious complications that plague these immunocompromised hosts.

In an era that offers little time for scholarship, we are tremendously grateful to the authors who contributed works of the highest caliber, providing thoughtfully distilled but still comprehensive summaries of complex topics. We are also grateful to Sarah Barth, Editor of the *Clinics in Chest Medicine*, for her guidance and, when necessary, prompting. It is our hope that the knowledge conveyed in this issue will impart upon the reader a sense of confidence in dealing with the often daunting task of caring for transplant recipients.

Robert M. Kotloff, MD
*Section of Advanced Lung Disease and
Lung Transplantation
Pulmonary, Allergy, and Critical Care Division
University of Pennsylvania Medical Center
838 West Gates Building
3400 Spruce Street
Philadelphia, PA 19104, USA*
E-mail address: kotloff@mail.med.upenn.edu

Vivek N. Ahya, MD
*Pulmonary, Allergy, and Critical Care Division
University of Pennsylvania Medical Center
832 West Gates Building
3600 Spruce Street
Philadelphia, PA 19104, USA*
E-mail address: ahyav@uphs.upenn.edu

ELSEVIER
SAUNDERS

Clin Chest Med 26 (2005) 517 – 527

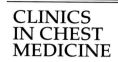

CLINICS
IN CHEST
MEDICINE

An Overview of Hematopoietic Stem Cell Transplantation

Corey Cutler, MD, MPH, FRCP(C)[a,b,c,*], Joseph H. Antin, MD[a,b,c]

[a]Harvard Medical School, Boston, MA, USA
[b]Division of Medical Oncology, Dana-Farber Cancer Institute, 44 Binney Street, D1B30, Boston, MA 02115, USA
[c]Brigham and Women's Hospital, Boston, MA, USA

Hematologic malignancy is the main clinical indication for hematopoietic stem cell transplantation (HSCT). Nonhematologic malignancies, including testicular cancer and pediatric neuroblastoma, and nonmalignant disorders, including the hemoglobinopathies, some autoimmune conditions, and the inborn errors of immunity and metabolism, can be treated with stem cell transplantation. Because the nonhematologic malignancies and the nonmalignant disorders are less common indications for transplantation, they are not discussed in this article.

Stem cell transplantation: background and indications

A great deal of progress has been made in clinical stem cell transplantation since the time Thomas and colleagues attempted to treat hematologic malignancies in 1957 [1]. An understanding of the human leukocyte antigen (HLA) system for donor selection, immunosuppression for prevention and treatment of graft-versus-host disease (GVHD), and significant advances in infectious disease therapy and supportive care have made HSCT commonplace in the era of modern medicine. Nonetheless, there still are significant limitations that make HSCT a risky medical procedure.

The most fundamental decision in stem cell transplantation is whether or not an autologous (self) or allogeneic (nonself) stem cell source is used. Autologous transplantation is a moderate morbidity, low mortality procedure that can be performed with relative safety even in individuals in the seventh and eighth decades of life. It is used with curative intent in individuals who have non-Hodgkin's lymphoma or Hodgkin's disease in second remission and as remission consolidation for patients who have multiple myeloma in a minimal residual disease state, where the procedure is expected to prolong disease-free survival but not cure the disorder. Occasionally, individuals who have acute leukemia in second or greater remission undergo autologous transplantation, but generally only when a suitable allogeneic donor is not available. For acute myeloid leukemia (AML) in first remission, the value of autologous stem cell transplantation as consolidation is less clear.

Autologous transplantation relies solely on dose intensity as a therapeutic modality. Autologous stem cells are collected, or harvested, from the intended recipient before the administration of high-dose chemotherapy. The stored stem cells, therefore, are protected from the toxic effects of the chemotherapy, which generally cause long-term myelosuppression or even permanent failure of hematopoiesis (myeloablation). Once the chemotherapeutic agents are metabolized, the cryopreserved stem cells are reinfused into the transplant recipient and the original immune system gradually is reconstituted. There are no alloimmune effects of autologous stem cell transplantation; these effects are seen uniquely in allogeneic transplantation.

Supported by grant no. P01 HL070149-01A1 from the National Heart, Lung and Blood Institute. Dr. Cutler is a recipient of a Rising Stars Award from the Dunkin Donuts Foundation and the Dana-Farber Cancer Institute.

* Corresponding author. Division of Medical Oncology, Dana-Farber Cancer Institute, 44 Binney Street, D1B30, Boston, MA 02115.

E-mail address: corey_cutler@dfci.harvard.edu (C. Cutler).

Allogeneic transplantation is the therapy of choice for individuals who have relapsed or refractory AML or high-risk AML in first remission. Similarly, it is the therapeutic modality of choice for the myelodysplastic disorders and myeloproliferative syndromes, including chronic myeloid leukemia (CML). Acute lymphoblastic leukemia (ALL) is treated with allogeneic stem cell transplantation in clinical scenarios similar to those for AML. Advanced lymphoid malignancies, including Hodgkin's and non-Hodgkin's lymphomas and chronic lymphocytic leukemia, often are treated with allogeneic transplantation after fail-

ure of a prior autologous procedure or earlier, in the case of advanced chemorefractory disease. Similarly, multiple myeloma is treated with allogeneic transplantation in young patients or in patients who have chemorefractory disease.

There are several important advantages of allogeneic transplantation over autologous transplantation. By using an allogeneic stem cell source, the recipient is guaranteed to receive a stem cell product that is free of tumor cell contamination. More importantly, allogeneic transplantation is associated with an allogeneic graft-versus-leukemia (GVL) or, more generically, a graft-versus-tumor effect that cannot be obtained with autologous transplantation. In keeping with the allogeneic response against host antigens, however, is the syndrome of GVHD. Analogous to acute rejection after solid organ transplantation, GVHD is a donor-derived, T-cell–mediated attack on host tissues, most notably the skin, gastrointestinal tract, and liver. Each organ system involved is staged individually, and a composite grade is generated for clinical use (Box 1) [2,3]. Clinically significant grades II–IV acute GVHD occur in 30% to 40% of recipients of sibling donor transplants and in 40% to 50% of unrelated donor transplants [4,5]. Although grade I disease often requires no therapy, grades II–IV acute GVHD represent a systemic condition that requires systemic therapy.

The actual allogeneic transplant is similar to the autologous procedure, using stem cells that are delivered once conditioning chemoradiotherapy is completed. Cryopreservation of stem cells often is not required if the stem cell harvest is performed on the day of the planned infusion of the stem cells. The recovery after allogeneic transplantation is longer, often requiring several weeks to months, and is associated with higher mortality at 100 days from transplantation.

Box 1. Modified Glucksberg staging system for acute graft-versus-host disease

Skin

  0 No rash
  1 0%–25% body surface area (BSA) involvement
  2 25%–50% BSA involvement
  3 >50% BSA involvement
  4 Diffuse erythroderma with bulla formation

Gut

  0 No diarrhea
  1 500–1000 mL/d
  2 1000–1500 mL/d
  3 1500–2000 mL/d
  4 >2000 mL/d or ileus

Liver

  0 Normal bilirubin
  1 Bilirubin 2.0–3.0 mg/dL
  2 Bilirubin 3.1–6.0 mg/dL
  3 Bilirubin 6.1–15.0 mg/dL
  4 Bilirubin >15.0 mg/dL

Overall grade

  0 No GVHD
  I Stage 1–2 skin only
  II Stage 1–3 skin or stage 1 gut or stage 1 liver
  III Stage 0–3 skin and stage 2–4 gut or stage 2–3 liver
  IV Stage 4 skin or stage 4 liver

Donor selection, stem cell source, and preparative regimens

Donor selection is a critical decision in stem cell transplantation. The decision to use autologous stem cells is made based on the nature of the hematologic malignancy being treated and the stage of the malignancy (discussed previously). Once the decision to use allogeneic stem cells is made, an appropriate donor must be identified. Donors are selected primarily based on HLA typing, although other factors, such as age, sex, parity, and cytomegalovirus (CMV) serostatus are considerations.

The HLA gene complex, located on the short arm of chromosome 6, is comprised of three clusters of genes—class I genes (including HLA-A, HLA-B, and HLA-C), class II genes (HLA-DR, HLA-DQ, and HLA-DP), and class III genes (functional genes, including some complement genes and β_2-microglobulin) [6,7]. Class III genes are not used in HLA matching and are not discussed further. The HLA complex, present on all antigen-presenting cells, is required for recognition of alloantigen in the context of self-protein. Traditionally, matching has been considered critical at six loci: the two HLA-A, HLA-B, and HLA-DRβ1 genes. More recently, mismatching at HLA-C has been demonstrated also to be relevant clinically [8]. The class I and class II genes are pleomorphic; hundreds of allelic variations are noted with high-resolution DNA typing within each gene. This heterogeneity, theoretically, makes HLA matching difficult, if not for the fact that the HLA complex generally is inherited as a complete haplotype. Siblings, therefore, either are perfectly matched (25% probability), matched at half of the HLA loci (haploidentical, 50% probability), or entirely HLA disparate (25% probability).

When an acceptable related donor is unavailable, a suitable volunteer unrelated donor is identified through registries of volunteer donors, such as the National Marrow Donor Program. The likelihood of identifying a perfectly matched donor is related partially to ethnicity, as many ethnic minorities are under-represented in the registry. As techniques in HLA matching improve, so do clinical outcomes after unrelated donor transplantation [9]. When necessary, however, partially mismatched stem cells are used, at the expense of increased rates of GVHD and poorer long-term outcome (discussed later) [8,10]. The degree of mismatch is important, as mismatches that can be detected serologically (antigenic mismatch) are associated more frequently with GVHD and worse clinical outcome than mismatches noted only when direct DNA sequencing of the HLA gene complex is used (allelic matching) [8]. At the allelic level, the location and particular amino acid substitutions may be important predictors for GVHD.

Despite seemingly perfect HLA matching, the use of HLA-identical unrelated donors is associated with a higher incidence of acute and chronic GVHD and lower overall survival rates compared with HLA-identical sibling transplantation. Minor histocompatibility antigens, oligopeptides presented by the HLA complex to immune effector cells, are more disparate between nonsibling donor-recipient pairs than sibling donor-recipient pairs, and likely account for the increased rates of GVHD in unrelated donor transplantation.

Two stem cell sources are available for autologous transplantation: bone marrow stem cells and mobilized peripheral blood stem cells. The former are obtained by direct aspiration of bone marrow from the pelvis under anesthesia. The latter are obtained by pretreating the donor with recombinant human granulocyte colony-stimulating factor (rhG-CSF; filgrastim) or chemotherapy. Treatment with rhG-CSF and chemotherapy causes a release of stem cells from the bone marrow stroma into the peripheral circulation, where they can be collected by specialized apheresis machines. Mobilized peripheral blood stem cells almost always are chosen as the preferred stem cell source for autologous transplantation, as they are more convenient to obtain and, in the case of diseases where marrow involvement is prominent (ie, myeloma or acute leukemia), have a lower chance of tumor cell contamination of the stem cell product. In addition, randomized trials demonstrate that peripheral blood stem cells engraft several days earlier than bone marrow–derived stem cells and are associated with a more favorable outcome [11,12].

In North America, peripheral blood stem cells are the most common stem cell source for autologous and allogeneic stem cell transplantation [13]. Umbilical cord stem cells are available for use in allogeneic recipients and, in this context, can be considered a special case of peripheral blood stem cells. Cord blood stem cells, collected at the time of delivery, represent more than 10% of all unrelated stem cell transplants facilitated by the National Marrow Donor Program.

There are important differences in bone marrow, peripheral blood, and cord blood–derived stem cells. In comparison with bone marrow–derived stem cells, peripheral blood stem cell products contain a higher proportion of CD34$^+$ cells, a known marker for pluripotent stem cells. On average, however, they also contain tenfold more T cells. These two factors result in quicker time to engraftment, albeit at the expense of increased rates of acute and chronic GVHD [14]. Cord blood products, conversely, contain far fewer CD34$^+$ cells and mature effector immune cells. As the number of stem cells is an important determinant of engraftment after transplantation, engraftment after single unit cord blood transplantation is delayed, and many cord blood units are of insufficient size for use in adult recipients. One important difference noted with the use of cord blood transplantation is a lower incidence of GVHD, allowing greater degrees of donor-recipient HLA mismatching [15,16].

Some form of conditioning therapy is a prerequisite to successful HSCT for malignant disorders. The goal of the conditioning therapy is twofold: first, the conditioning agents possess potent tumoricidal activity and second, the immunosuppression provided by conditioning therapy helps prevent rejection of the transplanted stem cells by the host immune system. Conditioning therapy consists of single agent or combination chemotherapy that is delivered alone or in association with total body irradiation (TBI). Many individual regimens exist; those used most commonly in the autologous setting are the cyclophosphamide, carmustine, and etoposide (CBV) regimen; the carmustine, etoposide, cytosine arabinoside, and melphalan (BEAM) regimen; and the single agent, melphalan (used only for multiple myeloma), although many others exist. Irradiation generally is omitted from autologous conditioning regimens because of concerns of late toxicity, including secondary myeloid malignancies [17,18].

In allogeneic HSCT, most myeloablative regimens are based on the chemotherapeutic agent, cyclophosphamide (Cy), which is administered either with busulfan (Bu) (the Bu/Cy regimen) or TBI (Cy/TBI). Up to 14 Gy of fractionated radiotherapy is delivered, usually with minimal shielding of the lung parenchyma. High doses of the chemotherapeutic agents are administered during brief periods of exposure, as opposed to prolonged exposure of moderate doses in the case of conventional chemotherapy, in an attempt to exploit the steep dose-response curves that most hematologic malignancies exhibit. The most important dose-limiting toxicity of these intense chemotherapy regimens, myelosuppression, is overcome by the subsequent administration of nonexposed healthy donor stem cells.

In autologous and allogeneic settings, there is no convincing evidence to suggest that one conditioning regimen is superior to another, and the choice of the conditioning regimen often is determined by institutional preference and the availability of TBI.

Newer, less intense preparative regimens have been developed to reduce the toxicity profile associated with myeloablative regimens [19,20]. These "reduced intensity," "minitransplantation," or "nonmyeloablative" regimens generally consist of a purine analog (such as fludarabine) delivered with one or more immunosuppressive chemotherapeutic agents, low-dose TBI or total lymphoid irradiation, or antithymocyte globulin or other antibody preparation. These regimens do not ablate host hematopoiesis; rather, their goal is to immunosuppress the transplant recipient sufficiently to allow engraftment of the donor hematopoietic stem cells. Whereas in traditional myeloablative transplantation, eradication of the host hematopoiesis and the hematologic malignancy is accomplished via the tumoricidal activity of

the conditioning regimen in conjunction with immunologic destruction of residual host malignant hematopoiesis, in nonmyeloablative transplantation, the expectation is that the GVL reaction is sufficient to eradicate all malignant cells. Because of the lower toxicity profile of the nonmyeloablative preparative regimen, these transplants can be offered to older patients, patients who have previously undergone myeloablative transplantation, and patients who have significant comorbid diseases who otherwise would not be candidates for traditional HSCT.

Manipulation of the stem cell product also can be used to minimize toxicity associated with transplantation. Strategies that selectively enrich $CD34^+$ progenitor cells (positive selection), deplete T cells (negative selection), or a combination of the two are used to reduce the incidence of acute GVHD; however, these methods often come at the expense of increased relapse after transplantation and more impaired immunologic recovery [21].

Mechanisms of injury in stem cell transplantation

Injury to the stem cell transplant recipients occurs through a variety of mechanisms. The high-dose conditioning chemoradiotherapy used is directly toxic to all rapidly dividing cells, including several nonhematopoietic lineages, whereas the ensuing inflammatory "cytokine storm" occurring as a result of conditioning-related injury may be responsible for the pathogenesis of several toxic complications, including acute lung injury and GVHD.

Nonhematopoietic epithelial surfaces, most notably the buccal and gastrointestinal mucosa, are sensitive to the toxic effects of chemoradiotherapy, and ulceration of the mucosa leads to a loss of the protective immunologic barrier normally afforded by the gut. This in turn can lead to translocation of intestinal bacteria from the lumen of the intestine to the bloodstream and result in septicemia. (The implications of the loss of gastrointestinal integrity and the association with acute GVHD are discussed later.)

The liver is a commonly affected organ, with rates of veno-occlusive disease (VOD) that range from 10% to 60% in published series [22]. The inciting injury is believed to be damage to the hepatic sinusoidal endothelium related to conditioning therapy and circulating inflammatory cytokines. Varying degrees of severity are noted, with attributable mortality as high as 67% and severe VOD resulting from concomitant multisystem organ failure [23]. Supportive measures are standard therapy, but a novel agent, defibrotide, seems promising for the therapy for this disorder [24].

Renal injury after transplantation often is associated with the toxic effects of GVHD prophylaxis agents, particularly the calcineurin inhibitors. A syndrome of thrombotic microangiopathy may occur after transplantation. When it occurs early after transplant (within 100 days) it often is the result of calcineurin inhibitors, particularly when given with sirolimus [25]. Late thrombotic microangiopathy often is attributed to the late effects of radiation therapy.

The lungs are a less common but important target of conditioning-related injury. Diffuse alveolar hemorrhage and idiopathic pneumonia syndrome occur in less than 10% of related and unrelated transplants, but the attributable mortality to these disorders is great. The etiology and pathophysiology of these forms of acute lung injury are discussed elsewhere in this article; however, it is worthwhile noting the contribution to these disorders of inflammatory cytokines [26,27] and chemotherapy administered as GVHD prophylaxis [28] and the possibility that lung injury after transplantation may represent a form of acute GVHD [29]. Other forms of lung injury (discussed later) include bronchiolitis obliterans, with or without organizing pneumonia, and recurrent pulmonary infection, with resultant bronchiectasis related to poor immunologic recovery and hypogammaglobulinemia after transplantation.

Other organ systems affected less commonly as a result of conditioning-related injury include the eyes and lacrimal tissues, the heart and pericardium, and the central and peripheral nervous system. Acute and chronic injury can occur to any of these organ systems.

Acute GVHD is the result of a donor-derived, T-cell–mediated attack on host tissues that occurs within 100 days of transplantation. Characterized by the triad of skin rash, liver function abnormalities, and watery diarrhea, acute GVHD is a major source of morbidity and mortality after transplantation. GVHD is an anticipated occurrence if the transplanted immune system develops any amount of immunocompetence, because donor and recipient pairs are expected to be disparate for many presented antigens (with the exception of syngeneic twins). The presence of some amount of GVHD correlates with the most favorable survival after transplantation, likely the result of a GVL effect. With excessive amounts of GVHD, however, mortality from GVHD itself outweighs the potential benefits of GVL [30].

The hypothesis that there is interplay between mucosal injury, infection, and acute GVHD initially was proposed by Antin and Ferrara [31]. In this hypothesis, mucosal injury from cytotoxic conditioning therapy is responsible for the weakening of the intestinal mucosal barrier. Translocation of microorganisms from the gut causes the transcription and release of inflammatory cytokines, which, in turn, in the context of allogeneic antigen, activate donor T cells (Fig. 1). Other mechanisms to initiate this inflammatory cytokine cascade certainly exist, because conditioning-related injury after nonmyeloablative transplantation is relatively benign in comparison with traditional, myeloablative transplantation.

Prophylaxis and treatment of acute GVHD necessarily implies further immunosuppression of an already immature and dysfunctional immune system. For this reason, therapy of advanced GVHD, even when effective, is associated most frequently with poor clinical outcomes, largely because of infectious complications of therapy [32–34].

Some attempts at altering GVHD prophylaxis to reduce the incidence of acute GVHD have led to substantial decreases in pulmonary toxicity after transplantation. Ho and colleagues demonstrate that the use of T-cell depletion is associated with severe pulmonary complications in only 8% of transplants, although this is likely the result of the omission of methotrexate as a GVHD prophylaxis agent rather than graft manipulation [28]. The use of reduced intensity conditioning, initially incorrectly believed to reduce GVHD but clearly associated with reduced transplant-associated morbidity, is associated with a reduced incidence of pulmonary complications after transplantation [35].

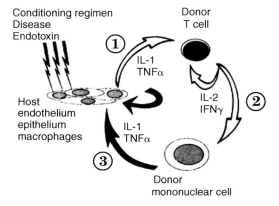

Fig. 1. Interplay between conditioning-related mucosal injury, infection, and acute GVHD, as originally proposed by Antin and Ferrara. (*From* Antin JH, Ferrara JL. Cytokine dysregulation and acute graft-versus-host disease. Blood 1992;80:2964–8; with permission.)

Immunologic reconstitution after stem cell transplantation

Recovery of granulopoiesis after stem cell transplantation is rapid, occurring between 14 and 21 days after transplantation, depending on the stem cell source used. This in no way, however, is an adequate measure of immunologic reconstitution after transplantation. A mature immunocompetent system can take more than a year to develop and even long-term survivors of allogeneic transplantation have persistent gaps in immunologic diversity when examined by sensitive molecular techniques [36]. Immunologic recovery after autologous transplantation generally is quicker and more complete than after allogeneic transplantation, because the environment in which immune reconstitution occurs is more favorable, being unhindered by immune suppression, GVHD, and other factors (discussed later).

There are many ways to measure immunologic reconstitution after transplantation. The absolute number or immunophenotypic characteristics of circulating immune cells are insufficient measures of their function. In vitro testing for activity against pathogens is artificial and may not represent in vivo functionality. The two best laboratory measures of immunologic diversity, T-cell receptor V_β gene spectatyping and T-cell rearrangement excision circle (TREC) analysis, are available; however, they generally are performed only in the context of research studies. Therefore, the best estimates of immunologic reconstitution after transplantation remain clinical outcomes, including infection, and death rates.

Examination of the variable (V_β gene) regions of the T-cell receptor gives a glimpse of the immunologic gaps in immune reconstitution after transplantation. As part of the normal gene rearrangements at the T-cell receptor during immune education, variable DNA segment lengths can be identified. Fig. 2 demonstrates the oligoclonal T-cell diversity of a stem cell transplant recipient 3 months after transplant in comparison with a normal individual [37]. Similar estimates of B cell immunity can be obtained by looking at immunoglobulin electrophoretic patterns.

Another measure of T-cell neogenesis is the measurement of TRECs. TRECs are short sequences of circularized DNA formed by the rearrangement of T-cell receptor genes during thymic education. These DNA fragments are not duplicated during T-cell proliferation and, therefore, are passed only to one daughter cell during cell division. The measurement of the frequency of these fragments in a population of T cells provides a measure of T-cell neogenesis [38].

There are many factors that influence the pace of immune reconstitution, including the source of stem cells, manipulation of the stem cells, the ages of donors and recipients, and the presence of GVHD. The source of stem cells influences the graft composition and, therefore, can influence immunologic recovery. Steady state bone marrow has sixfold more T cells than umbilical cord blood, whereas peripheral blood stem cell products have almost 10 times more T cells than bone marrow [39]. Most of the umbilical cord T cells are naive and, thus, less likely to provide passively transferred immunity. In contrast, passively transferred bone marrow and peripheral blood mature T cells play an important role in early lymphocyte immunity after transplantation. A similar situation exists for B cells, where the number of transferred cells is sevenfold higher in marrow products than cord products and threefold higher in peripheral blood products than in marrow stem cell products.

There are clinical correlates of the differences seen in graft composition. In a recent retrospective review, 35% of all deaths occurring more than 3 months after cord blood transplantation were the result of infectious causes [15]. Similarly, the incidence of CMV reactivation after transplantation was higher with use of cord blood compared with bone marrow, again implicating the relative naiveté of cord blood products and their inability to protect against viral pathogens after transplantation [40]. When peripheral blood and bone marrow products are compared, peripheral blood stem cell products are more reactive to nonspecific mitogens and to infectious antigens, including candida and tetanus [41]. A randomized trial that compared peripheral blood stem cell with bone marrow transplantation also demonstrates that the rate of bacterial, viral, and fungal infections was lower after peripheral blood stem cell transplantation than marrow transplantation [42].

Occasionally, stem cell grafts are manipulated at the time of transplantation, most commonly by the removal of T cells from the graft. These manipulations can occur in vitro, using antibodies in a cell separating column device or in vivo, using monoclonal or polyclonal antibodies administered to recipients or to the stem cell product itself. The resultant T-cell depleted transplant is associated with less GVHD and transplant-related mortality (TRM), but increased rates of graft loss (as T cells are important for engraftment) and relapse (loss of the T-cell–mediated GVL) are unfortunate consequences. Furthermore, T-cell depletion is associated with delayed immune reconstitution with an inverted CD4 to CD8 ratio for up to 2 years after transplantation, with a concomitant increase in opportunistic viral infections [21].

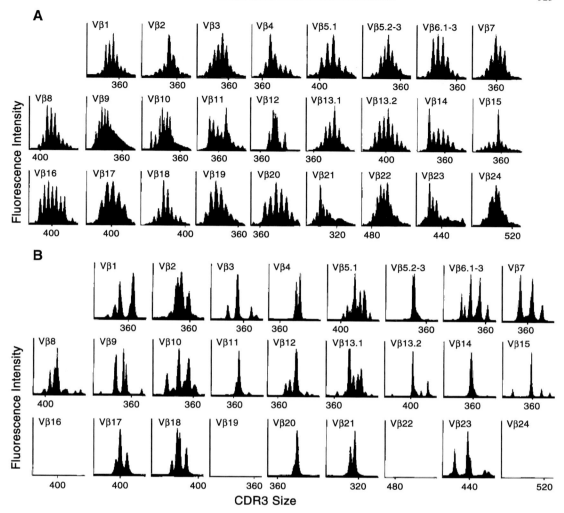

Fig. 2. V$_\beta$ spectratype from a normal (*A*) and a transplant (*B*) patient demonstrating marked gaps in V$_\beta$ repertoire. (*From* Wu CJ, Chillemi A, Alyea EP, et al. Reconstitution of T-cell receptor repertoire diversity following T-cell depleted allogeneic bone marrow transplantation is related to hematopoietic chimerism. Blood 2000;95:352–9; with permission.)

The ages of the patient and the donor correlate significantly with immunologic reconstitution after transplantation. Younger individuals have more rapid and more complete immune reconstitution when similar stem cell sources are used [43,44]. This difference may be attributable partly to the contribution of the thymus, which often is functionally absent by the fourth decade of life. The role of the thymus also may account for differences in immune reconstitution when ablative, TBI-containing regimens, and non-ablative regimens are compared. Because TBI invariably damages thymic epithelium, critical for T-cell education, it has been shown that immune reconstitution is more rapid with a nonablative regimen.

The immunologic milieu in which the developing immune system is placed plays a critical role in immunologic reconstitution. Normal immune function after transplant implies a brisk donor inflammatory response against all host tissues, which clinically is consistent with severe, acute GVHD. As such, some amount of immune suppression is required to limit this process, with care used not to completely suppress all immune function and inevitably induce fatal opportunistic infections. T-cell immunosuppression, usually with a calcineurin inhibitor, is required after transplantation, and measured doses of the antiproliferative agent methotrexate are given to selectively kill alloreactive T cells early after transplantation. GVHD, when present, has significant implications for immune function beyond what is attributed to administered immunosuppressive drugs. T-cell neogenesis, as measured by TREC analysis, is impaired in the context of chronic GVHD and infection [44]. Therefore, both the drugs used to prevent GVHD and GVHD itself have significant detrimental effects on immunologic reconstitution after transplantation.

Outcome of stem cell transplantation

There are many factors that influence the outcome of stem cell transplantation, including the nature of the malignancy for which transplant was indicated, the degree of donor-recipient match, the stem cell product used, the nature of the conditioning regimen, and comorbid conditions present in the recipients. Finally, the year in which transplantation is performed is an important predictor of outcome, as improvements in transplantation technology and the emergence of new supportive measures, including new antifungal and antiviral agents and experimental therapy for veno-occlusive disease of the liver and idiopathic pneumonia syndrome, have had a substantial impact on long-term survival, as have refinements in HLA matching techniques.

The most important variables that influence outcome are the disease that is being transplanted and at what stage of disease the transplant occurs. The Center for International Blood and Marrow Transplantation Research (CIBMTR) has captured data from approximately 40% of all stem cell transplants

performed worldwide since 1970. An analysis of their data from 1996 through 1991 on the outcomes of matched, sibling transplantation performed for CML during the first year of stable phase, AML in first remission, and ALL in first remission is shown in Fig. 3. Outcomes for CML are the most favorable, with long-term survival achieved in approximately 70%. The outcomes in AML are intermediate, with approximately 60% long-term survival, and for ALL, long-term survival is seen in only 45%.

The stage of the disease also is a critical variable in predicting outcomes from transplantation. Approximately 60% survival is expected for AML transplanted in first remission. In contrast, a 5-year survival rate of only 35% is demonstrated in a retrospective study of 310 patients who underwent transplant in second or subsequent complete remission. This rate was significantly better than the outcomes for patients transplanted in untreated or refractory relapse (14% and 11%, respectively) [45].

It is clear that survival after transplantation is affected by any degree of donor-recipient mismatch. Flomenberg and colleagues demonstrate that a single mismatch at HLA-A, HLA-B, HLA-C, or HLA-DR is associated with an increased hazard rate for acute GVHD (1.19–1.41), chronic GVHD (1.01–1.35), and death after transplantation (1.21–1.33) [8].

Whether or not the stem cell source influences overall survival remains uncertain. Many studies comparing the differences between peripheral blood and bone marrow for matched, related transplantation demonstrate only subtle differences in outcomes favoring peripheral blood, particularly in advanced disease [46]. Whether or not these differences persist

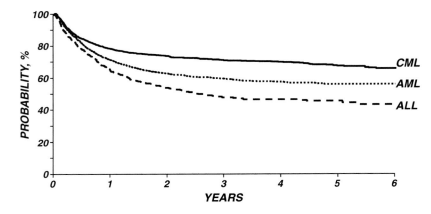

Fig. 3. Survival probability for matched, sibling transplantation for CML transplanted in first stable less than 1 year from diagnosis (n = 2720), AML in first remission (n = 3193), and ALL in first remission (n = 886). (*Data from* Center for International Blood and Marrow Transplant Research (CIBMTR). CIBMTR summary slide set 2003. Available at: http://www.ibmtr.org/newsletter/newsletter_sums.html.)

in the unrelated setting currently is unknown. Comparisons with cord blood and adult-derived stem cells are difficult, because cord blood transplantation for adults is reserved for individuals who do not have a sibling donor or, often, who do not have a fully histocompatible unrelated donor. Two recent analyses suggest that matched bone marrow is slightly superior to cord blood transplantation but that mismatched unrelated bone marrow and cord blood are equivalent stem cell sources [15,16].

TRM continues to be a major concern, with rates of nonrelapse mortality ranging from 18% to 28%, the majority of which occur with the first 100 days after transplantation [47]. As such, the approach of nonmyeloablative transplantation is used to eliminate much of this early mortality. Rates of nonrelapse mortality generally are lower after nonmyeloablative transplantation, even when applied to patients of advanced age and who have more comorbidity. In a comparison of myeloablative and nonmyeloablative stem cell transplants performed at the Fred Hutchinson Cancer Research Center, 100-day TRM was 3% in the nonmyeloablative group compared with 23% in the group that underwent full, ablative conditioning [48]. To compare the influence of comorbidity on older adults undergoing transplantation, Alyea and colleagues examined a cohort of individuals over age 50, the majority of whom had AML. No differences in overall outcome were noted; however, although the predominant cause of death in the myeloablative regimens was treatment related, the major cause of death in the nonmyeloablative regimens was relapse [49]. Whether or not the application of nonmyeloablative regimens to populations of patients generally considered fit enough for fully ablative transplantation will result in enhanced long-term survival with less TRM is one of the more important questions in transplantation currently examined.

There is a suggestion that outcomes after transplantion improve over time. Using CML as an example, the Seattle group reports 4-year overall survival in the range of 60% to 66% when HLA-identical siblings were used as bone marrow donors in the late 1980s [50] but reports a markedly improved 3-year survival of 87% in 2005 [51]. Although similar examples exist for other malignancies, these historical comparisons often are difficult to make, given recent trends to offer transplantation to patients who are in more advanced stages of disease.

Another time-related factor is the influence of HLA typing, which has improved in recent years. Results in unrelated donors are approaching those seen when related donors are used. For example, in ALL, transplantation with matched, related donors

and matched, unrelated donors yield similar results in a cohort of 221 individuals transplanted for various stages of the disease (42% versus 45% 5-year disease-free survival) [52]. In the unrelated setting, however, mismatching of donor-recipient pairs still carries considerable risk and causes a decrement in survival [8,10].

Future directions

Transplantation of human stem cells has realized considerable progress in the past 50 years. Nonetheless, predicting the behavior of the transplanted immune system remains a challenge. GVHD, an expected but unwanted complication of transplantation, remains an important clinical problem. The ramifications of GVHD, most notably infection, continue to be leading causes of morbidity and mortality after transplantation. Strategies to improve and control graft function after transplantation include more sophisticated methods of graft engineering, such as selective depletion of alloreactive T cells, the enrichment of regulatory T cells, and the addition of mesenchymal marrow cells. Novel agents in GVHD prophylaxis may reduce GVHD without causing an undue increase in immunosuppression. Ultimately, a better understanding of the pathophysiology of chronic GVHD may improve long-term immune reconstitution after transplantation.

References

[1] Thomas E, Lochte Jr H, Lu W, et al. Intravenous infusion of bone marrow in patients receiving radiation and chemotherapy. N Engl J Med 1957;257:491–6.

[2] Glucksberg H, Storb R, Fefer A, et al. Clinical manifestations of graft-versus-host disease in human recipients of marrow from HL-A-matched sibling donors. Transplantation 1974;18:295–304.

[3] Przepiorka D, Weisdorf D, Martin P, et al. 1994 Consensus Conference on Acute GVHD Grading. Bone Marrow Transplant 1995;15:825–8.

[4] Nash RA, Antin JH, Karanes C, et al. Phase 3 study comparing methotrexate and tacrolimus with methotrexate and cyclosporine for prophylaxis of acute graft-versus-host disease after marrow transplantation from unrelated donors. Blood 2000;96:2062–8.

[5] Ratanatharathorn V, Nash RA, Przepiorka D, et al. Phase III study comparing methotrexate and tacrolimus (prograf, FK506) with methotrexate and cyclosporine for graft-versus-host disease prophylaxis after HLA-identical sibling bone marrow transplantation. Blood 1998;92:2303–14.

[6] Klein J, Sato A. The HLA system. First of two parts. N Engl J Med 2000;343:702–9.

[7] Klein J, Sato A. The HLA system. Second of two parts. N Engl J Med 2000;343:782–6.

[8] Flomenberg N, Baxter-Lowe LA, Confer D, et al. Impact of HLA class I and class II high-resolution matching on outcomes of unrelated donor bone marrow transplantation: HLA-C mismatching is associated with a strong adverse effect on transplantation outcome. Blood 2004;104:1923–30.

[9] Shaw BE, Madrigal JA, Potter M. Improving the outcome of unrelated donor stem cell transplantation by molecular matching. Blood Rev 2001;15:167–74.

[10] Petersdorf EW, Kollman C, Hurley CK, et al. Effect of HLA class II gene disparity on clinical outcome in unrelated donor hematopoietic cell transplantation for chronic myeloid leukemia: the US National Marrow Donor Program Experience. Blood 2001;98:2922–9.

[11] Vellenga E, van Agthoven M, Croockewit AJ, et al. Autologous peripheral blood stem cell transplantation in patients with relapsed lymphoma results in accelerated haematopoietic reconstitution, improved quality of life and cost reduction compared with bone marrow transplantation: the Hovon 22 study. Br J Haematol 2001;114:319–26.

[12] Vose JM, Sharp G, Chan WC, et al. Autologous transplantation for aggressive non-Hodgkin's lymphoma: results of a randomized trial evaluating graft source and minimal residual disease. J Clin Oncol 2002;20:2344–52.

[13] Center for International Blood and Marrow Transplantation Registry. Report on State of the Art in Blood and Marrow Transplantation. Available at: http://www.ibmtr.org/newsletter/sums_update.html.

[14] Cutler C, Giri S, Jeyapalan S, et al. Acute and chronic graft-versus-host disease after allogeneic peripheral-blood stem-cell and bone marrow transplantation: a meta-analysis. J Clin Oncol 2001;19:3685–91.

[15] Laughlin MJ, Eapen M, Rubinstein P, et al. Outcomes after transplantation of cord blood or bone marrow from unrelated donors in adults with leukemia. N Engl J Med 2004;351:2265–75.

[16] Rocha V, Labopin M, Sanz G, et al. Transplants of umbilical-cord blood or bone marrow from unrelated donors in adults with acute leukemia. N Engl J Med 2004;351:2276–85.

[17] Krishnan A, Bhatia S, Slovak ML, et al. Predictors of therapy-related leukemia and myelodysplasia following autologous transplantation for lymphoma: an assessment of risk factors. Blood 2000;95:1588–93.

[18] Metayer C, Curtis RE, Vose J, et al. Myelodysplastic syndrome and acute myeloid leukemia after autotransplantation for lymphoma: a multicenter case-control study. Blood 2003;101:2015–23.

[19] Khouri IF, Keating M, Körbling M, et al. Transplant-lite: induction of graft-versus-malignancy using fludarabine-based nonablative chemotherapy and allogeneic blood progenitor-cell transplantation as treatment for lymphoid malignancies. J Clin Oncol 1998;16:2817–24.

[20] Slavin S, Nagler A, Naparstek E, et al. Nonmyeloablative stem cell transplantation and cell therapy as an alternative to conventional bone marrow transplantation with lethal cytoreduction for the treatment of malignant and nonmalignant hematologic Diseases. Blood 1998;91:756–63.

[21] Ho VT, Soiffer RJ. The history and future of T-cell depletion as graft-versus-host disease prophylaxis for allogeneic hematopoietic stem cell transplantation. Blood 2001;98:3192–204.

[22] Richardson P, Guinan E. Hepatic veno-occlusive disease following hematopoietic stem cell transplantation. Acta Haematol 2001;106:57–68.

[23] Carreras E, Bertz H, Arcese W, et al. Incidence and outcome of hepatic veno-occlusive disease after blood or marrow transplantation: a prospective cohort study of the European Group for Blood and Marrow Transplantation. European Group for Blood and Marrow Transplantation Chronic Leukemia Working Party. Blood 1998;92:3599–604.

[24] Richardson PG, Murakami C, Jin Z, et al. Multi-institutional use of defibrotide in 88 patients after stem cell transplantation with severe veno-occlusive disease and multisystem organ failure: response without significant toxicity in a high-risk population and factors predictive of outcome. Blood 2002;100: 4337–43.

[25] Cutler C, Henry N, Magee C, et al. Sirolimus and thrombotic microangiopathy after allogeneic hematopoietic stem cell transplantation. Biol Blood Marrow Transplant 2005;11(7):551–7.

[26] Hildebrandt GC, Olkiewicz KM, Choi S, et al. Donor T cell-production of RANTES significantly contributes to the development of idiopathic pneumonia syndrome after allogeneic stem cell transplantation. Blood 2005; 104(2):586–93.

[27] Hildebrandt GC, Olkiewicz KM, Corrion LA, et al. Donor-derived TNF-{alpha} regulates pulmonary chemokine expression and the development of idiopathic pneumonia syndrome after allogeneic bone marrow transplantation. Blood 2004;104:586–93.

[28] Ho VT, Weller E, Lee SJ, et al. Prognostic factors for early severe pulmonary complications after hematopoietic stem cell transplantation. Biol Blood Marrow Transplant 2001;7:223–9.

[29] Cooke KR, Yanik G. Acute lung injury after allogeneic stem cell transplantation: is the lung a target of acute graft-versus-host disease? Bone Marrow Transplant 2004;34:753–65.

[30] Horowitz MM, Gale RP, Sondel PM, et al. Graft-versus-leukemia reactions after bone marrow transplantation. Blood 1990;75:555–62.

[31] Antin JH, Ferrara JL. Cytokine dysregulation and acute graft-versus-host disease. Blood 1992;80:2964–8.

[32] Carpenter PA, Appelbaum FR, Corey L, et al. A humanized non-FcR-binding anti-CD3 antibody, visilizumab, for treatment of steroid-refractory acute graft-versus-host disease. Blood 2002;99:2712–9.

[33] Ho VT, Zahrieh D, Hochberg E, et al. Safety and

efficacy of denileukin diftitox in patients with steroid-refractory acute graft-versus-host disease after allogeneic hematopoietic stem cell transplantation. Blood 2004;104:1224–6.

[34] Marty FM, Lee SJ, Fahey MM, et al. Infliximab use in patients with severe graft-versus-host disease and other emerging risk factors of non-Candida invasive fungal infections in allogeneic hematopoietic stem cell transplant recipients: a cohort study. Blood 2003;102:2768–76.

[35] Fukuda T, Hackman RC, Guthrie KA, et al. Risks and outcomes of idiopathic pneumonia syndrome after nonmyeloablative and conventional conditioning regimens for allogeneic hematopoietic stem cell transplantation. Blood 2003;102:2777–85.

[36] Storek J, Joseph A, Espino G, et al. Immunity of patients surviving 20 to 30 years after allogeneic or syngeneic bone marrow transplantation. Blood 2001;98:3505–12.

[37] Wu CJ, Chillemi A, Alyea EP, et al. Reconstitution of T-cell receptor repertoire diversity following T-cell depleted allogeneic bone marrow transplantation is related to hematopoietic chimerism. Blood 2000;95:352–9.

[38] Hochberg EP, Chillemi AC, Wu CJ, et al. Quantitation of T-cell neogenesis in vivo after allogeneic bone marrow transplantation in adults. Blood 2001;98:1116–21.

[39] Theilgaard-Monch K, Raaschou-Jensen K, Palm H, et al. Flow cytometric assessment of lymphocyte subsets, lymphoid progenitors, and hematopoietic stem cells in allogeneic stem cell grafts. Bone Marrow Transplant 2001;28:1073–82.

[40] Tomonari A, Iseki T, Ooi J, et al. Cytomegalovirus infection following unrelated cord blood transplantation for adult patients: a single institute experience in Japan. Br J Haematol 2003;121:304–11.

[41] Ottinger HD, Beelen DW, Scheulen B, et al. Improved immune reconstitution after allotransplantation of peripheral blood stem cells instead of bone marrow. Blood 1996;88:2775–9.

[42] Storek J, Dawson MA, Storer B, et al. Immune reconstitution after allogeneic marrow transplantation compared with blood stem cell transplantation. Blood 2001;97:3380–9.

[43] Small TN, Papadopoulos EB, Boulad F, et al. Comparison of immune reconstitution after unrelated and related T-cell-depleted bone marrow transplantation: effect of patient age and donor leukocyte infusions. Blood 1999;93:467–80.

[44] Lewin SR, Heller G, Zhang L, et al. Direct evidence for new T-cell generation by patients after either T-cell-depleted or unmodified allogeneic hematopoietic stem cell transplantations. Blood 2002;100:2235–42.

[45] Michallet M, Thomas X, Vernant JP, et al. Long-term outcome after allogeneic hematopoietic stem cell transplantation for advanced stage acute myeloblastic leukemia: a retrospective study of 379 patients reported to the Societe Francaise de Greffe de Moelle (SFGM). Bone Marrow Transplant 2000;26:1157–63.

[46] Stem Cell Trialists Group. Allogeneic peripheral blood stem cell transplant vs. bone marrow transplant in the management of hematological malignancies: an individual patient data meta-analysis of 9 randomized trials. Hematol J 2004;5:s89.

[47] Champlin RE, Schmitz N, Horowitz MM, et al. Blood stem cells compared with bone marrow as a source of hematopoietic cells for allogeneic transplantation. Blood 2000;95:3702–9.

[48] Diaconescu R, Flowers CR, Storer B, et al. Morbidity and mortality with nonmyeloablative compared with myeloablative conditioning before hematopoietic cell transplantation from HLA-matched related donors. Blood 2004;104:1550–8.

[49] Alyea EP, Kim H, Cutler C, et al. Similar Outcome of non-myeloablative and myeloablative allogeneic hematopoietic cell transplantation for patients greater than fifty years of age. Blood 2005;105:1810–4.

[50] Clift RA, Buckner CD, Appelbaum FR, et al. Allogeneic marrow transplantation in patients with chronic myeloid leukemia in the chronic phase: a randomized trial of two irradiation regimens. Blood 1991;77:1660–5.

[51] Oehler VG, Radich JP, Storer B, et al. Randomized trial of allogeneic related bone marrow transplantation versus peripheral blood stem cell transplantation for chronic myeloid leukemia. Biol Blood Marrow Transplant 2005;11:85–92.

[52] Kiehl MG, Kraut L, Schwerdtfeger R, et al. Outcome of allogeneic hematopoietic stem-cell transplantation in adult patients with acute lymphoblastic leukemia: no difference in related compared with unrelated transplant in first complete remission. J Clin Oncol 2004;22:2816–25.

Clin Chest Med 26 (2005) 529 – 543

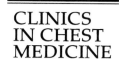

CLINICS
IN CHEST
MEDICINE

An Overview of Solid Organ Transplantation

Roy D. Bloom, MD[a], Lee R. Goldberg, MD, MPH[b],
Andrew Y. Wang, MD[c], Thomas W. Faust, MD[c], Robert M. Kotloff, MD[d],*

[a]Renal, Electrolyte, and Hypertension Division, University of Pennsylvania Medical Center, 3400 Spruce Street,
Philadelphia, PA 19104, USA
[b]Cardiovascular Disease Division, University of Pennsylvania Medical Center, 3400 Spruce Street,
Philadelphia, PA 19104, USA
[c]Gastroenterology Division, University of Pennsylvania Medical Center, 3400 Spruce Street, Philadelphia, PA 19104, USA
[d]Pulmonary, Allergy, and Critical Care Division, University of Pennsylvania Medical Center, 3400 Spruce Street,
Philadelphia, PA 19104, USA

The era of solid organ transplantation was inaugurated in 1954 with the performance of the first successful kidney transplantation. This success was followed by a series of technical achievements that expanded the field to heart, liver, pancreas, and lung transplantation. The introduction of cyclosporine in the early 1980s revolutionized immunosuppressive strategies and further propelled the field forward. Once a medical curiosity, solid organ transplantation is now a commonplace occurrence, with more than 27,000 procedures performed in the United States in 2004 alone [1]. This article offers an overview of the various solid organ transplant procedures to provide a context within which subsequent articles on pulmonary complications can be viewed.

Heart transplantation

Status of heart transplantation in the United States

Heart transplantation remains the treatment of choice for younger patients who have intractable heart failure despite maximal medical and device therapy who are otherwise healthy. In the United States for the 365-day period ending June 30, 2004, 1997 cardiac transplants were performed. On that same date, 3494 patients were on the waiting list for cardiac transplantation [2]. Since 1993, the number of patients being listed for transplant has been decreasing gradually because of improved medical and surgical management of advanced heart failure that has led to a 1-year survival approaching that of transplantation [3]. In addition, a new status system has shifted the distribution of donor organs to sicker patients, making early listing less imperative [4]. The annual mortality rate for patients listed and awaiting cardiac transplantation is approximately 18%. This statistic may be underestimated, because 2.6% of listed patients are removed from the list because of deterioration before death. The median time from initial listing to cardiac transplantation in adults is about 9.4 months [2]. The times can vary significantly depending on the urgency status of the patient (1A, 1B, or 2), blood group, body size, and geographic location [5]. As an example, for blood group O recipients the median waiting time in the United States was 290 days; blood group AB patients waited a median of 47 days [1]. Patients who are listed as status 1A had a median time to transplantation of 49 days; those listed as status 2 waited a median of 392 days [1].

Indications and contraindications

The primary indications for cardiac transplantation include refractory heart failure despite maximal medical support, refractory ventricular arrhythmias,

---

* Corresponding author.
E-mail address: kotloff@mail.med.upenn.edu (R.M. Kotloff).

and refractory angina [6]. The 1-year survival of patients after transplantation is about 86%; therefore, patients listed for transplantation should have an estimated 1-year risk of mortality without transplantation of greater than 15% [2]. Several risk models have been proposed to help risk stratify patients who have heart failure using both invasive and noninvasive methods [6]. The most potent predictor of outcome in ambulatory patients who have heart failure is a symptom-limited metabolic stress test to calculate peak oxygen consumption (VO_2). Several studies have indicated that a peak VO_2 of less than 10 mL/kg/min indicates a poor prognosis with a survival that is less than that of transplantation. Patients who have a peak VO_2 of less than 12 mL/kg/min and refractory symptoms of heart failure also have been shown to have an improved quality of life after transplantation [6]. Nonambulatory patients who require continuous intravenous administration of inotropes and who cannot be weaned or who require mechanical support to maintain an adequate cardiac index are also considered potential candidates for cardiac transplantation. In rare instances, refractory ventricular arrhythmias or refractory angina that persist despite maximal medical and surgical therapies are also indications for transplantation [7].

The contraindications for cardiac transplantation include any medical condition that would be expected to limit life expectancy after transplantation. Recent or active malignancies, active infections, or other chronic life-threatening diseases typically exclude a patient from being considered for transplantation. In addition, evidence of end-organ damage, including advanced pulmonary disease, renal insufficiency, hepatic insufficiency, or severe vascular disease, also precludes transplantation. Age greater than 65 years has become a relative contraindication, because patients above this age have been shown to have worse outcomes [4,6]. Psychosocial factors, including inability to follow a rigorous medical regimen after transplantation, can also be contraindications. Pulmonary hypertension with a pulmonary vascular resistance of greater than 4 Wood units that cannot be reduced by medical means or through the placement of a ventricular-assist device is considered an absolute contraindication for isolated cardiac transplantation. In the setting of fixed pulmonary hypertension, the donor right ventricle often fails, leading to a high risk of perioperative mortality [6].

Allocation system

In January of 1999, the United Network for Organ Sharing (UNOS) implemented an acuity status system for patients awaiting cardiac transplantation in the United States. Under this system, donor hearts are to be allocated to the sickest patients first to maximize waiting list survival. The current acuity system includes three levels. Patients who are at the greatest risk of death are listed as status 1A; patients who are status 2 are considered to have a lower risk. Within an ABO blood group and recipient size range, donor organs are offered first to the highest priority patients and then to the lower risk groups until the organs are matched with a recipient. Hearts are offered geographically using the location of the donor. Hearts are offered first to local transplant centers and then to centers outside the region in a series of concentric circles of 500 miles in diameter until an organ is matched [8]. The ischemic time of approximately 4 hours limits the distance from which a heart can be harvested.

For each acuity status, a number of objective criteria must be met. The criteria for being listed as status 1A include

> Mechanical circulatory support (intra-aortic balloon pump, total artificial heart, or extracorporeal membrane oxygenation)
> Implantation of a ventricular-assist device (for 30 days once the center has determined the patient is stable)
> Complications involving a ventricular-assist device including mechanical failure or infection, or
> High-dose or multiple inotropes (dobutamine, dopamine, or milrinone) with an indwelling pulmonary artery catheter

IA status can also be obtained through an exception review process in each region. This system is used when the patient has a high risk of death within 1 to 2 weeks without transplantation but does not fit any of the established criteria [8]. The 30-day period of 1A time after placement of a ventricular-assist device can be applied at any time after implantation. This provision allows the patient to recover from the initial surgery as well as from heart failure. Several studies have indicated that waiting several weeks for end-organ function to normalize after ventricular-assist device surgery improves cardiac transplantation outcomes. Therefore, many centers wait to activate the 30 days of 1A time at 2 to 6 weeks after implantation [9].

1B status is for patients who are being treated with a single inotrope that does not meet the criteria of high dose. Patients can be ambulatory and in the community or hospitalized. 1B status can also be obtained either before or after the 30-day period after placement of a ventricular-assist device. Status 2 patients are those who meet the indications for transplantation and have an expected 1-year mortality risk of more than 15% but are not taking continuous inotropes or do not have a mechanical support device [8].

Pretransplantation care

Patients awaiting cardiac transplantation are managed with a variety of heart failure therapies including neurohormonal blocking agents (angiotensin-converting enzyme inhibitors, beta blockers, aldosterone antagonists, angiotensin receptor blockers) and diuretics. In addition, eligible patients may receive a biventricular pacemaker, and almost all these patients have an implantable defibrillator to protect against sudden cardiac death before transplantation [10]. It is important that clinicians re-evaluate patients being considered for cardiac transplantation, because several of the newer therapies can promote positive remodeling of the ventricle over time, precluding or at least delaying the need for transplantation.

Intravenous inotropic therapy is often initiated for patients who remain in a low cardiac output state or who have refractory symptoms of congestion despite maximal medical support and, if appropriate, biventricular pacing. The most commonly used chronic inotropes include milrinone and dobutamine. Inotropes can significantly improve cardiac index, decrease symptoms, and improve end-organ perfusion. Inotropes also significantly increase the risk of arrhythmias, including potentially fatal ventricular arrhythmias. In the past, patients receiving continuous inotropes remained hospitalized until a suitable organ became available. Recent studies have shown that with the use of an implantable defibrillator to treat dangerous ventricular arrhythmias, patients awaiting transplantation can be managed safely as outpatients [11].

Patients who have acute hemodynamic compromise or have a chronic low cardiac output state despite inotropic support may be candidates for placement of a ventricular-assist device. These devices can supplement or replace the cardiac output from the right, left, or both ventricles. Ventricular-assist devices have been used to bridge patients to transplantation, and there is evidence that in the appropriate population these devices can reverse end-organ dysfunction and allow improved outcomes after transplantation [9]. Certain ventricular-assist devices allow patients to be managed successfully as outpatients while awaiting transplantation.

Surgical techniques

Three surgical techniques are commonly in use for cardiac transplantation: the standard, bicaval, or total technique [12]. In the standard or biatrial technique, cuffs of the recipient atria, including the orifices of the pulmonary veins, are left intact and then are sewn to the donor atria. Advantages of this technique include a shorter surgical time and no need to re-implant the pulmonary veins. During the past several years, the bicaval approach has gained favor, because it has reduced atrial arrhythmias, sino-atrial nodal dysfunction, and tricuspid regurgitation. In this technique, the recipient pulmonary veins are excised in a cuff of left atrium and then are attached to the donor left atrium. The entire recipient right atrium is removed. The superior and inferior vena cavae are attached, as are the aorta and pulmonary arteries. Several studies have shown that this technique, although it adds ischemic time, has led to improved short- and long-term outcomes. The total technique involves removal of the entire recipient heart with the exception of two small "buttons" of left atrial tissue containing the four pulmonary veins. The remainder of the anastomoses are identical to the bicaval technique, except that there are two anastomoses in the left atrium. Limited studies have suggested that this technique adds significant ischemic time but does not lead to improved outcomes [6,12].

Cardiac transplantation outcomes

The outcomes in cardiac transplantation have improved over time, with the 1-year survival rate for patients undergoing transplantation from January 1, 2001 through June 30, 2003 being 86.7%. The 3-year survival rate is 78.6% [2]. At 1 year, 90% of surviving patients report no functional limitations, and approximately 36% return to work [13]. In the first year, the most common cause of death includes graft dysfunction. After the first year, infections and graft dysfunction are the most common causes. Late causes of death include graft vasculopathy and malignancies [13].

Graft vasculopathy is one of the major limitations to long-term survival after cardiac transplantation. Several donor and recipient factors can influence the development of vasculopathy and lead to graft dysfunction and death. Graft vasculopathy differs from typical coronary disease in that it is diffuse in nature and can affect the small vessels first, making it difficult to detect with coronary angiography. Intravascular ultrasound has become the criterion standard for detecting and monitoring graft coronary disease but is not available routinely outside research protocols. Most researchers agree that this form of vasculopathy is immune mediated, and several small studies have shown regression with newer or augmented immunosuppression. The routine use of 3-hydroxy-3-methylglutaryl coenzyme A reductase inhibitors in all cardiac transplant recipients, regardless of lipid profile, has become the standard of care because of evidence suggesting that the anti-inflammatory property of statins may help prevent or delay vasculopathy [14].

Liver transplantation

Background

The first successful human liver transplantation was performed in 1967 by Starzl and colleagues [15]. As of November 30, 2004, more than 68,000 liver transplantations have been performed in 142 institutions across the United States; 5670 liver transplants were performed in 2003 alone [1]. More than 16,000 patients await liver transplantation each year, and median times on the waiting list range from 210 to 1243 days, depending on blood type. Because of the shortage of suitable donor organs, 1818 patients died in 2002 while awaiting liver transplantation [16].

Indications for liver transplantation

Orthotopic liver transplantation may be indicated for acute or chronic liver failure from any cause [17]. In the United States, alcohol-induced liver disease and chronic hepatitis C infection are the most common indications for liver transplantation [15,18,19]. Hepatic decompensation is associated with high short-term morbidity and mortality. Two-year survival in patients who have cirrhosis complicated by ascites is only 50% [20]. Similarly, patients who have cirrhosis and are admitted with variceal hemorrhage have an inpatient mortality of 30% to 50% [21,22]. Renal failure, which is common in patients who have fulminant hepatic failure (FHF) or advanced cirrhosis, is associated with increased short- and long-term pretransplantation mortality [23]. Patients who have type 1 hepatorenal syndrome (HRS) have a 2-week mortality of 80%, and only 10% of these patients survive longer than 3 months [24]. Hepatic encephalopathy, spontaneous bacterial peritonitis, and hepatopulmonary syndrome are other late manifestations of chronic liver disease that are associated with significant morbidity and should

prompt referral to a liver transplant center [25]. Hepatocellular carcinoma is common in patients who have cirrhosis but also may be found in patients who have chronic replicative hepatitis B infection in the absence of significant fibrosis. Patients who have a single, isolated hepatocellular carcinoma measuring between 2 and 5 cm in diameter or patients who have fewer than three lesions, each less than 3 cm in diameter, should be referred for liver transplantation.

Patients hospitalized for FHF resulting from viral or autoimmune hepatitis, Wilson's disease, acute Budd-Chiari syndrome, or drug hepatotoxicity should be referred to a transplant center for expedited transplant evaluation. Patients who have FHF are listed separately from those with chronic liver disease. In response to the severity of acute liver injury, patients who have FHF are given status 1 priority, which places them at the top of the waiting list.

Last, liver transplantation may be indicated in patients who have intractable pruritus, metabolic bone disease, recurrent bacterial cholangitis, or progressive malnutrition. Although these patients may not have decompensated cirrhosis or FHF, transplantation should be considered to treat the extremely poor quality of life associated with these conditions.

Listing criteria and organ allocation

Although a topic of recent debate, there are no minimal listing criteria for liver transplantation at this time [26]. Donor livers are allocated based on ABO blood type, and acutely ill patients who are listed as status 1 are transplanted first. After status 1, livers are allocated by the modified Model for End-stage Liver Disease (MELD) score, which is used in patients who have chronic liver disease. The MELD score originally was developed to predict outcomes in cirrhotic patients undergoing transjugular intrahepatic portosystemic shunt [27]. The MELD score (range: 6–40) is derived from three widely available and easily repeatable laboratory values: total bilirubin, creatinine, and international normalized ratio. Studies have found the MELD score to be highly predictive of 3-month mortality in hospitalized patients who have cirrhosis. MELD scores between 20 and 35 are associated with 10% to 60% 3-month mortality, whereas MELD scores greater than 35 are associated with 80% mortality at 3 months [28,29]. At present, MELD exception points are conferred to patients who have stage 2 hepatocellular carcinoma or hepatopulmonary syndrome [1,26]. When two or more patients of the same blood group have the same MELD score, patients who have the longest waiting-list time are given priority.

Contraindications

Problems that absolutely preclude liver transplantation include active extrahepatic infections, poor social support, untreated psychiatric disorders, significant coronary artery disease, advanced chronic obstructive or restrictive pulmonary disease, and active alcohol or drug abuse [15]. Untreated HIV infection has been considered an absolute contraindication. Patients who have well-controlled HIV, however, should be considered for clinical trials that will assess the role of transplantation in stable patients receiving highly active antiretroviral therapy. Other contraindications to orthotopic liver transplantation include extrahepatic malignancies, cholangiocarcinoma, and anatomic abnormalities that make transplantation unfeasible.

Advanced age is a negative risk factor, because patients older than 65 years have worse outcomes than patients who are 60 to 65 years of age or younger [30]. Despite these findings, advanced age alone should not exclude patients from transplantation but should necessitate a thorough pretransplantation evaluation. Although patients who have diabetes are at higher risk for adverse outcomes after transplantation, liver transplantation is not contraindicated in patients who have well-controlled diabetes [31,32].

Renal failure, irrespective of its cause, does not exclude patients from liver transplantation. As mentioned previously, type 1 HRS is an indication for transplantation. Patients who have HRS of prolonged duration (likely type 2 HRS) or with chronic renal failure from other causes should be evaluated by a transplant nephrologist and considered for combined liver-kidney transplantation.

Deceased-donor versus living-donor liver transplantation

Most transplanted livers come from deceased donors. In 2003, 5348 deceased-donor liver transplants (DDLT) were performed, whereas only 322 living-donor liver transplants (LDLT) were done during the same period [1]. The concept of LDLT originated from renal transplantation, and LDLT was found to be particularly applicable to pediatric patients because left lateral segment transplants could provide sufficient hepatic mass for small children. Because of the increasing demand for donor organs and a static deceased-donor pool, LDLT has been increasingly recognized as a viable option for patients in need of transplantation. Unlike the pediatric patient, an adult recipient requires a larger liver volume, which may include a right hepatic lobe resection or a full left graft in smaller adult recipients [33–35].

Despite the usefulness of LDLT, the risk to the donor is significant. Nine percent to 19% of donors may develop complications [36]. Complications include wound infection, small-bowel obstruction, and incisional hernias. Approximately 10% of donors develop bile leaks and neurapraxia. Although morbidity is possible, donors have demonstrated general acceptance of the procedure and have had favorable outcomes [36].

Surgical procedure

The technical aspects of surgery involving DDLT and LDLT are beyond the scope of this article. The three major phases of surgery include native liver dissection (1 to 2 hours), the anhepatic phase (1.5 to 3 hours), and revascularization of the liver [15]. The most commonly used surgical technique was described by Starzl and colleagues in 1963 [37]. Earlier operations included removal of the retrohepatic vena cava causing decreased venous return to the heart and hemodynamic instability [38]. One of the major modifications in transplant surgery has included preservation of the retrohepatic vena cava to maintain venous return to the heart, minimizing hemodynamic instability and eliminating the need for venovenous bypass [39]. This "piggyback" technique is now commonly used in most transplant centers and has been found to be safe and associated with few surgical complications [15,38].

Certain perioperative factors are of potential consequence in the posttransplantation period. Prolonged cold-ischemia time is associated with primary nonfunction and hepatic artery thrombosis [15]. Cold-ischemia times longer than 15 hours are significantly associated with higher rates of acute cellular rejection [40].

Immediate postoperative complications

Many of the immediate complications after transplantation are related to the surgical procedure. The most common postoperative surgical complication is intra-abdominal bleeding, which may occur in 10% to 15% of patients [41]. Although a picture of ischemic liver injury is common immediately after transplantation, the liver-associated enzymes usually normalize by 2 to 3 days after transplantation. Evidence of cholestasis after this time requires further investigation. It is appropriate to begin with an ultrasound examination to evaluate for biliary ductal dilation, which may signal a biliary stricture. Simultaneous

Doppler imaging should be obtained to evaluate for hepatic artery thrombosis, portal and hepatic vein thrombosis, or inferior vena cava obstruction. If a stricture is found, or if the ultrasound is unrevealing, endoscopic retrograde cholangiopancreatography should be considered the criterion standard to evaluate the biliary tree. Biliary stents may be required for strictures or leaks. Liver biopsy is recommended for patients who have persistently abnormal liver-associated enzymes to evaluate for acute cellular rejection or other causes of hepatic injury and dysfunction, such as drug-induced hepatotoxicity or infection.

Outcomes

Patient survival rates among DDLT recipients are 88% at 1 year and 74% at 5 years after transplantation [16]. Virtually identical patient survival rates are associated with LDLT [16]. Graft survival rates, however, seem to be somewhat lower for LDLT (64.4% for LDLT versus 73.3% for DDLT at 2 years) [42]. Nonetheless, LDLT is a reasonable option for patients who are unlikely to receive DDLT in a timely fashion.

Kidney transplantation

Background and history

Chronic kidney disease is associated with debilitating consequences and a reduction in life expectancy. Chronic kidney disease commonly progresses to end-stage renal disease (ESRD), in which renal replacement therapy is required to prevent death from uremic complications. Dialysis and transplantation are the two treatment options for ESRD. Compared with dialysis, transplantation is associated with significant improvement in quality of life and in overall longevity [43]. At the same time, annualized per patient costs of transplant-related care of around $17,000 pale in comparison with the $53,000 for dialysis [44].

The first kidney transplantation was successfully performed by Joseph Murray and colleagues in Boston in 1954, between a pair of identical twins receiving no immunosuppression [45]. After these pioneering efforts, kidney transplantation expanded globally, and Murray received the Nobel Prize in Medicine in 1990. Currently, there are around 350,000 ESRD patients in the United States, although with population aging and the escalation of diabetes

and hypertension, this number is projected to exceed 650,000 by the end of the decade [46]. The increased success of transplantation and mounting ESRD rates have culminated in a greater demand–supply disparity and a surge in the number of patients waitlisted for a kidney. Although 200,000 kidney transplantations have been performed in the United States since 1988, nearly 65,000 patients remain on the national waiting list for a kidney, more than double the number a decade ago [1].

Indications for kidney transplantation

Any patient whose quality of life or lifespan is likely to be improved after transplantation should be considered a potential candidate. The remarkably few contraindications to kidney transplantation alone are related mostly to excessive comorbidity, when the risks of sustaining harm with surgery and immunosuppression outweigh the benefits of transplantation. Such conditions include advanced liver or lung disease, intractable or advanced infection, or unremitting malignancy. Cardiovascular disease, for which kidney disease is a major risk factor, is the leading cause of mortality in ESRD patients [47,48]. Special emphasis therefore is placed on evaluation of cardiovascular disease in kidney candidates, but its presence does not preclude transplantation unless it is active and not amenable to any intervention. It is recommended that waitlisted kidney candidates be periodically rescreened for cardiovascular disease until they receive a transplant [49].

Types of kidney transplants

Both living and deceased donors are used as sources of kidneys for renal transplantation. Living donors are either genetically related (parent, child, sibling) or unrelated (friend, spouse, altruistic donor) to the recipient. Living donation avoids ischemia-reperfusion injury associated with procurement, storage, transportation, and implantation of kidneys from deceased donors; moreover, living donors are healthy at the time of donation. For all these reasons, living-donor kidneys are typically superior in quality and function. In particular, the best outcomes are observed with kidneys transplanted between human leukocyte antigen (HLA)-identical siblings. Survival rates for all types of non–HLA-identical living-donor transplants are similar regardless of the donor–recipient genetic relationship and, importantly, exceed results with even the best-matched deceased-donor kidneys. Living-donor kidney transplantation can also be performed on an elective basis and can be timed to minimize or even avoid the need for any dialysis in the recipient.

With the burgeoning waiting list and increasingly poor quality of available deceased-donor kidneys, the emphasis on living donation has magnified during the past decade. Coupled with the advent of laparoscopic nephrectomy technology and the observed outcome benefits of living-kidney donation alluded to previously, living donation in the United States has expanded from about 2500 in 1992 to more than 6000 in 2001 [50]. During this same time, the deceased-donor count changed only from 4500 to 5500 per year [50]. Because two recipients can receive kidneys from each deceased donor, there still are more deceased-donor transplantations performed overall each year. For the living donor, living with one remaining kidney has no effect on life expectancy or lifestyle, childbearing potential, or access to medical care or insurability.

Timing of waitlist placement and transplantation

Current UNOS policy mandates that patients can be waitlisted for a transplant only when their glomerular filtration rate is less than 20 mL/min. Once listed, median waiting times range between 3 and 4 years, although this time varies regionally and according to patient blood type [50]. Professional guidelines recommend referral of patients for transplantation well in advance of their needing dialysis, to help identify potential living donors and to also gain lead-time on the waitlist [51]. Because dialysis duration before transplantation is related inversely to survival after transplantation, transplantation before starting dialysis is desirable [52,53]. Because of lengthening waiting times, however, transplantation before dialysis seldom occurs in patients who do not have living donors.

Human leukocyte antigen matching and allocation

Acute rejection occurs with increasing degree of HLA mismatch [54]. Because zero-mismatched kidneys experience the lowest rates of acute rejection, a national policy for sharing of such organs from deceased donors has been developed and refined during the past 2 decades [55]. At present, 17% of deceased-donor kidneys are shared nationally by this policy, although there is evidence that the benefits of optimal HLA matching may be mitigated by increased ischemia-reperfusion injury associated with shipment of such organs [56].

Another enormous challenge facing the kidney transplant community is the growing pool of patients who have acquired anti-HLA antibodies because of sensitization from prior blood transfusions or transplants or through pregnancy. In many cases, the high levels of sensitization render it almost impossible to find suitable donors for affected individuals. There is growing interest in the use of pretransplantation immunosuppressive protocols to lower or eliminate anti-HLA antibodies in such patients to facilitate future transplantation. Similar experimental strategies also are being investigated for the transplantation of kidneys across ABO-incompatible barriers. Preliminary results with these novel regimens are encouraging, although their longer-term safety and efficacy remain unknown [44,57].

Kidney transplant surgery and the perioperative period

The transplanted kidney is placed extraperitoneally in the right or left lower abdominal quadrant. The transplant renal artery and veins generally are anastomosed to the external iliac artery and vein, respectively. The transplanted ureter usually is reimplanted to the recipient bladder using a technique to prevent urine reflux. Although immediate function of the transplanted kidney is desirable, it often does not occur. Many transplant centers obtain imaging studies (ultrasound with Doppler; nuclear isotope flow scan) of the kidney in the immediate postoperative period to assess blood flow and allograft function. Technical factors related to vascular anastomoses or immunologic catastrophes such as hyperacute rejection may, rarely, result in immediate graft failure within hours of transplantation and the need for transplant nephrectomy. More commonly, most deceased-donor and some live-donor recipients experience early transient graft dysfunction. The term "delayed graft function" is defined as the requirement for dialysis within the first week after transplantation. Although this term does not capture patients who have early graft dysfunction who do not require dialysis and includes patients who have immediate function who are dialyzed for an indication such as hyperkalemia, it has persisted as a universal standard for clinical trial purposes. Delayed graft function usually is caused by acute tubular necrosis; the reported frequency ranges from 2% to 50% [58]. Factors such as deceased-donor source, procurement injury, ischemia-reperfusion injury, drug nephrotoxicity, volume depletion, and acute rejection all predispose to delayed graft function [58]. Although functional recovery is the rule, long-term graft survival may be compromised. Strategies to mitigate delayed graft function include trimming ischemic times by expediting the transplantation, aggressive perioperative volume expansion, and avoiding or minimizing calcineurin inhibitors and other nephrotoxic agents in the peritransplantation setting. When delayed graft function persists despite these strategies, kidney transplant biopsy is commonly performed within the first 2 to 3 weeks after transplantation to optimize therapy.

Outcomes after kidney transplantation

One-year patient survival rates exceed 95%, whereas 1-year graft survival rates are now over 91% overall [50]. Current 5-year patient and graft survival rates are 92% and 79% for living-donor and 86% and 65% for deceased-donor recipients, respectively [50]. Long-term, graft half-life beyond the first year after transplantation has improved only marginally, with graft loss in this setting caused mainly by chronic allograft nephropathy, a process characterized by an inexorable decline in kidney function resulting from progressive scarring [59]. Both immunologic (eg, acute rejection, HLA mismatching) and nonimmunologic factors (eg, ischemia-reperfusion injury, hypertension, calcineurin-inhibitor toxicity) have been implicated in predisposing to chronic allograft nephropathy. With an improving immunosuppressive arsenal, chronic allograft nephropathy now is being replaced by death, most commonly in the setting of cardiovascular disease, as the leading cause of chronic graft failure [48,59].

Lung transplantation

Background/current status

Human lung transplantation was attempted first in 1963, but it was not until 2 decades later that extended survival was achieved. After the initial technical successes of the 1980s, the field of lung transplantation realized dramatic growth in both the number of procedures performed and the number of candidates placed on waiting lists for organs. Since the latter part of the 1990s, however, lung transplant activity has leveled to an approximate rate of 1000 procedures annually in the United States, representing one half the volume of heart transplants and one fifth the volume of liver transplants performed [16]. The constraints on lung transplantation reflect in large part the severe scarcity of suitable allografts; only approximately 15% of cadaveric donors capable of donating at least one solid organ have lungs suitable for transplantation. There has been a modest increase in the number of lung donors in the past several years, but this increase has been offset by a growing trend favoring bilateral over single-lung transplantation [16]. Because of the current constraints, the number of registered candidates awaiting lung transplantation in the United States now exceeds the annual number of procedures by almost fourfold. Additionally, the median waiting time has escalated to approximately 3 years, although it is anticipated that this waiting period will change with implementation of the new allocations system (discussed later).

Candidate selection

Lung transplantation is a therapeutic option for a broad spectrum of chronic, debilitating pulmonary disorders of the airways, parenchyma, and vasculature [60]. Chronic obstructive pulmonary disease (COPD) is the leading indication for lung transplantation, accounting for approximately half of all procedures performed worldwide [61]. Other leading indications include idiopathic pulmonary fibrosis (17% of cases) and cystic fibrosis (16% of cases). Once a common indication for transplantation, primary pulmonary hypertension now accounts for less than 5% of procedures, reflecting major advances in the medical management of these patients [16,61]. Transplantation of patients who have lung involvement caused by collagen vascular disease (eg, scleroderma) remains controversial because of concerns that extrapulmonary manifestations of the systemic disease could compromise the posttransplantation course. Nonetheless, short-term functional outcomes and survival after transplantation are comparable with other patient populations, and most centers are willing to offer transplantation to carefully selected patients who do not have significant extrapulmonary organ dysfunction [62]. In contrast, lung transplantation for bronchoalveolar carcinoma, a subtype of lung cancer that tends to remain localized to the lung parenchyma, largely has been abandoned because of an unacceptably high rate of cancer recurrence [63].

Listing for transplantation is considered when the lung disease is deemed to pose a high risk of death within several years. Disease-specific guidelines for timely referral and listing of patients, based on available predictive indices, have been published [64]. The imprecise nature of these predictive indices must be acknowledged, particularly with respect to COPD and Eisenmenger's syndrome, which tend to follow highly variable and often protracted courses even in the advanced stages. The patient's perception of an unacceptably poor quality of life is an important additional factor to consider but should not serve as the sole justification for referral of a patient whose disease is not deemed to be at a life-threatening stage.

The scarcity of organs and the somewhat inferior outcomes achieved with increasing age have prompted the establishment of recommended age cutoffs: 55 years for heart-lung, 60 years for bilateral lung, and 65 years for single-lung transplantation. Candidates should be functionally disabled (New York Heart Association class III or IV) but still ambulatory. Many programs screen for and exclude profoundly debilitated patients by requiring a minimum distance on a standard 6-minute walk test, most frequently 600 feet [65]. The presence of significant renal, hepatic, or left ventricular dysfunction precludes isolated lung transplantation, but multiorgan transplantation can be considered in highly select patients. Other absolute contraindications include active infection with HIV, hepatitis B virus, or hepatitis C virus with histologic evidence of significant liver damage; active or recent cigarette smoking, drug or alcohol abuse; recent malignancy (other than nonmelanotic skin cancers); and extremes of weight. The risk posed by other chronic medical conditions such as diabetes mellitus, osteoporosis, gastroesophageal reflux, and limited coronary artery disease should be assessed individually based on severity of disease, presence of end-organ damage, and ease of control with standard therapies. Among candidates who have cystic fibrosis, airways colonization with *Burkholderia cepacia* is considered a strong contraindication to lung transplantation by the majority of centers, because of the demonstrated propensity of this organism to cause lethal infections after transplantation [65,66]. Transplantation of patients receiving mechanical ventilation is associated with an increased risk of mortality at 1 year and therefore is not commonly performed [61,65].

Allocation system

From 1990 to 2005, lung allocation in the United States was based on a seniority system that prioritized candidates by the amount of time they had accrued on the waiting list, without regard to severity of illness. This system ultimately was called into question because it failed to accommodate patients who have a more rapidly progressive course, who often could not tolerate the prolonged waiting times to transplantation and who were likely to die before receiving an organ. Indeed, excessive wait list mortality was documented among certain patient populations, such as those with idiopathic pulmonary

fibrosis and cystic fibrosis, as compared with patients who have COPD [67]. In response to the perceived inequities of the time-based system, and under mandate of the federal government, a new system was implemented in May of 2005 that allocates lungs on the basis of both medical urgency (ie, risk of death without a transplant) and net transplantation benefit (the difference between predicted survival after transplantation and survival with continued waiting) [8]. By incorporating this latter concept, the system attempts to avoid the pitfall of preferentially allocating the scarce donor organ pool to desperately ill patients who have an unacceptably high posttransplantation mortality rate.

The new model, derived from a multivariate analysis of data from the comprehensive UNOS national database, identifies 10 factors independently predictive of death on the waiting list and seven predictive of death after transplantation. For each patient, these factors are used to calculate predicted 1-year survival with and without transplantation. Patients who demonstrate a large net difference in survival (predicted posttransplantation − pretransplantation survival) in conjunction with a high degree of medical urgency (low predicted pretransplantation survival) receive the highest priority scores. Several concerns have been raised about the new system that will have to be addressed in an ongoing evaluation of its merits:

1. The predictive model employed has not been prospectively validated.
2. The calculation of net transplant benefit is based on predicted 1-year posttransplantation survival, which is heavily influenced by differences in disease-specific perioperative mortality rates and does not truly reflect long-term outcomes.
3. Net transplant benefit is defined exclusively in terms of survival and does not acknowledge dramatically improved functional status and quality of life as a net benefit.

Surgical procedures

Heart-lung transplantation was the first procedure to be performed successfully, but it has largely been supplanted by techniques to replace the lungs alone. Heart-lung transplantation now is principally restricted to Eisenmenger's syndrome with surgically irreparable cardiac lesions and advanced lung disease with concurrent left ventricular dysfunction or severe coronary artery disease. Previously, the presence of severe right ventricular dysfunction was deemed an indication for heart-lung transplantation. Subsequent experience with isolated lung transplantation, however, has demonstrated the remarkable ability of the right ventricle to recover once pulmonary artery pressures are normalized.

Single-lung transplantation is the procedure of choice for pulmonary fibrosis and for older patients who have chronic obstructive pulmonary disease but is contraindicated in patients who have suppurative lung disorders such as cystic fibrosis. Most centers also consider severe pulmonary hypertension to be a contraindication to single-lung transplantation. In this setting, single-lung transplantation would result in diversion of nearly the entire cardiac output through the allograft, because of the high vascular resistance in the remaining native lung, and this diversion can contribute to exaggerated reperfusion pulmonary edema in the allograft. Major advantages of single-lung transplantation are its technical ease and its efficient use of the limited donor pool, permitting two recipients to benefit from a single donor.

Bilateral sequential lung transplantation involves the performance of two single-lung transplantation procedures in succession during a single operative session. In the absence of severe pulmonary hypertension, cardiopulmonary bypass often can be avoided by sustaining the patient on the contralateral lung during implantation of each allograft. The primary indications for this procedure are cystic fibrosis, other forms of bronchiectasis, and pulmonary vascular disorders. Additionally, some programs have advocated its use in younger patients who have emphysema, arguing that it offers functional and survival advantages over single-lung transplantation [68].

Living-donor bilateral lobar transplantation is the newest procedure to be introduced and is still uncommonly performed. It involves the implantation of right and left lower lobes harvested from two living, blood group–compatible donors. The procedure generally has been reserved for candidates whose deteriorating status does not permit them to wait for a cadaveric donor. Given the inherently undersized nature of the grafts, it is preferable that the donors be considerably taller than the recipient. Patients who have cystic fibrosis are particularly well suited as a target population because even as adults they tend to be of small stature. Concerns about excessive risk to the donor have thus far proven to be unfounded. In the largest experience reported to date, there were no deaths among 253 donors, and there were only eight complications of sufficient magnitude to warrant surgical re-exploration [69]. Donation of a lobe results in an average decrement in vital capacity of 17%.

Outcomes

Current 1-, 3-, and 5-year survival rates are 80%, 61%, and 46%, respectively [16]. Primary graft failure and infection are the most common causes of early deaths; bronchiolitis obliterans is the leading cause of late deaths. There has been a modest improvement in 1-year survival during the past decade [16]. Unfortunately, 5-year survival rate has not changed and remains considerably below the 70% 5-year survival achieved after liver and heart transplantation.

For patients who have COPD, survival for recipients younger than 60 years of age is superior after bilateral than after single-lung transplantation [70], but the converse has been demonstrated for those who have pulmonary fibrosis. Survival after living-donor transplantation is comparable with that achieved after cadaveric transplantation [71].

Pancreas transplantation

Background and history

Pancreas transplantation has evolved during the past 40 years for the treatment of type I diabetes. The first pancreas transplants were performed in 1966 and were associated with dismal results because of technical limitations and ineffective immunosuppression [72]. Increasing experience, coupled with procedural refinement and the emergence of superior immunosuppression, resulted in improving outcomes and, ultimately, the wider acceptance of pancreas transplantation as an effective treatment option. Since the late 1980s, the field has enjoyed unabated growth [73]. In total, 18,843 pancreas transplantations had been performed worldwide as of October 2002. The annual number of pancreas transplantations has increased from approximately 200 in 1988 to more than 1400 in 2002 [73].

Transplantation options for patients who have diabetes

Pancreas transplantation almost always is reserved for patients who have type I diabetes, although it has occasionally been performed in type II diabetics as well. Pancreatic allografts usually are procured from deceased donors because the reduction in residual islet mass in living donors may increase the subsequent risk of glucose intolerance in such individuals. Pancreas transplantation takes place in one of three settings:

1. Simultaneous pancreas-kidney transplantation (SPK), in which the pancreas and a kidney from the same donor are transplanted into a recipient with advanced kidney disease during one operation
2. Pancreas after kidney transplantation (PAK), in which a pancreas is transplanted into a patient who has previously received a kidney from a different living or deceased donor
3. Pancreas transplantation alone (PTA), usually reserved for patients who have hyperlabile glycemic control and well-preserved renal function

Currently more than 2400 patients are waitlisted for SPK, and about 1700 patients are listed for isolated pancreas transplantation, either as PAK or PTA [1].

Goals and rationale of pancreas transplantation

Studies have demonstrated that intensive insulin therapy in type I diabetics is associated with fewer long-term complications and, thereby, enhanced life expectancy [74]. Pancreas transplantation represents an alternative to chronic insulin therapy, with goals of effecting chronic euglycemia while simultaneously eliminating the need for exogenous insulin administration. In this way, successfully transplanted pancreas recipients experience an improvement in quality of life and eliminate both the need for chronic glucose monitoring and the life-threatening risks of hypoglycemic unawareness. Additional benefits of pancreas transplantation include the prevention and reversal of diabetic nephropathy as well as some amelioration of sensory, motor, and autonomic neuropathy [75].

Indications for pancreas transplantation

As a rule, all pancreas transplant candidates should be C-peptide deficient. Patients who have advanced diabetic kidney disease are potentially eligible for SPK transplantation. Indications for isolated pancreas transplantation are less well established, although the widely endorsed American Diabetes Association's position is that this procedure should be reserved for patients who have life-threatening hypoglycemic unawareness, frequent acute metabolic complications associated with hy-

perlabile glycemic control, or failure of conventional insulin therapies to prevent acute complications [76]. Historically, older candidate age (above 45 years) and the presence of cardiovascular disease were relative contraindications to pancreas transplantation, based on their association with worse outcomes [77]. Ongoing experience during the past decade and improving results have seen an increase in age, as well as comorbidity, of potential pancreas recipients [73].

Surgical considerations in pancreas transplantation

Several surgical issues require consideration in pancreas transplantation. The transplant pancreas, together with a small segment of the adjacent duodenum (containing the sphincter of Oddi), is procured en bloc from the donor. Although transplantation of the whole pancreas serves as the source of abundant functioning islets, the graft's exocrine drainage through the pancreatic duct must be accommodated. The first widely adopted technique involved pancreatic duct drainage into the urinary bladder through a pancreaticoduodenocystostomy, but this procedure was associated with frequent complications [78]. Enteric drainage was developed as an alternative option to the bladder route [79]. With enteric drainage, the segment of transplant duodenum is attached to the small bowel either with a Roux-en-Y anastomosis or directly end-to-side [79,80].

Another surgical issue is the method of venous drainage for the transplant pancreas. Initially, most procedures were performed with venous drainage through the iliac vessels. With this technique, insulin released from the pancreas enters the systemic circulation directly, avoiding the physiologic first-pass effect in the liver. This technique results in systemic hyperinsulinemia, although there is no evidence that this form of chronic hyperinsulinemia has any adverse consequence [81]. During the past decade, the technique of draining the venous outflow directly into the portal vein has become increasingly common [82]. Although this approach approximates the normal trafficking of insulin through the liver, registry data do not demonstrate any outcome differences between the two routes of venous drainage [73].

The immediate posttransplantation course typically is characterized by rapid improvements in blood glucose levels. Failure of such improvement should prompt a high index of suspicion for an early complication, such as graft thrombosis, rejection, pancreatitis, duct leaks, or infection. International Registry data continue to indicate a technical failure rate of 7% to 14%, depending on the technique involved and type of pancreas transplantation performed [73].

Monitoring for pancreas rejection remains imprecise. Hyperglycemia is a late marker, developing only after most of the islet mass has been damaged. Elevations in amylase and lipase levels raise the suspicion of graft dysfunction and warrant imaging studies and consideration for biopsy.

Outcomes after pancreas transplantation

Historically, pancreas outcomes after SPK transplantation were superior to those after either PAK or PTA. This difference was attributed to increased immunologic problems observed in isolated-pancreas transplantation and to the ability of the creatinine to serve as a reliable surrogate of graft function in patients receiving SPK [83]. With superior immunosuppression and greater expertise, 1-year pancreas graft survival rates are now similar for all three types of transplantation, although by 5 years SPK recipients continue to exhibit the best pancreas outcomes at 69% [50]. Registry analyses further indicate that, compared with remaining on the waiting list, SPK transplantation is associated with lower mortality rates, although this advantage has not been established unequivocally for PAK or PTA recipients [84,85]. SPK transplantation is also associated with better patient and kidney graft survival than transplantation of a deceased-donor kidney alone but offers no advantage over a kidney from a living donor [86,87]. Based on these data, the following clinical approach to type I diabetics with advanced chronic kidney disease is recommended. Pre-emptive transplantation should be pursued if at all possible to minimize or avoid the need for dialysis, a poor outcome determinant. For patients who have acceptable comorbidity, a living-donor kidney should be used if available, followed by subsequent PAK; patients without living donors should be waitlisted and transplanted with a deceased-donor SPK. Patients in whom pancreas transplantation is contraindicated should receive a kidney alone, from either a living (preferable) or deceased donor.

Long-term pancreas graft failure is characterized by hyperglycemia and the need to restart conventional glucose-lowering therapies. In this setting, hyperglycemia may be a manifestation of either (1) islet failure (low C-peptide and insulin levels) secondary to alloimmune (acute or chronic rejection) or recurrent autoimmune-mediated injury, or (2) insulin resistance (high C-peptide and insulin levels), associated with posttransplantation weight gain and some immunosuppressive therapies.

References

[1] The organ procurement and transplantation network database. Available at: http://www.optn.org/latestData/viewDataReports.asp. Accessed April 17, 2005.

[2] Scientific registry of transplant recipients: fast facts about transplants, July 1, 2003 through June 30, 2004. Available at: http://www.ustransplant.org/csr_0105/facts.php. Accessed April 17, 2005.

[3] Pierson III RN, Barr ML, McCullough KP, et al. Thoracic organ transplantation. Am J Transplant 2004; 9:93–105.

[4] Deng MC. Orthotopic heart transplantation: highlights and limitations. Surg Clin North Am 2004;84: 243–55.

[5] Ellison MD, Edwards LB, Edwards EB, et al. Geographic differences in access to transplantation in the United States. Transplantation 2003;76:1389–94.

[6] Kirklin JK, McGiffin DC, Pinderski LJ, et al. Selection of patients and techniques of heart transplantation. Surg Clin North Am 2004;84:257–87.

[7] Shanewise J. Cardiac transplantation. Anesthesiol Clin North America 2004;22:753–65.

[8] Organ distribution: Allocation of thoracic organs (policy 3.7). Available at: http://www.unos.org/policiesandbylaws/policies.asp?resources=true. Accessed April 17, 2005.

[9] Stevenson LW, Rose EA. Left ventricular assist devices: bridges to transplantation, recovery, and destination for whom? Circulation 2003;108:3059–63.

[10] Hunt SA, Baker DW, Chin MH, et al. ACC/AHA guidelines for the evaluation and management of chronic heart failure in the adult: executive summary. A report of the American College of Cardiology/American Heart Association Task Force on Practice Guidelines. Circulation 2001;104:2996–3007.

[11] Brozena SC, Twomey C, Goldberg LR, et al. A prospective study of continuous intravenous milrinone therapy for status IB patients awaiting heart transplant at home. J Heart Lung Transplant 2004;23: 1082–6.

[12] Roselli EE, Smedira NG. Surgical advances in heart and lung transplantation. Anesthesiol Clin North America 2004;22:789–807.

[13] Taylor DO, Edwards LB, Boucek MM, et al. The Registry of the International Society for Heart and Lung Transplantation: twenty-first official adult heart transplant report–2004. J Heart Lung Transplant 2004; 23:796–803.

[14] Valantine H. Cardiac allograft vasculopathy after heart transplantation: risk factors and management. J Heart Lung Transplant 2004;23(5 Suppl):S187–93.

[15] Everson GTTJ. Transplantation of the liver. In: Schiff ER, Sorrell MF, Maddrey WC, editors. Schiff's

diseases of the liver. 9th edition. Philadelphia: Lippin-cott Williams & Wilkins; 2002. p. 1585–614.

[16] 2004 OPTN/SRTR annual report. Available at: http://www.optn.org/AR2004/default.htm. Accessed April 17, 2005.

[17] Carithers Jr RL. Liver transplantation. American Association for the Study of Liver Diseases. Liver Transpl 2000;6:122–35.

[18] Curry MP. Hepatitis B and hepatitis C viruses in liver transplantation. Transplantation 2004;78:955–63.

[19] Everson G, Bharadhwaj G, House R, et al. Long-term follow-up of patients with alcoholic liver disease who underwent hepatic transplantation. Liver Transpl Surg 1997;3:263–74.

[20] D'Amico G, Morabito A, Pagliaro L, et al. Survival and prognostic indicators in compensated and decom-pensated cirrhosis. Dig Dis Sci 1986;31:468–75.

[21] D'Amico G, Pagliaro L, Bosch J. The treatment of portal hypertension: a meta-analytic review. Hepatol-ogy 1995;22:332–54.

[22] Smith JL, Graham DY. Variceal hemorrhage: a criti-cal evaluation of survival analysis. Gastroenterology 1982;82:968–73.

[23] Nair S, Verma S, Thuluvath PJ. Pretransplant renal function predicts survival in patients undergoing orthotopic liver transplantation. Hepatology 2002;35:1179–85.

[24] Gines A, Escorsell A, Gines P, et al. Incidence, predictive factors, and prognosis of the hepatorenal syndrome in cirrhosis with ascites. Gastroenterology 1993;105:229–36.

[25] Hoeper MM, Krowka MJ, Strassburg CP. Portopul-monary hypertension and hepatopulmonary syndrome. Lancet 2004;363:1461–8.

[26] Olthoff KM, Brown Jr RS, Delmonico FL, et al. Summary report of a national conference: evolving concepts in liver allocation in the MELD and PELD era. December 8, 2003, Washington, DC, USA. Liver Transpl 2004;10(Suppl 2):A6–22.

[27] Schepke M, Roth F, Fimmers R, et al. Comparison of MELD, Child-Pugh, and Emory model for the pre-diction of survival in patients undergoing transjugular intrahepatic portosystemic shunting. Am J Gastro-enterol 2003;98:1167–74.

[28] Kamath PS, Wiesner RH, Malinchoc M, et al. A model to predict survival in patients with end-stage liver disease. Hepatology 2001;33:464–70.

[29] Wiesner RH, McDiarmid SV, Kamath PS, et al. MELD and PELD: application of survival models to liver allocation. Liver Transpl 2001;7:567–80.

[30] Keswani RN, Ahmed A, Keeffe EB. Older age and liver transplantation: a review. Liver Transpl 2004;10:957–67.

[31] John PR, Thuluvath PJ. Outcome of liver trans-plantation in patients with diabetes mellitus: a case-control study. Hepatology 2001;34:889–95.

[32] Yoo HY, Thuluvath PJ. The effect of insulin-dependent diabetes mellitus on outcome of liver transplantation. Transplantation 2002;74:1007–12.

[33] Bak T, Wachs M, Trotter J, et al. Adult-to-adult living donor liver transplantation using right-lobe grafts: results and lessons learned from a single-center experience. Liver Transpl 2001;7:680–6.

[34] Marcos A, Ham JM, Fisher RA, et al. Single-center analysis of the first 40 adult-to-adult living donor liver transplants using the right lobe. Liver Transpl 2000;6:296–301.

[35] Sorrell M. Transplantation. In: Schiff ER, Sorrell MF, Maddrey WC, editors. Schiff's diseases of the liver. 9th edition. Philadelphia: Lippincott Williams & Wil-kins; 2002. p. 1581–3.

[36] Trotter JF, Talamantes M, McClure M, et al. Right hepatic lobe donation for living donor liver trans-plantation: impact on donor quality of life. Liver Transpl 2001;7:485–93.

[37] Starzl TE, Marchioro TL, Vonkaulla KN, et al. Homo-transplantation of the Liver in Humans. Surg Gynecol Obstet 1963;117:659–76.

[38] Parrilla P, Sanchez-Bueno F, Figueras J, et al. Analy-sis of the complications of the piggy-back technique in 1,112 liver transplants. Transplantation 1999;67:1214–7.

[39] Tzakis A, Todo S, Starzl TE. Orthotopic liver trans-plantation with preservation of the inferior vena cava. Ann Surg 1989;210:649–52.

[40] Wiesner RH, Demetris AJ, Belle SH, et al. Acute hepatic allograft rejection: incidence, risk factors, and impact on outcome. Hepatology 1998;28:638–45.

[41] Lebeau G, Yanaga K, Marsh JW, et al. Analysis of surgical complications after 397 hepatic transplanta-tions. Surg Gynecol Obstet 1990;170:317–22.

[42] Thuluvath PJ, Yoo HY. Graft and patient survival after adult live donor liver transplantation compared to a matched cohort who received a deceased donor transplantation. Liver Transpl 2004;10:1263–8.

[43] Wolfe RA, Ashby VB, Milford EL, et al. Compari-son of mortality in all patients on dialysis, patients on dialysis awaiting transplantation, and recipients of a first cadaveric transplant. N Engl J Med 1999;341:1725–30.

[44] Jordan S, Cunningham-Rundles C, McEwan R. Util-ity of intravenous immune globulin in kidney trans-plantation: efficacy, safety, and cost implications. Am J Transplant 2003;3:653–64.

[45] Merrill JP, Murray JE, Harrison JH, et al. Successful homotransplantation of the human kidney between identical twins. JAMA 1956;160:277–82.

[46] Xue JL, Ma JZ, Louis TA, et al. Forecast of the num-ber of patients with end-stage renal disease in the United States to the year 2010. J Am Soc Nephrol 2001;12:2753–8.

[47] Go AS, Chertow GM, Fan D, et al. Chronic kidney disease and the risks of death, cardiovascular events, and hospitalization. N Engl J Med 2004;351:1296–305.

[48] Ojo AO, Hanson JA, Wolfe RA, et al. Long-term survival in renal transplant recipients with graft func-tion. Kidney Int 2000;57:307–13.

[49] Gaston RS, Danovitch GM, Adams PL, et al. The re-

port of a national conference on the wait list for kidney transplantation. Am J Transplant 2003;3:775–85.

[50] Gaston RS, Alveranga DY, Becker BN, et al. Kidney and pancreas transplantation. Am J Transplant 2003; 3(Suppl 4):64–77.

[51] Kasiske BL, Cangro CB, Hariharan S, et al. The evaluation of renal transplantation candidates: clinical practice guidelines. Am J Transplant 2001;1(Suppl 2):3–95.

[52] Mange KC, Joffe MM, Feldman HI. Effect of the use or nonuse of long-term dialysis on the subsequent survival of renal transplants from living donors. N Engl J Med 2001;344:726–31.

[53] Meier-Kriesche HU, Port FK, Ojo AO, et al. Effect of waiting time on renal transplant outcome. Kidney Int 2000;58:1311–7.

[54] Held PJ, Kahan BD, Hunsicker LG, et al. The impact of HLA mismatches on the survival of first cadaveric kidney transplants. N Engl J Med 1994;331: 765–70.

[55] Takemoto S, Terasaki PI, Cecka JM, et al. Survival of nationally shared, HLA-matched kidney transplants from cadaveric donors. The UNOS Scientific Renal Transplant Registry. N Engl J Med 1992;327:834–9.

[56] Mange KC, Cherikh WS, Maghirang J, et al. A comparison of the survival of shipped and locally transplanted cadaveric renal allografts. N Engl J Med 2001;345:1237–42.

[57] Sonnenday CJ, Warren DS, Cooper M, et al. Plasmapheresis, CMV hyperimmune globulin, and anti-CD20 allow ABO-incompatible renal transplantation without splenectomy. Am J Transplant 2004;4:1315–22.

[58] Perico N, Cattaneo D, Sayegh MH, et al. Delayed graft function in kidney transplantation. Lancet 2004;364: 1814–27.

[59] Pascual M, Theruvath T, Kawai T, et al. Strategies to improve long-term outcomes after renal transplantation. N Engl J Med 2002;346:580–90.

[60] Arcasoy SM, Kotloff RM. Lung transplantation. N Engl J Med 1999;340:1081–91.

[61] Trulock EP, Edwards LB, Taylor DO, et al. The Registry of the International Society for Heart and Lung Transplantation: twenty-first official adult lung and heart-lung transplant report–2004. J Heart Lung Transplant 2004;23(7):804–15.

[62] Rosas V, Conte JV, Yang SC, et al. Lung transplantation and systemic sclerosis. Ann Transplant 2000;5:38–43.

[63] Garver Jr RI, Zorn GL, Wu X, et al. Recurrence of bronchioloalveolar carcinoma in transplanted lungs. N Engl J Med 1999;340:1071–4.

[64] Maurer JR, Frost AE, Estenne M, et al. International guidelines for the selection of lung transplant candidates. The International Society for Heart and Lung Transplantation, the American Thoracic Society, the American Society of Transplant Physicians, the European Respiratory Society. J Heart Lung Transplant 1998;17:703–9.

[65] Levine SM. A survey of clinical practice of lung transplantation in North America. Chest 2004;125: 1224–38.

[66] Chaparro C, Maurer J, Gutierrez C, et al. Infection with Burkholderia cepacia in cystic fibrosis: outcome following lung transplantation. Am J Respir Crit Care Med 2001;163:43–8.

[67] Hosenpud JD, Bennett LE, Keck BM, et al. Effect of diagnosis on survival benefit of lung transplantation for end-stage lung disease. Lancet 1998;351:24–7.

[68] Pochettino A, Kotloff RM, Rosengard BR, et al. Bilateral versus single lung transplantation for chronic obstructive pulmonary disease: intermediate-term results. Ann Thorac Surg 2000;70:1813–8.

[69] Bowdish ME, Barr ML, Schenkel FA, et al. A decade of living lobar lung transplantation: perioperative complications after 253 donor lobectomies. Am J Transplant 2004;4:1283–8.

[70] Meyer DM, Bennett LE, Novick RJ, et al. Single vs bilateral, sequential lung transplantation for end-stage emphysema: influence of recipient age on survival and secondary end-points. J Heart Lung Transplant 2001;20:935–41.

[71] Meyer DM, Edwards LB, Torres F, et al. Impact of recipient age and procedure type on survival after lung transplantation for pulmonary fibrosis. Ann Thorac Surg 2005;79:950–7.

[72] Kelly WD, Lillehei RC, Merkel FK, et al. Allotransplantation of the pancreas and duodenum along with the kidney in diabetic nephropathy. Surgery 1967;61: 827–37.

[73] Gruessner AC, Sutherland DE. Pancreas transplant outcomes for United States (US) and non-US cases as reported to the United Network for Organ Sharing (UNOS) and the International Pancreas Transplant Registry (IPTR) as of October 2002. Clin Transpl 2002;41–77.

[74] The Diabetes Control and Complications Trial Research Group. The effect of intensive treatment of diabetes on the development and progression of long-term complications in insulin-dependent diabetes mellitus. N Engl J Med 1993;329:977–86.

[75] Larsen JL. Pancreas transplantation: indications and consequences. Endocr Rev 2004;25:919–46.

[76] Robertson P, Davis C, Larsen J, et al. Pancreas transplantation in type 1 diabetes. Diabetes Care 2004; 27(Suppl 1):S105.

[77] Manske CL, Thomas W, Wang Y, et al. Screening diabetic transplant candidates for coronary artery disease: identification of a low risk subgroup. Kidney Int 1993;44:617–21.

[78] Sollinger HW, Stratta RJ, D'Alessandro AM, et al. Experience with simultaneous pancreas-kidney transplantation. Ann Surg 1988;208:475–83.

[79] Stephanian E, Gruessner RW, Brayman KL, et al. Conversion of exocrine secretions from bladder to enteric drainage in recipients of whole pancreaticoduodenal transplants. Ann Surg 1992;216:663–72.

[80] Bloom RD, Olivares M, Rehman L, et al. Long-term pancreas allograft outcome in simultaneous pancreas-kidney transplantation: a comparison of enteric and bladder drainage. Transplantation 1997;64:1689–95.

[81] Robertson RP, Abid M, Sutherland DE, et al. Glucose homeostasis and insulin secretion in human recipients of pancreas transplantation. Diabetes 1989; 38(Suppl 1):97–8.

[82] Kuo PC, Johnson LB, Schweitzer EJ, et al. Simultaneous pancreas/kidney transplantation–a comparison of enteric and bladder drainage of exocrine pancreatic secretions. Transplantation 1997;63:238–43.

[83] Humar A, Ramcharan T, Kandaswamy R, et al. Pancreas after kidney transplants. Am J Surg 2001;182: 155–61.

[84] Gruessner RW, Sutherland DE, Gruessner AC. Mortality assessment for pancreas transplants. Am J Transplant 2004;4:2018–26.

[85] Venstrom JM, McBride MA, Rother KI, et al. Survival after pancreas transplantation in patients with diabetes and preserved kidney function. JAMA 2003;290: 2817–23.

[86] Bunnapradist S, Cho YW, Cecka JM, et al. Kidney allograft and patient survival in type I diabetic recipients of cadaveric kidney alone versus simultaneous pancreas kidney transplants: a multivariate analysis of the UNOS database. J Am Soc Nephrol 2003;14:208–13.

[87] Reddy KS, Stablein D, Taranto S, et al. Long-term survival following simultaneous kidney-pancreas transplantation versus kidney transplantation alone in patients with type 1 diabetes mellitus and renal failure. Am J Kidney Dis 2003;41:464–70.

Clin Chest Med 26 (2005) 545 – 560

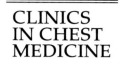

Pulmonary Complications of Transplantation: Radiographic Considerations

Rosita M. Shah, MD*, Wallace Miller, Jr, MD

Division of Thoracic Radiology, Hospital of the University of Pennsylvania, 3400 Spruce Street, Philadelphia, PA 19107, USA

The spectrum of pulmonary disorders arising as a complication of solid organ and hematopoietic stem cell transplantation (HSCT) is diverse, reflecting varying pathogenic mechanisms, which include systemic immune suppression, surgical insults, toxicity of preconditioning regimens, and alloimmune mechanisms [1,2]. Not surprisingly, a wide range of pulmonary imaging findings can be expected on chest radiography and CT. When approached as isolated imaging abnormalities, these findings are often as nonspecific as the presenting clinical symptoms, with a long list of differential possibilities. By using a pattern approach in conjunction with knowledge of the clinical setting, however, one may individually tailor the differential diagnosis and subsequently provide more assistance to the clinical work-up.

After transplantation, radiographic abnormalities in the chest often take the form of significant parenchymal disease. The commonly encountered radiographic patterns of parenchymal disease include (1) airspace consolidation, (2) ground-glass opacification, and (3) nodules [3]. Although these imaging abnormalities usually are readily apparent on chest radiographs, CT allows earlier detection and is extremely useful in providing additional information regarding the type of pattern and the extent and distribution of an abnormality, all factors that affect the reader's ability and confidence in rendering a specific diagnosis [4].

The principle aim of the following discussion is to clarify radiographic definitions associated with common parenchymal patterns encountered in the transplant population and to discuss the most common pathologic causes responsible for each pattern. The article also touches on radiographic findings signifying complications of other intrathoracic structures, including the airways, pleural space, and mediastinum.

Airspace consolidation

Airspace consolidation is defined by increased opacity of sufficient density to obscure underlying lung architecture [5]. In other words, when airspace consolidation is present, the normal vascular pattern is not visualized. Important diagnostic considerations when airspace consolidation is present include (1) chronicity of the radiographic abnormality and associated patient symptomatology; (2) characterization of the consolidation as focal, multifocal, or diffuse; and (3) the presence of additional findings including nodularity and cavitation.

Airspace consolidation results from pathologic processes that produce alveolar filling and may occur in acute or chronic settings. The rapidity of the onset is an important factor in deciding the likelihood of a given diagnosis. Acute airspace filling most often develops in the setting of pulmonary edema, pneumonia, and alveolar hemorrhage, with patients exhibiting abrupt onset of symptoms [6]. Chronic airspace filling is encountered much less frequently and, in the setting of transplantation, is seen most often in indolent infections and posttransplantation lympho-

---

* Corresponding author.
  E-mail address: Rosita.shah@uphs.upenn.edu (R.M. Shah).

proliferative disorder (PTLD) [7,8]. In these instances, the consolidative abnormality frequently
displays nodular features.

Acute airspace consolidation

Pulmonary edema: general comments

Both hydrostatic and permeability edema are frequent pulmonary complications after transplantation
[1]. Hydrostatic pulmonary edema often is precipitated
by overaggressive administration of intravenous fluids
and blood product support. The risk is compounded by
the presence of cardiac or renal impairment, caused by
factors such as the cardiotoxic effects of chemotherapeutic agents and radiation, dysfunction of the
cardiac or renal allograft, and acute renal failure resulting from intraoperative hypotension or nephrotoxic
drugs (eg, calcineurin inhibitors) [1,9]. Imaging features of advanced cardiogenic edema include diffusely distributed, central, and gravity-dependent
consolidations [10]. On occasion, a batwing configuration may be observed, in which the perihilar regions are consolidated with sparing of the lung
periphery [11]. A rapid response to diuresis is expected
in most cases.

As in other critically ill patients, permeability
edema in transplant recipients may follow a wide
range of local pulmonary and systemic insults, which
include sepsis, aspiration, transfusion reactions, and
drug toxicities [12]. Some forms of permeability
edema (eg, transfusion-related acute lung injury) tend
to be self limited, with rapid radiographic clear-
ing over several days. More commonly, severe and
widespread injury results in diffuse alveolar damage
and the clinical correlate, acute respiratory distress
syndrome (ARDS) [13,14]. With the development of
ARDS, there is persistence of imaging abnormalities.
Exudative ARDS is characterized by patchy consolidation and ground-glass opacities, often with a
gravitational component [15]. Significant pleural
effusions are observed in one third of patients on
CT scans but are rarely recognized on portable chest
radiographs [16]. In patients sustaining direct lung
injuries (eg, aspiration), airspace consolidations are
the dominant abnormalities, typically multifocal but
occasionally seen in a unilateral distribution on initial films [17]. In contrast, lung injury occurring in
association with systemic insults (eg, sepsis) more
commonly produces widespread ground-glass opacification [17]. In the fibroproliferative phase of ARDS,
there is frequent improvement in the degree of air
space consolidation, with greater amounts of ground-
glass opacity seen. Traction type bronchiectasis and

subpleural cystic changes denote development of
fibrosis [18].

Reperfusion edema in the lung transplant recipient

Among the various transplant populations, lung
transplant recipients are uniquely predisposed to the
development of noncardiogenic pulmonary edema
caused by ischemia-reperfusion injury arising from
harvest, ex vivo cold storage, and reimplantation of
the allograft [19]. Reperfusion edema of varying
degree occurs in almost all patients. Chest radiographs typically demonstrate areas of airspace consolidation in the transplanted lung; the native lung is
uninvolved after single-lung transplantation [20,21].
The appearance of opacities within the first day or
two after transplantation distinguishes reperfusion
edema from acute rejection, which does not develop
until day 5 or beyond. Typically, the opacities associated with reperfusion edema are mild in extent
and present predominantly in the basilar and perihilar
regions of the allograft. Pulmonary opacities may
increase for the first few days after transplantation but
should not progress after the sixth postoperative day.
Worsening pulmonary opacities after the sixth day
should be assumed to represent another phenomenon,
such as pneumonia or rejection. The peak severity of
parenchymal involvement was observed by day 4 in
43 of 44 patients who had reperfusion edema studied
by Kundu and colleagues [21], who noted poor
correlation between clinical severity and the extent of
radiographic findings. After peaking in intensity
within the first few days, reperfusion edema typically
resolves slowly over the course of a week or more.

In approximately 12% of lung transplant recipients, ischemia-reperfusion injury is severe, resulting
in an ARDS-like picture termed "primary graft
failure" [22]. Patients who have primary graft failure
manifest severe hypoxemia and often require prolonged mechanical ventilatory support. Mortality
rates of up to 60% have been reported. On chest
radiographs, primary graft failure is characterized by
diffuse consolidation of the entire allograft within the
first 3 days after transplantation [22]. Unlike the more
common reperfusion edema, the lung typically
remains consolidated for weeks to months, as in diffuse alveolar damage from other causes. Among survivors, the radiographic abnormalities ultimately
resolve, with associated partial or complete recovery
of respiratory function.

Noncardiogenic edema in other transplant recipients

Noncardiogenic edema and ARDS are common in
patients undergoing often complicated organ transplant surgery. The incidence of ARDS is highest after

liver transplantation, where it is encountered in up to 15% of patients and is associated with mortality rates as high as 80% [23].

In up to 50% of patients who have diffuse alveolar consolidation after HSCT, an infectious cause is not documented, and pathologic findings consist of edema associated with diffuse alveolar damage. Depending on the clinical scenario, some of these patients are diagnosed as having idiopathic pneumonia syndrome, diffuse alveolar hemorrhage, or engraftment syndrome [24–26]. Imaging findings parallel those seen in association with ARDS (Fig. 1).

Acute allograft rejection after lung transplantation

Acute cellular rejection of the lung allograft is an exceedingly common phenomenon after lung transplantation, occurring in 50% to 75% of recipients at some time within the first year. In many cases, acute rejection is detected clinically or by surveillance lung biopsies, without change in the chest radiograph [27]. Chest radiographic abnormalities include consolidation (Fig. 2), interstitial opacities including septal lines, and small pleural effusions [27]. The presence of a stable heart size and normal width of the vascular pedicle favor a diagnosis of acute rejection rather than cardiogenic edema [27]. Imaging findings on high-resolution CT (HRCT) associated with acute rejection include consolidation, ground-glass opacification, septal and peribronchovascular thickening, volume loss, and pleural fluid [28]. Based on the presence of these findings, the CT literature has demonstrated a sensitivity of 35% to 65%, a specificity of 73% to 85%, a positive predictive value of 60%, and a negative predictive value of 50% for the

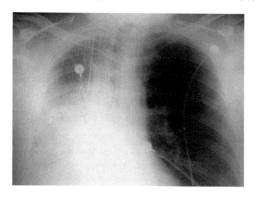

Fig. 2. Acute rejection. The patient manifested increasing dyspnea and hypoxemia 5 days after single-lung transplantation for emphysema. Chest radiograph demonstrates near-complete consolidation of the right lung allograft. Grade 3 acute cellular rejection was documented by transbronchial biopsy.

diagnosis of acute rejection [28,29]. In most cases, acute rejection is identified with clinical and histologic parameters without the need to resort to CT scanning.

Pneumonia

Despite widespread and improved prophylaxis, pulmonary infections remain a leading source of morbidity and mortality in all posttransplantation populations. Bacterial pneumonias prevail among the various causes and typically present radiographically as rapidly evolving focal areas of consolidation. Unfortunately, there is a significant degree of overlap in the imaging features of pneumonia caused by a wide spectrum of infectious organisms, and radiographic features alone cannot be used to predict the causative organism with certainty. For example, in a review of 45 episodes of pneumonia in lung transplant recipients, Collins and colleagues [30] found that there was no characteristic pattern of findings that permitted distinction among the cases of bacterial, Cytomegalovirus (CMV), and *Aspergillus* pneumonia. The imaging findings should always be correlated with the time elapsed since transplantation, the magnitude of immunosuppression, and the presence and pace of onset of clinical symptoms accompanying the radiographic abnormalities, because these factors may influence the likelihood of a given infectious cause.

In the initial days after the operative procedure, all solid organ transplant recipients, like other surgical patients, are subject to an increased risk of nosocomial bacterial pneumonias, most commonly caused by *Pseudomonas aeruginosa*, other gram-negative

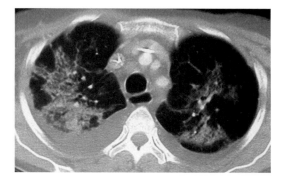

Fig. 1. Idiopathic pneumonia syndrome. The patient displayed worsening oxygenation 3 weeks after HSCT. Bronchoalveolar lavage results were negative for an infectious diagnosis. Thin-section CT reveals extensive bilateral alveolar consolidation and moderate pleural effusions. Open lung biopsy revealed findings of diffuse alveolar damage.

organisms, and *Staphylococcus aureus* [31]. HSCT recipients are also at increased risk for nosocomial pneumonia caused by these organisms in the pre-engraftment period characterized by profound and sustained neutropenia. These organisms most commonly produce bronchopneumonia patterns [32]. Radiographic findings may be more subtle after HSCT, presumably because of the attenuated inflammatory response in the neutropenic patient. Bacterial infections with community-acquired pathogens, including *Streptococcus pneumoniae* and *Legionella* species, become more common in the later stages of transplantation, often manifesting with lobar pneumonia patterns [33]. Although both the native and transplanted lungs are at an increased risk of developing pneumonia after single-lung transplantation, the frequency of infection is greater in the transplanted lung [34].

The two radiographic patterns of bacterial pneumonia, lobar and lobular (ie, bronchopneumonia), have distinct imaging features when imaged early in the course of an infection and in patients who have normal lung architecture. Imaging features of lobar pneumonias include nonsegmental, homogeneous, and coalescent areas of consolidation, maintained lung volume with minimal atelectasis, and prominent air bronchograms [35]. In contrast, imaging features of a bronchopneumonia include patchy, heterogeneous consolidations with significant atelectasis and peribronchial thickening [36]. The consolidations in a bronchopneumonia can have a prominent nodular component that is often bronchocentric or centrilobular in distribution on CT, reflecting peribronchial inflammation and involvement of acini surrounding the affected small airways in the central portions of secondary lobules [37]. Sublobular consolidations are characteristic in bronchopneumonia, contrasting with the more extensive, nonsegmental consolidation of lobar pattern pneumonias. The nodular opacities of a bronchopneumonia, which demonstrate a bronchocentric distribution, should be distinguished from randomly distributed, often discrete and peripherally located nodules seen in fungal infection (Fig. 3).

CT scans offer a number of advantages over standard chest radiography in the diagnosis and evaluation of pneumonia. Foremost is the greater sensitivity of CT in detecting subtle abnormalities. This sensitivity is particularly relevant in cases of early bronchopneumonia, in which centrilobular nodules and early patchy consolidation are unlikely to be radiographically apparent on standard chest radiographs. The increased sensitivity of CT is also important in diagnosing pneumonia in neutropenic patients. In one study of febrile neutropenic patients, HRCT was able

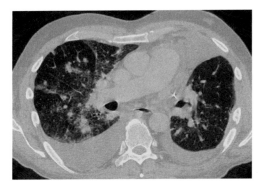

Fig. 3. *Legionella* pneumonia. The patient developed fever after HSCT. Thin-section CT demonstrates a bronchopneumonia pattern consisting of poorly defined bronchocentric nodules in the right upper lobe with an associated moderate effusion. Legionella urinary antigen was positive.

to demonstrate findings of pneumonia up to 5 days earlier than standard chest radiography [38]. CT also may be beneficial in demonstrating additional findings that point away from a routine bacterial infection (eg, cavitation, pleural reaction, intrathoracic lymphadenopathy), in determining the preferred route of biopsy, and in recognizing complications of infection requiring treatment such as pleural or mediastinal collections.

Alveolar hemorrhage

Diffuse alveolar hemorrhage occurs in 5% to 20% of HSCT recipients in the first month after transplantation and is associated with mortality rates as high as 80% to 100% with supportive care alone [39]. In addition to intra-alveolar hemorrhage, patients have pathologic evidence of diffuse alveolar damage. Imaging features consist of localized or widespread alveolar consolidations, often with prominent centrilobular nodular features (Fig. 4) [40]. On follow-up radiographs, the airspace opacities may be replaced by an interstitial pattern, reflecting resorption of alveolar blood and interstitial accumulation of hemosiderin-laden macrophages.

Chronic airspace consolidation

Metastatic calcification

Abnormalities in calcium metabolism are common in the hepatic and renal transplant populations, frequently leading to soft tissue deposition, often in the lung parenchyma. Metastatic pulmonary calcification usually manifests as focal areas of airspace consolidation on chest radiographs; CT scans often

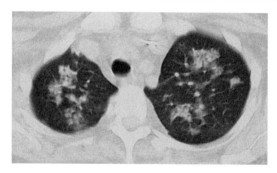

Fig. 4. Diffuse alveolar hemorrhage. The patient developed dyspnea after HSCT. Thin-section CT demonstrates widespread patchy alveolar consolidation. Bronchoalveolar lavage revealed progressively bloody aspirates with negative cultures.

reveal a nodular quality to these areas (Fig. 5) [41]. Findings may be slowly progressive over time. It is important to recognize the chronicity of these infiltrates in distinguishing metastatic calcification from infection. Imaging with CT can show foci of significantly increased attenuation (>100 Hounsfeld units), which would strongly support the diagnosis [42]. In some cases, calcification of the walls of chest wall vessels is also apparent. Other parenchymal abnormalities, pleural effusions, and adenopathy are typically absent. Active calcium deposition can also be confirmed by uptake in the lungs on radionuclide bone scans.

Neoplasm

Focal chronic airspace consolidation is an occasional manifestation of neoplastic lung disease, either

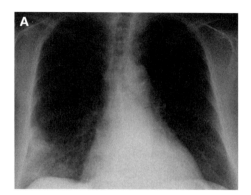

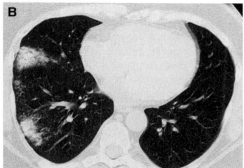

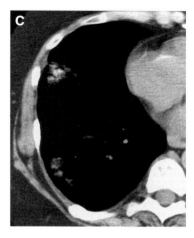

Fig. 5. Pulmonary metastatic calcification. The patient was evaluated for symptoms suggestive of an upper respiratory tract infection 3 months after successful renal transplantation. (A) Chest radiograph reveals right basilar air space consolidation, unchanged from prior studies. (B) CT (lung windows) confirms consolidative features. (C) CT (soft tissue windows) reveals high-density foci suggestive of calcification.

secondary to an infiltrative mass with consolidative features, typical of PTLD, or secondary to post-obstructive changes, which can accompany the development of bronchogenic carcinoma. Both these neoplastic processes occur most frequently in lung transplant and heart transplant recipients [43]. Both more commonly present as nodules or masses and are discussed later as causes of nodular parenchymal disorders.

Ground-glass opacity

Ground-glass opacity, defined at CT by increased parenchymal attenuation insufficiently dense to obscure normal lung architecture, may occur in the setting of isolated interstitial disease, isolated alveolar disease, or, most commonly, with disease processes affecting both interstitial and alveolar compartments [5]. Simply put, any parenchymal abnormality below the resolution threshold of HRCT can produce ground-glass opacity. In the case of alveolar filling, any of the disease processes leading to airspace consolidation can also produce ground-glass opacity, especially if imaged early, before complete alveolar opacification. Therefore, components of ground-glass opacity frequently are encountered with and accompany the consolidative features of edema and alveolar hemorrhage.

Infection

Ground-glass opacity can also be a manifestation of pulmonary infection, most commonly associated with the opportunistic pneumonias encountered in this patient population. Ground-glass opacity is the most common finding in pneumonia caused by *Pneumocystis jeroveci* and CMV, as well as other respiratory viruses [44–46].

In patients who have not received or tolerated prophylaxis, *Pneumocystis* pneumonia (PCP) is most common within the initial months after solid organ transplantation or HSCT [47]. Radiographically, this infection is characterized by ground-glass opacities that typically occur in a geographic pattern, with alternating areas of normal and abnormal lung parenchyma [44]. This pattern reflects the underlying lobular anatomy of the lung, in which entire secondary pulmonary lobules are uniformly opacified and seen adjacent to normal or less affected lobules. Ground-glass opacities may also be diffusely homogeneous or can be associated with reticular interstitial abnormalities (Fig. 6) [44]. Adenopathy and pleural effusions are uncommon. Although cavitary and

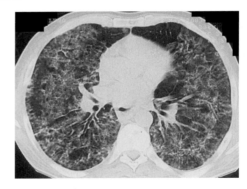

Fig. 6. Pneumocystis pneumonia. The patient developed fever and dyspnea after renal transplantation. Thin-section CT reveals extensive ground-glass opacity with prominent reticular interstitial component. Bronchoalveolar lavage results confirmed PCP.

noncavitary nodular infiltrates have, rarely, been described in PCP, the presence of nodules should strongly suggest an alternative or coexisting infectious diagnosis [48].

With the use of antiviral prophylaxis, the onset of CMV pneumonia is delayed, and most cases now are seen more than 3 months after transplantation [49]. CT imaging features are dominated by ground-glass opacity and may be accompanied by a prominent nodular component, uncommon in PCP (Fig. 7) [7,45,50].

In the past, the most common infectious causes of ground-glass opacity were PCP and CMV pneumonia. With the increasing use of prophylactic medications, these infections are becoming less common. As a consequence, some other, more unusual viral infections now account for a greater proportion of infectious causes of ground-glass opacity in transplant recipients. These include Herpes simplex viruses and some community-acquired viruses, such as adenovirus, parainfluenza, and respiratory syncytial virus [46].

Drug-induced pulmonary toxicity

Ground-glass opacity is a common manifestation of drug-induced pulmonary toxicity and may reflect a variety of underlying insults, including permeability edema, diffuse alveolar damage, hypersensitivity pneumonitis, and nonspecific or usual interstitial pneumonitis [51,52]. The diagnosis of drug toxicity should always be considered in patients presenting with "pneumonia" that fails to respond promptly to antibiotics. It may also present more insidiously over weeks to months. Drug toxicity is a frequent consid-

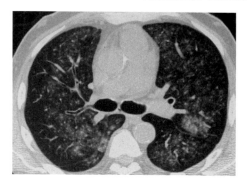

Fig. 7. CMV pneumonia. Patient presented with fever 3 months after renal transplantation. Thin-section CT reveals extensive ground-glass opacity with a prominent centrilobular nodular morphology. Transbronchial biopsy demonstrated changes of CMV pneumonia.

eration in HSCT recipients because of the numerous agents with potential pulmonary toxicity often given as part of pretransplantation conditioning regimens. Breast cancer patients treated with high-dose chemotherapy regimens followed by autologous HSCT seem to be particularly predisposed to a syndrome of drug-induced lung injury. Termed the "delayed pulmonary toxicity syndrome," this entity is characterized radiographically by ground-glass opacities and physiologically by a fall in the diffusing capacity [53]. In the past, solid organ transplant recipients were not commonly exposed to agents causing pulmonary toxicity. The recent introduction of sirolimus for use as an immunosuppressive agent has been accompanied by numerous reports of drug-induced pneumonitis, which may be characterized radiographically by the appearance of ground-glass opacities [54].

Diffuse alveolar hemorrhage

Alveolar hemorrhage most often appears as diffuse consolidation within the lung parenchyma. When the extent of hemorrhage is less severe, however, the radiographic presentation can be that of diffuse ground-glass opacities on CT scans [40].

Acute allograft rejection

As discussed previously, acute allograft rejection after lung transplantation is associated with a multitude of radiographic findings. In one series, the most common CT finding associated with biopsy-proven

acute rejection was ground-glass attenuation, present in 65% of cases overall [29]. Ground-glass opacities were seen in all cases of high-grade rejection (grade 3 and 4) but in only a minority of those with lower grades. The overall sensitivity, specificity, and positive and negative predictive value of ground-glass attenuation in the diagnosis of acute rejection were 65%, 85%, 54%, and 90%, respectively.

Mosaic attenuation and air trapping

HRCT of the lungs commonly demonstrates heterogeneous density, termed "mosaic attenuation" (Fig. 8). The mosaic pattern of lung attenuation is comprised of small polygonal areas of alternating lung density, representing normal and abnormal adjoining secondary pulmonary lobules [55]. A mosaic pattern of lung attenuation on HRCT signifies one of three processes: (1) true infiltrative parenchymal disease, in which areas of ground-glass opacity represent the abnormality; (2) pulmonary vascular disease, in which lucent zones represent areas of underperfused parenchyma; and (3) airway disease, in which lucent zones correspond to air trapping [56]. One finding useful in distinguishing among these three possibilities is assessment of vessel size, which is normal in infiltrative parenchymal disease producing ground-glass opacity but is diminished in vascular and airway disease. A second valuable method of differentiation is the comparison of images obtained during the inspiratory and expiratory phases of the respiratory cycle. Normal areas of lung become denser at end expiration as they empty their gaseous contents. In contrast, persistent areas of decreased

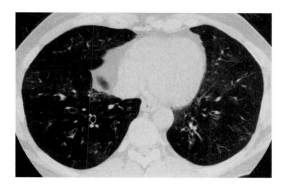

Fig. 8. Mosaic attenuation pattern. Thin-section CT reveals heterogeneous lung density that is geographic in distribution.

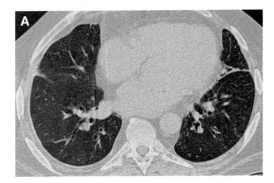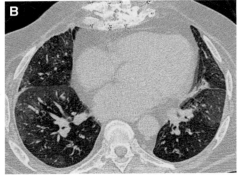

Fig. 9. Air trapping in bronchiolitis obliterans syndrome. (*A*) Inspiratory CT is unremarkable. (*B*) Expiratory CT optimally demonstrates a mosaic attenuation pattern consistent with air trapping.

attenuation reflect air trapping, the cardinal feature of small airways disease.

Air trapping is the most recognized and reliable imaging sign of bronchiolitis obliterans syndrome (BOS), a fibroproliferative disorder of the small airways that is the chief manifestation of chronic allograft rejection after lung transplantation and a presumed manifestation of chronic graft-versus-host disease after HSCT [57]. Because the finding of air trapping may be evident only on imaging obtained during expiration, assessment of the lung and HSCT recipient with respiratory symptoms should routinely include HRCT with expiratory images (Fig. 9). The utility of HRCT in diagnosing BOS has been most extensively studied in lung transplant recipients and extrapolated to the HSCT population. The reported sensitivity of air trapping for the diagnosis of established BOS ranges from 74% to 91%, and the specificity ranges from 67% to 94% [57–59]. Because scattered areas of air trapping are common, almost universal findings in most asymptomatic patients, including normal healthy volunteers, use of a threshold minimum of 32% for the amount of involved parenchyma seems to increase the diagnostic accuracy for distinguishing patients who do or do not have BOS [60]. The extent of air trapping seems to correlate with the severity of airflow obstruction measured by spirometry [60]. In addition to air trapping, more longstanding and severe cases of BOS are associated with the presence of peribronchial thickening and bronchiectasis (Fig. 10) [61].

The role of HRCT as a screening tool in the detection of early BOS, before the onset of clinical symptoms or pulmonary function abnormalities, is debatable. In one recent study, demonstration of air trapping had a sensitivity of only 50% and positive and negative predictive values of only 70% and 60%,

respectively, in identifying asymptomatic patients who would go on to develop BOS [62]. Additionally, the detection of air trapping was a reversible finding in 43% of patients, raising questions about the significance of this finding on isolated examinations [62]. Other investigators have reported somewhat better performance statistics with use of a computer-determined mean lung attenuation score at end expiration, but this technique is not widely available at present [63].

Nodules

The presence of parenchymal nodules in the transplant recipient has been most closely associated with opportunistic fungal infections [64]. The reality,

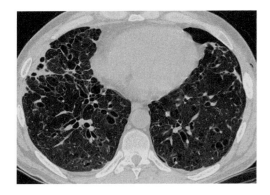

Fig. 10. Late BOS. The patient was a bilateral lung transplant recipient with advanced BOS. CT reveals extensive bronchiectasis. Incidentally noted is a spontaneous left pneumothorax.

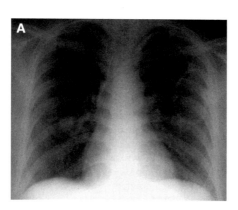
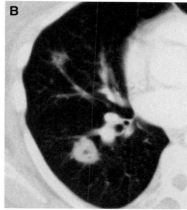

Fig. 11. Nocardiosis. Patient was evaluated 2 years after orthotopic liver transplantation. (*A*) Chest radiograph demonstrates poorly defined lung nodule. (*B*) CT reveals multiple, focal, cavitary and noncavitary right lung nodules. Positive cultures were obtained by fine-needle aspiration.

however, is that nodules constitute a common component of the imaging findings seen in many posttransplantation disorders. Often, characterization of the nodules according to morphology and distribution can prevent the over-reporting of possible fungal infection and can generate a more accurate differential diagnosis. Single or multifocal discrete nodules are most commonly associated with fungal and nocardial infections (Fig. 11) [65] and neoplastic disease [66]. On the other hand, profuse centrilobular or tree-in-bud nodular opacities are encountered commonly in the setting of infectious and inflammatory bronchiolitis. More focal regions of poorly defined centrilobular and bronchocentric nodules are characteristic of bacterial bronchopneumonias [67].

Discrete nodules representing infections

Fungal pneumonias, most commonly caused by *Aspergillus*, and bacterial infections caused by *Nocardia* species are characterized by discrete nodular abnormalities. Typical imaging features include one or several 1- to 3-cm, discrete, cavitary or noncavitary nodules of varying sizes and extent of consolidation [64,68,69]. When solitary they typically appear masslike and resemble a bronchogenic carcinoma.

Angioinvasion, typically a complication of invasive aspergillosis and mucormycosis, results in parenchymal hemorrhage, which often manifests as ground-glass opacity. The finding of a rim of ground-glass opacity surrounding a nodule is well known as the halo sign (Fig. 12) [70]. More commonly, ground-glass opacities are adjacent to areas of segmental consolidation, a finding present in 80% of neutropenic

patients who have angioinvasive pulmonary aspergillosus [64]. This finding is not specific to fungal infections and has been reported in association with hemorrhagic metastases and vasculitic lesions [71]. A peripheral distribution with involvement of the subpleural lung parenchyma is most common.

Subsequent necrosis of infarcted lung parenchyma may produce a nondependently situated central nodule surrounded by a crescentic lucency; this finding is termed the "air-crescent sign" (Fig. 13) [72]. Although strongly suggestive of *Aspergillus* infection

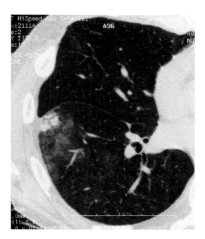

Fig. 12. Invasive aspergillosis with CT halo sign. Patient with hemoptysis status after bilateral lung transplantation. CT reveals a poorly defined, peripheral right lower lobe nodule. Surrounding ground-glass opacity constitutes the radiographic halo sign.

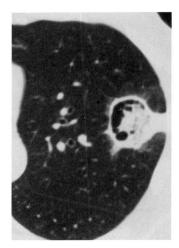

Fig. 13. Invasive aspergillosis with CT air-crescent sign. The patient developed fever after HSCT. CT demonstrates a left upper lobe cavitary nodule. The cavity demonstrates a crescentic configuration after necrosis of infarcted lung parenchyma.

in the transplant population, identification of the air crescent in invasive aspergillosis is a relatively late finding, limiting its utility as a diagnostic sign. In previously neutropenic patients, development of the air-crescent sign is associated with the return of granulocyte function [73].

Septic emboli, arising as a complication of bacteremia, commonly present with focal nodular abnormalities that mimic opportunistic fungal infection. A peripheral distribution is characteristic, and cavitation is common [74].

Discrete nodules representing neoplastic disease

PTLD, which encompasses a spectrum of B-cell proliferative disorders ranging from benign polyclonal proliferation to non-Hodgkins lymphomas, can involve a variety of extranodal sites [75]. Intrathoracic involvement is highest among lung transplant recipients, occurring in 50% to 80% of cases, but can be seen in all solid organ transplant populations [76]. Among HSCT recipients, PTLD usually presents as a widely disseminated process; pulmonary involvement as a component of this presentation occurs in approximately 20% of patients. Imaging plays an important role in the early recognition of this disorder, when therapeutic responses may be greatest, and is useful in demonstrating the extent of intrathoracic involvement as well as in identifying extrathoracic sites of disease. Among lung transplant recipients, the presence of a single pulmonary nodule at presentation has been associated with a more favorable prognosis than multifocal lung disease [77].

The most common imaging findings include single or multiple pulmonary nodules (Fig. 14). The nodules are randomly distributed and noncavitary [77,78]. The presence of a surrounding ground-glass rim mimicking fungal infection has been reported. After single-lung transplantation, PTLD characteristically involves the allograft and spares the native lung. Adenopathy, when present, is a minor part of the radiographic picture in most cases. Pleural effusions are uncommon.

Primary bronchogenic carcinoma has been reported in up to 4% of single-lung transplant recipients

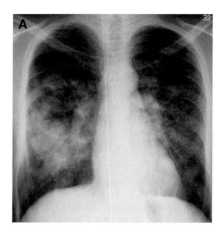
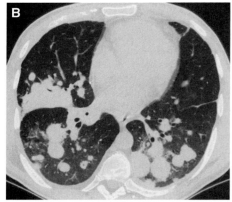

Fig. 14. PTLD in an asymptomatic patient after bilateral lung transplantation. (*A*) Chest radiograph demonstrates confluent bilateral lung nodules. (*B*) HRCT confirms an extensive nodular abnormality.

who have underlying emphysema or idiopathic pulmonary fibrosis. Prior cigarette smoking is the prevailing risk factor in both groups, but the presence of widespread pulmonary fibrosis is an underappreciated risk factor in the idiopathic pulmonary fibrosis population. Consequently, a solitary nodule or mass in the native lung has a high likelihood of representing a bronchogenic carcinoma. Bronchogenic carcinoma has been reported with similar frequency in the heart transplant population and should be considered in the differential diagnosis of a lung nodule or mass. Among liver transplant recipients who have a prior history of hepatocellular carcinoma, recurrent tumor often presents as single or multiple pulmonary nodules, usually within 2 years of transplantation.

Diffuse (centrilobular) nodules

Centrilobular nodules, often with a prominent tree-in-bud pattern, are generally characteristic of disorders of the small airway, including infectious and inflammatory bronchiolitis (Fig. 15) [67,79]. A tree-in-bud pattern is considered present when small, distinct centrilobular nodules are clustered in relation to branching peripheral airways. Pulmonary pathogens associated with bronchiolitis and of concern in the posttransplantation population include the community respiratory viruses (respiratory syncytial virus, adenovirus, influenza, and parainfluenza) and mycobacteria. There can confusion between the

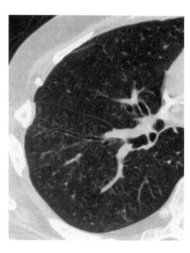

Fig. 15. Follicular bronchiolitis. Patient with dyspnea and skin findings of graft-versus-host disease after HSCT. HRCT reveals an extensive centrilobular nodular abnormality with tree-in-bud morphology.

imaging features of bronchiolitis and bronchopneumonia. In general, the nodules of a bronchopneumonia are larger and less distinct.

Tree-in-bud opacities may also be a manifestation of BOS. When present in BOS, they are usually associated with areas of bronchiectasis and air trapping. Diffuse tree-in-bud opacities occasionally may be the only imaging manifestation of BOS, however.

Miscellaneous radiographic abnormalities

Mediastinal fluid collections

Mediastinal fluid collections may be encountered in patients after heart, lung, or heart-lung transplantation. Within 10 days of sternotomy, the finding of mediastinal fluid is nonspecific [80]. The longer a fluid collection persists, the greater is the likelihood of postoperative infection. Periaortic fluid collections and pseudoaneurysms may be a manifestation of aortic dehiscence secondary to rejection of the aortic graft component of the cardiac allograft [81].

Coronary allograft vasculopathy

Advanced coronary artery disease in the transplanted heart represents the most significant late cause of death in this population. Demonstration of significant calcification by electron beam CT was strongly associated with the presence of coronary artery stenosis of greater than 50% in one recent study [82]. Conversely, the absence of coronary artery calcification had a negative predictive value of 97% for coronary artery stenosis of this degree.

Hyperinflation of the transplanted lung

Acute hyperinflation of the native lung has been demonstrated in up to 31% of emphysema patients undergoing single-lung transplantation, but in only half of these instances was it associated with compromised hemodynamics or graft function [83]. The problem typically occurs while the patient is receiving positive-pressure mechanical ventilation and can be rapidly rectified by early extubation or by insertion of a double-lumen endotracheal tube and use of independent lung ventilation. Beyond the perioperative period, some patients who have emphysema demonstrate exaggerated or progressive native lung hyperinflation associated with suboptimal or deteriorating pulmonary function caused by extrinsic compression of the allograft. In such cases, performance of lobectomy or lung-volume reduction surgery on the native lung has resulted in improvement in lung function. Imaging findings in both acute and chronic cases include markedly reduced volume in the transplanted lung, herniation of the native lung

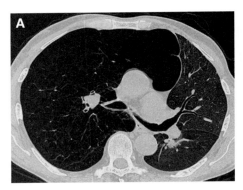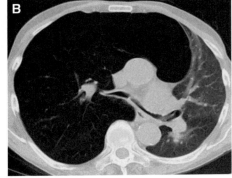

Fig. 16. Hyperinflation of native lung after single-lung transplantation. Routine follow-up was performed subsequent to left lung transplant. (*A*) Initial HRCT reveals severe centrilobular emphysema in the native right lung and moderate contralateral mediastinal shift. (*B*) Follow-up CT obtained 12 months later reveals progressive native lung hyperinflation, with markedly reduced volume of the left lung allograft volume and compression of the left main stem bronchus. There is mucus plugging distal to the site of narrowing.

across the midline, and severe mediastinal shift toward the allograft (Fig. 16).

Detection of disease recurrence

Radiographic surveillance may demonstrate recurrence of disease in the transplanted lung, which occurs most frequently in patients who have sarcoidosis but which has also been documented with lymphangiomyomatosis, Langerhans' cell histiocytosis, giant cell pneumonitis, panbronchiolitis, bronchoalveolar cell carcinoma, desquamative interstitial pneumonitis, emphysema secondary to alpha-1 antitrypsin deficiency, and alveolar proteinosis [84]. The imaging findings parallel those seen with the original disease. In contrast, cystic fibrosis does not have the potential to recur after transplantation, because respiratory epithelial cells in the transplanted lungs are of donor lineage and therefore possess the normal rather than mutated genes responsible for the disease. Thus, the finding of bronchiectasis in the allografts of a transplant recipient who had underlying cystic fibrosis is caused by chronic infection or BOS and not by recurrent disease.

Pleural effusions

The development of pleural fluid on the side of the allograft is an expected finding after lung transplantation, persisting for up to 2 weeks after surgery [85]. The accumulation of pleural fluid beyond this time, or an increase in size of a previously stable effusion, may be an indicator of infection or rejection. Recurrent chylous effusions are well recognized in patients undergoing lung transplantation for lymphangiomyomatosis [86]. Chylous effusions rarely

may also occur in the perioperative period in any lung transplant recipient because of surgical trauma to the thoracic duct. Finally, patients who have had prior pleurodesis or thoracic surgery or who have extensive pleural adhesions resulting from the underlying lung disease are at risk for perioperative hemothorax. The risk of hemothorax is increased further when cardiopulmonary bypass is required, because of the attendant requirement for systemic anticoagulation.

Perioperative pleural effusions are also common after liver transplantation and have been attributed to disruption of diaphragmatic lymphatics. These effusions are either right-sided or bilateral but are never solely on the left. They may enlarge during the initial postoperative week but usually resolve by the third week.

Bronchial anastomotic complications

The incidence of bronchial anastomotic complications after lung transplantation has fallen, reflecting improved surgical and immunosuppressive techniques, but airway dehiscence, stenosis, and infection continue to plague a significant minority of patients. CT, especially when multiplanar reconstructions are used, plays a significant role in the diagnosis of airway complications [87]. It is important not to confuse the normal appearance of the telescoping surgical anastomosis with airway stenosis. The membranous portions of the native and transplanted bronchi are attached end to end, but the cartilaginous aspects of the bronchi are overlapped by one or two cartilaginous rings to buttress the anastomosis [88]. As a result, a small cartilaginous shelf extends into the bronchial lumen, appearing as a thin band protrud-

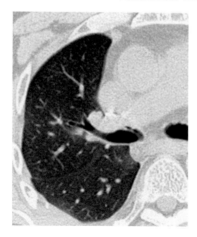

Fig. 17. Anastomotic dehiscence. HRCT demonstrates extraluminal gas adjacent to the right bronchial anastomosis. Partial anastomotic dehiscence was confirmed by bronchoscopy.

ing into the mainstem bronchus on CT scans. The accuracy of diagnosing bronchial stenosis is enhanced with use of three-dimensional endobronchial reconstruction images [89].

Findings of airway dehiscence include focal extraluminal gas collections and pneumomediastinum (Fig. 17). Additionally, detection on chest radiography of a new spontaneous pneumothorax or abrupt worsening of a pre-existent small postoperative pneumothorax in the absence of instrumentation (eg, central line insertion) should raise suspicion for bronchial dehiscence. Because the pleural spaces may be in communication after bilateral lung transplantation, unilateral dehiscence can result in development of bilateral pneumothoraces.

A unique complication of lung transplantation is infection of the bronchial anastomosis with *Aspergillus* species, a complication seen in the context of ischemic injury to the airway early after transplantation [90]. Instead of the normally thin band of tissue representing the wall of the telescoped bronchus, CT scans may show a polypoid mass extending from the wall of the bronchus at the level of the anastomosis. In severe cases, this finding can be accompanied by evidence of associated airway dehiscence, with small collections of extraluminal gas adjacent to the anastomosis.

Summary

Pulmonary complications occur frequently among solid organ and HSCT recipients. Thoracic imaging is an essential tool in detecting these complications and

in generating a differential diagnosis. Although the array of possibilities can sometimes be bewildering, a systematic approach to interpretation of radiographic patterns can be valuable in narrowing the differential to a few leading diagnostic considerations. In particular, the categorization of parenchymal abnormalities as airspace consolidation, ground-glass opacities,

---

Box 1. Radiographic patterns of disease in transplant recipients

Diffuse consolidation

    Hydrostatic pulmonary edema
    ARDS
    Reperfusion edema/primary graft
        failure (lung transplant)
    Diffuse alveolar hemorrhage (HSCT)
    Acute rejection (lung transplant)

Focal consolidation

Acute
    Bacterial pneumonia
    Acute rejection (lung transplant)
Chronic
    Metastatic calcification
        (liver, kidney transplant)
    Neoplasm
Ground-glass opacities
    Opportunistic infection
        PCP
        CMV
        Other viruses
    Drug toxicity
    Diffuse alveolar hemorrhage (HSCT)
    Acute rejection (lung transplant)
Discrete nodules
    Infections
        Invasive aspergillosis
        Nocardiosis
    Tumors
        PTLD
        Lung cancer (lung transplant)
Centrilobular nodules
    Infections
        Viral
        Bacterial (bronchopneumonia)
    BOS
Air trapping
    BOS (lung transplant, HSCT)

or nodules (both discrete and centrilobular) has important diagnostic implications. Additionally, distinguishing air trapping from other causes of a mosaic perfusion pattern is critical in the diagnosis of diseases of the small airways. The main patterns of parenchymal disease and the most commonly associated pathologic diagnoses are summarized in Box 1.

References

[1] Kotloff RM, Ahya VN, Crawford SW. Pulmonary complications of solid organ and hematopoietic stem cell transplantation. Am J Respir Crit Care Med 2004; 170:22–48.

[2] Jules-Elysee K, Stover DE, Yahalom J, et al. Pulmonary complications in lymphoma patients treated with high-dose therapy and autologous bone marrow transplantation. Am Rev Respir Dis 1992;146:485–91.

[3] Murata K, Khan A, Herman PG. Pulmonary parenchymal disease: evaluation with high-resolution CT. Radiology 1989;170:629–35.

[4] Mathieson JR, Mayo JR, Staples CA, et al. Chronic diffuse infiltrative lung disease: comparison of diagnostic accuracy of CT and chest radiography. Radiology 1989;171:111–6.

[5] Austin JHM, Muller NI, Friedman PJ, et al. Glossary of terms for CT of the lungs: recommendations of the Nomenclature Committee of the Fleischner Society. Radiology 1996;200:327–31.

[6] Brown MJ, Miller RR, Muller NI. Acute lung disease in the immunocompromised host: CT and pathologic examination findings. Radiology 1994;190:247–54.

[7] Leung AN, Gosselin MV, Napper CH, et al. Pulmonary infections after bone marrow transplantation: clinical and radiographic findings. Radiology 1999;210: 699–710.

[8] Collins J, Muller NL, Leung AN, et al. Epstein-Barr virus associated lymphoproliferative disease of the lung: CT and histologic findings. Radiology 1998;208: 749–59.

[9] Soubani AO, Miller KB, Hassoun PM. Pulmonary complications of bone marrow transplantation. Chest 1996;109:1066–77.

[10] Pistolesi M, Mniati M. The radiologic distinction of cardiogenic and non cardiogenic edema. AJR Am J Roentgenol 1985;144:879–94.

[11] Wiener-Kronish JP, Webb WR, Matthay MA. Hydrostatic versus increased permeability pulmonary edema: diagnosis based on radiographic criteria in critically ill patients. Radiology 1988;168:73–9.

[12] Tomashefski Jr JF. Pulmonary pathology of the adult respiratory distress syndrome. Clin Chest Med 1990; 11:593–619.

[13] Bachofen M, Weibel ER. Structural alterations of lung parenchyma in the adult respiratory distress syndrome. Clin Chest Med 1982;3:35–56.

[14] Snyder LS, Hertz MI, Harmon KR, et al. Failure of lung repair following acute lung injury: regulation of he fibroproliferative response (Part 2). Chest 1990;4: 989–93.

[15] Desai SR, Wells AU, Suntharalingam G, et al. Acute respiratory distress syndrome caused by pulmonary and extrapulmonary injury: a comparative CT study. Radiology 2001;218:689–93.

[16] Gluecker T, Capasso P, Schnyder P, et al. Clinical and radiologic features of pulmonary edema. Radiographics 1999;19:1507–31.

[17] Goodman LR, Fumagalli R, Tagliabue P, et al. Adult respiratory distress syndrome due to pulmonary and extrapulmonary causes: CT, clinical, and functional correlations. Radiology 1999;213:545–52.

[18] Desai SR, Wells AU, Rubens MB, et al. Acute respiratory distress syndrome. CT abnormalities at long-term follow-up. Radiology 1999;210:29–35.

[19] Siegelman SS, Sinha SB, Veith FJ. Pulmonary reimplantation response. Ann Surg 1971;177:30–6.

[20] Anderson DC, Glazer HS, Semenkovich JW, et al. Lung transplant edema: chest radiography after lung transplantation—the first 10 days. Radiology 1995; 195:275–81.

[21] Kundu K, Herman SJ, Winton TL. Reperfusion edema after lung transplantation: radiographic manifestations. Radiology 1998;206:75–80.

[22] Christie JD, Kotloff RM, Pochettino A, et al. Clinical risk factors for primary graft failure following lung transplantation. Chest 2003;124:1232–41.

[23] O'Brien JD, Ettinger NA. Pulmonary complications of liver transplantation. Clin Chest Med 1996;17:99–114.

[24] Kantrow SP, Hackman RC, Boeckh M, et al. Idiopathic pneumonia syndrome: changing spectrum of lung injury after marrow transplantation. Transplantation 1997; 63:1079–86.

[25] Weisdorf DJ. Diffuse alveolar hemorrhage: an evolving problem? Leukemia 2003;17:1049–50.

[26] Spitzer TR. Engraftment syndrome following hematopoietic stem cell transplantation. Bone Marrow Transplant 2001;27:893–8.

[27] Bergin CJ, Castellino RA, Blank N, et al. Acute lung rejection after heart-lung transplantation: correlation of findings on chest radiographs with lung biopsy results. AJR Am J Roentgenol 1990;155:23–7.

[28] Gotway MB, Dawn SK, Sellami D, et al. Acute rejection following lung transplantation: limitations in accuracy of thin-section CT for diagnosis. Radiology 2001;221:207–12.

[29] Loubeyre P, Revel D, Delignette A, et al. High-resolution computed tomographic findings associated with histologically diagnosed acute lung rejection in heart-lung transplant recipients. Chest 1995;107: 132–8.

[30] Collins J, Muller NL, Kazerooni EA, et al. CT findings of pneumonia after lung transplantation. AJR Am J Roentgenol 2000;175:811–8.

[31] Montoya JG, Giraldo LF, Efron B, et al. Infectious complications among 620 consecutive heart transplant

patients at Stanford University Medical Center. Clin Infect Dis 2001;33:629–40.

[32] Heitzman ER. The radiological diagnosis of pneumonia in the adult: a commentary. Semin Roentgenol 1989;24:212–7.

[33] Torres A, Ewig S, Inausti J, et al. Etiology and microbial patterns of pulmonary infiltrates in patients with orthotopic liver transplantation. Chest 2000;117:494–502.

[34] Horvath J, Summer S, Loyd J, et al. Infection in the transplanted and native lung after single lung transplantation. Chest 1993;104:681–5.

[35] Genereux GP, Stilwell GA. The acute bacterial pneumonias. Semin Roentgenol 1980;15:9–16.

[36] Scanlon GT, Unger JD. The radiology of bacterial and viral pneumonias. Radiol Clin North Am 1973;11:317–38.

[37] Reittner P, Muller NL, Heyneman L, et al. Mycoplasma pneumoniae pneumonia: radiographic and high-resolution CT features in 28 patients. AJR Am J Roentgenol 2000;174:37–41.

[38] Heussel CP, Kauczor HU, Heussel G, et al. Early detection of pneumonia in febrile neutropenic patients: use of thin-section CT. AJR Am J Roentgenol 1997;169:1347–53.

[39] Agusti C, Ramirez J, Picado C, et al. Diffuse alveolar hemorrhage in allogeneic bone marrow transplantation: a postmortem study. Am J Respir Crit Care Med 1995;151:1006–10.

[40] Primack SL, Miller RR, Muller NL. Diffuse pulmonary hemorrhage: clinical, pathologic and imaging features. AJR Am J Roentgenol 1995;164:295–300.

[41] Hartman TE, Muller NL, Primack SL, et al. Metastatic pulmonary calcification in patients with hypercalcemia: findings on chest radiographs and CT scans. AJR Am J Roentgenol 1994;162:799–802.

[42] Kuhlman JE, Ren H, Hutchins GM, et al. Fulminant pulmonary calcification complicating renal transplantation: CT demonstration. Radiology 1989;173:459–60.

[43] Collins J, Kazerooni EA, Lacomis J, et al. Bronchogenic carcinoma after lung transplantation: frequency, clinical characteristics, and imaging findings. Radiology 2002;224:131–8.

[44] Kuhlman JE. Pneumocystis infections: the radiologist's perspective. Radiology 1996;198:623–35.

[45] McGuinness G, Scholes JV, Garay SM, et al. Cytomegalovirus pneumonitis: spectrum of parenchymal CT findings with pathologic correlation in 21 AIDS patients. Radiology 1994;192:451–9.

[46] Gasparetto EL, Escuissato DL, Marchiori E, et al. High-resolution CT findings of respiratory syncytial virus pneumonia after bone marrow transplantation. AJR Am J Roentgenol 2004;182:1133–7.

[47] Gordon SM, LaRosa SP, Kalmadi S, et al. Should prophylaxis for Pneumocystis carinii pneumonia in solid organ transplant recipients ever be discontinued? Clin Infect Dis 1999;28:240–6.

[48] Boiselle PM, Crans Jr CA, Kaplan MA. The changing face of Pneumocystis carinii pneumonia in AIDS patients. AJR Am J Roentgenol 1999;172:1301–9.

[49] Konoplev S, Champlin RE, Giralt S, et al. Cytomegalovirus pneumonia in adult autologous blood and marrow transplant recipients. Bone Marrow Transplant 2001;27:877–81.

[50] Kang EY, Patz Jr EF, Muller NL. Cytomegalovirus pneumonia in transplant patients: CT findings. J Comput Assist Tomogr 1996;20:295–9.

[51] Rossi SE, Erasmus JJ, McAdams P, et al. Pulmonary drug toxicity: radiologic and pathologic manifestation. Radiographics 2000;20:1245–59.

[52] Smith GJ. The histopathology of pulmonary reactions to drugs. Clin Chest Med 1990;11:95–117.

[53] Wilcznski SW, Erasmus JJ, Petros WP, et al. Delayed pulmonary toxicity syndrome following high-dose chemotherapy and bone marrow transplantation for breast cancer. Am J Respir Crit Care Med 1998;157:565–73.

[54] Pham PT, Pham PC, Danovitch GM, et al. Sirolimus-associated pulmonary toxicity. Transplantation 2004;77:1215–20.

[55] Primack SL, Remy-Jardin M, Remy J, et al. High resolution CT of the lung: pitfalls in the diagnosis of infiltrative lung disease. AJR Am J Roentgenol 1996;167:413–8.

[56] Stern EJ, Swensen SJ, Hartman TE, et al. CT mosaic pattern of lung attenuation: distinguishing different causes. AJR Am J Roentgenol 1995;165:813–6.

[57] Siegel MJ, Bhalla S, Gutierrez FR, et al. Post-lung transplantation bronchiolitis obliterans syndrome: usefulness of expiratory thin-section CT for diagnosis. Radiology 2001;220:455–62.

[58] Leung AN, Fisher K, Valentine V, et al. Bronchiolitis obliterans after lung transplantation: detection using expiratory HRCT. Chest 1998;113:365–70.

[59] Worthy SA, Park CS, Kim JS, et al. Bronchiolitis obliterans after lung transplantation: high-resolution CT findings in 15 patients. AJR Am J Roentgenol 1997;169:673–7.

[60] Bankier AA, Van Muylem AV, Knoop C, et al. Bronchiolitis obliterans syndrome in heart-lung transplant recipients: diagnosis with expiratory CT. Radiology 2001;218:533–9.

[61] Copley SJ, Wells AU, Muller NL, et al. Thin-section CT in obstructive pulmonary disease: discriminatory value. Radiology 2002;223:812–9.

[62] Konen E, Gutierrez C, Chaparo C, et al. Bronchiolitis obliterans syndrome in lung transplant recipients: can thin-section CT findings predict disease before its clinical appearance. Radiology 2004;231:467–73.

[63] Knollmann FD, Ewert R, Wundrich T, et al. Bronchiolitis obliterans syndrome in lung transplant recipients: use of spirometrically gated CT. Radiology 2002;225:655–62.

[64] Won HJ, Lee KS, Cheon JE, et al. Invasive pulmonary aspergillosis: prediction at thin-section CT in patients with neutropenia—a prospective study. Radiology 1998;208:777–82.

[65] Fegin DS. Nocardiosis of the lung: chest radiographic findings in 21 cases. Radiology 1986;159:9–14.

[66] Rappaport DC, Chamberlain DW, Shepherd FA, et al. Lymphoproliferative disorders after lung transplantation: imaging features. Radiology 1998;206:519–24.

[67] Gruden JF, Webb WR, Warnock M. Centrilobular opacities in the lung on high-resolution CT: diagnostic considerations and pathologic correlation. AJR Am J Roentgenol 1994;162:559–74.

[68] Kwong JS, Muller NL, Godwin JD, et al. Thoracic actinomycosis: CT findings in eight patients. Radiology 1992;183:189–92.

[69] Franquet T, Muller NL, Gimenez A, et al. Spectrum of pulmonary aspergillosis: histologic clinical and radiologic findings. Radiographics 2001;21:825–37.

[70] Hruban RH, Meziane EA, Zerhouni PS, et al. Radiologic-pathologic correlation of the CT halo sign in invasive pulmonary aspergillosis. J Comput Assist Tomogr 1987;11:534–6.

[71] Primack SL, Hartman TE, Lee KS, et al. Pulmonary nodules and the CT halo sign. Radiology 1994;190: 513–5.

[72] Abramson S. The air crescent sign. Radiology 2001; 218:230–2.

[73] Gefter WB, Albelda SM, Talbot GH, et al. Invasive pulmonary aspergillosis and acute leukemia. Radiology 1985;157:605–10.

[74] Huang R-M, Naidich DP, Lubat E, et al. Septic pulmonary emboli: CT-radiographic correlation. AJR Am J Roentgenol 1989;153:41–5.

[75] Nalesnik MA. Posttransplantation lymphoproliferative disorders (lymphoproliferative disease): current perspectives. Semin Thorac Cardiovasc Surg 1996;81: 139–48.

[76] Paranjothi S, Yusen RD, Kraus MD, et al. Lymphoproliferative disease after lung transplantation: comparison of presentation and outcome of early and late cases. J Heart Lung Transplant 2001;20:1054–63.

[77] Pickhardt PJ, Siegel MJ, Anderson DC, et al. Chest radiography as a predictor of outcome in posttransplantation lymphoproliferative disorder in lung allograft recipients. AJR Am J Roentgenol 1998;171: 375–82.

[78] Reynders CS, Whitman GJ, Chew FS. Post-transplant lymphoproliferative disorder of the lung. AJR Am J Roentgeonl 1995;14:214–21.

[79] Eisenhuber E. The tree-in-bud sign. Radiology 2002; 222:771–2.

[80] Templeton PA, Fishman EK. CT evaluation of post-sternotomy complications. AJR Am J Roentgenol 1992;159:45–50.

[81] Knollmann FD, Hummel M, Hetzer R, et al. CT of heart transplant recipients: spectrum of disease. Radiographics 2000;20:1637–48.

[82] Knollmann FD, Bocksch W, Speigelsberger S, et al. Electron-beam computed tomography in the assessment of coronary artery disease after heart transplantation. Circulation 2000;101:2078–82.

[83] Weill D, Torres F, Hodges TN, Olmos JJ, et al. Acute native lung hyperinflation is not associated with poor outcomes after single lung transplant for emphysema. J Heart Lung Transplant 1999;18:1080–7.

[84] Collins J, Hartman MJ, Warner TF, et al. Frequency and CT findings of recurrent disease after lung transplantation. Radiology 2001;219:503–9.

[85] Collins J, Kuhlman JE, Love RB. Acute life-threatening complications of lung transplantation. Radiographics 1998;18:21–43.

[86] Collins J, Muller NL, Kazerooni EA, et al. Lung transplantation for lymphangioleiomyomatosis: role of imaging in the assessment of complications related to the underlying disease. Radiology 1999;210:325–32.

[87] Quint LE, Whyte RI, Kazerooni EA, et al. Stenosis of the central airways: evaluation by using helical CT with multiplanar reconstructions. Radiology 1995;194: 871–7.

[88] Schroder C, Scholl F, Daon E, et al. A modified bronchial anastomosis technique for lung transplantation. Ann Thorac Surg 2003;75:1697–704.

[89] McAdams HP, Palmer SM, Erasmus JJ, et al. Bronchial anastomotic complications in lung transplant recipients: virtual bronchoscopy for noninvasive assessment. Radiology 1998;209:689–95.

[90] Logan PM, Primack SL, Miller RR, et al. Invasive aspergillosis of the airways: radiographic, CT and pathologic findings. Radiology 1994;193:383–8.

ELSEVIER
SAUNDERS

Clin Chest Med 26 (2005) 561 – 569

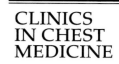

CLINICS
IN CHEST
MEDICINE

Acute Lung Injury After Hematopoietic Stem Cell Transplantation

Steve G. Peters, MD*, Bekele Afessa, MD

*Division of Pulmonary and Critical Care Medicine, Mayo Clinic College of Medicine, 200 First Street SW,
Rochester, MN 55905, USA*

Hematopoietic stem cell transplantation (HSCT) has emerged as a common therapeutic option for a variety of life-threatening disorders, especially hematologic malignancies. Pulmonary complications are reported in 30% to 60% of all recipients and represent a major cause of mortality [1,2]. A major proportion of these complications are the direct result of infection. This article addresses early, noninfectious causes of acute lung injury in the HSCT recipient. Early complications are usually defined as those occurring in the first 100 to 120 days after transplantation.

Upper airway injury

Box 1 summarizes early respiratory complications associated with HSCT and not attributed directly to infection. Oropharyngeal mucositis occurs in nearly all patients receiving HSCT [3–5]. High-dose chemotherapy regimens and total body irradiation (TBI) are associated with more severe mucosal injury. The severity of mucositis is associated with secondary infection, need for narcotics, duration of parenteral nutrition, hospital length of stay, and overall mortality [4].

Radiation pneumonitis

Radiation pneumonitis is usually an acute manifestation of direct pulmonary toxicity. A delayed inflammatory reaction and fibrosis also can be seen weeks after the exposure. Although TBI may be part of some conditioning regimens, it is difficult to distinguish the effects of radiation from those of high-dose chemotherapy, and synergistic effects are likely [6,7]. Interstitial pneumonitis has been observed more frequently in HSCT conditioning regimens that use TBI [6]. Radiation pneumonitis seems to be more common after high-dose chemotherapy, in patients who have pre-existing lung disease, and in those receiving localized chest wall therapy for breast cancer [7]. If other causes for interstitial pneumonitis are excluded, treatment typically includes corticosteroids. Morbidity and mortality are significant, although it is difficult to isolate the effects of the radiation from those of chemotherapy, prior infections, or other causes of acute lung injury. Chen and colleagues [6] reported 45% mortality related to interstitial pneumonitis in myeloma patients receiving high-dose chemotherapy and TBI before autologous HSCT.

Idiopathic pneumonia syndrome

Definition

Early after HSCT, it is common for patients to develop diffuse lung infiltrates. The differential

This work was supported by the Mayo Foundation.

* Corresponding author.

E-mail address: peters.steve@mayo.edu (S.G. Peters).

Box 1. Early noninfectious pulmonary complications of hematopoietic stem cell transplantation

Mucositis, upper airway injury
Radiation-induced lung disease
Pleural effusions
Drug toxicity
Idiopathic pneumonia syndrome
Engraftment syndrome, peri-engraftment
  respiratory distress
Diffuse alveolar hemorrhage

diagnosis may include infection, alveolar hemorrhage, lung injury as part of an engraftment syndrome (ES), or other noninfectious causes for acute lung injury. In an effort to reconcile the variable terms and clinical criteria used in this setting, consensus definitions for idiopathic pneumonia syndrome (IPS) were established by a National Institutes of Health workshop in 1993 (Box 2) [8]. IPS is defined by the presence of acute, bilateral pulmonary infiltrates, associated symptoms of cough and dyspnea, hypoxemia, and restrictive physiology, in the absence of infection or heart failure. Absence of infection usually is established by negative bronchoalveolar lavage (BAL) analyzed for pathogens and by the lack of clinical response to antimicrobial therapy. By this definition, IPS encompasses the entities of diffuse alveolar hemorrhage (DAH) and periengraftment respiratory distress syndrome (PERDS) [9,10]. Although many clinical features of these entities overlap, clinical presentation and outcomes may differ. Lung biopsies in IPS may show diffuse alveolar damage, organizing or acute pneumonia, and interstitial lymphocytic inflammation [11,12].

Incidence and risk factors

The incidence of IPS has ranged from approximately 2% to 5% in several reports, with most large series averaging 7% to 10% [12–17]. Clark and colleagues [8] reported median onset 42 to 49 days (range, 1–90 days) after allogeneic transplantation, with an early peak in the first 2 weeks and then relatively constant occurrence over the first 3 months. IPS can also occur as a late complication during the first 12 to 15 months after HSCT. Kantrow and colleagues [12] found a 7.7% actuarial incidence of IPS in HSCT recipients in the first 120 days after transplantation. Median time to onset was 21 days. Overall hospital mortality was 74%. Although inci-

dence was not significantly different between autologous (5.7%) and allogeneic (7.6%) recipients in the study by Kantrow and colleagues, the compiled data from many studies suggest that allogeneic transplantation is a risk factor for IPS [18]. Acute graft-versus-host disease (GVHD) has been associated with an approximately fivefold increased risk of IPS in allogeneic recipients [19]. Yanik and colleagues [20] reported that IPS was associated with acute GVHD in 72% of cases, and that hepatic veno-occlusive disease preceded IPS in 34%. Use of methotrexate after HSCT has also been identified as a risk factor for IPS [17]. Fukuda and colleagues [15] analyzed the occurrence of IPS after conventional conditioning, compared with nonmyeloablative regimens. The incidence of IPS was significantly lower after nonmyeloablative conditioning than after conventional induction therapy (2.2% versus 8.4%). IPS was also

Box 2. Consensus criteria for idiopathic pneumonia syndrome

Widespread alveolar injury

Multilobar infiltrates on chest
  radiograph or CT scan
New symptoms and signs of pneumonia (eg, cough, dyspnea, crackles)
Physiologic impairment; hypoxemia,
  restrictive ventilatory defect

Absence of infection

Bronchoalveolar lavage negative for bacterial pathogens or lack of clinical improvement after antibiotic therapy
BAL findings negative for nonbacterial pathogens (eg, viral, fungal, mycobacterial organisms)
Transbronchoscopic lung biopsy if patient's condition permits
If practical, a second confirmatory test to exclude infection within 2 to 14 days (eg, repeat BAL or open lung biopsy)

Adapted from Clark JG, Hansen JA, Hertz MI, et al. NHLBI workshop summary. Idiopathic pneumonia syndrome after bone marrow transplantation. Am Rev Respir Dis 1993;147:1601–6; with permission.

associated with greater patient age, diagnosis of leukemia, and severe GVHD. In the conventional conditioning group, TBI was associated with increased risk for IPS. These findings suggest that chemotherapy, radiation, and GVHD all contribute to the risk of IPS.

Clinical course and treatment

The overall mortality attributed to the development of IPS after HSCT has been approximately 70% to 80% [8,14,19–21]. Risks for death have included malignancy other than leukemia, and grade 4 GVHD [12]. Most patients require mechanical ventilation, and among those patients mortality has been approximately 90%. Death is usually caused by multiorgan dysfunction rather than by isolated respiratory failure [22]. There have been recent reports of better overall survival for HSCT patients requiring ICU admission and mechanical ventilation, but IPS remains a major cause of early mortality [23,24]. There have been limited reports of successful noninvasive ventilation in acute respiratory failure in neutropenic patients and after HSCT [25,26]. It is not known, however, whether early use of noninvasive ventilation might alter the course of IPS after HSCT.

Therapy of IPS is typically supportive, including supplemental oxygen and positive-pressure ventilator support as necessary. Many patients also are treated with antiviral, antifungal, and antibacterial agents because infection often cannot be excluded with certainty despite negative bronchoscopic studies. Treatment with high-dose corticosteroids (eg, methyl-prednisolone, 2 mg/kg daily) has been reported in several series. Because the entities of DAH and PERDS (discussed later) seem to show better response to corticosteroids than other causes of IPS, the data are difficult to interpret.

Pathophysiology

The pathophysiology of IPS reflects multiple pathways of diffuse acute lung injury. Humoral and cellular mediators of host and donor origin have been implicated. In nonimmunocompromised patients, the proposed pathogenesis of acute lung injury and acute respiratory distress syndrome has centered on the role of neutrophil products. Complement activation, leukocyte recruitment, neutrophilic alveolitis, and release of inflammatory mediators contribute to direct lung injury. It has been evident, however, that neutropenic patients can develop typical physiologic, clinical, and pathologic findings of acute respiratory distress syndrome [27].

Although the pathogenesis is not fully understood, the development of IPS in HSCT recipients has been attributed to inflammatory mediators including lipo-polysaccharide, interferon-gamma, and tumor-necrosis factor-alpha (TNF-alpha), and to the infiltration of donor T cells [28–32]. In mouse models of IPS after stem cell transplantation, BAL fluid shows elevated levels of TNF-alpha and of cytokines induced by interferon-gamma [28,29,33]. Monocyte chemoattractant protein is also expressed, and monocyte influx is implicated in the inflammatory lung injury [34]. Neutralization of monokines induced by interferon-gamma reduces the severity of lung injury in IPS models. Binding of TNF-alpha also mitigates the degree and progression of lung injury [29,35].

In human HSCT recipients, serum levels of interleukin-6, interleukin-8 and TNF-alpha have been correlated with transplant related complications including IPS [31]. In BAL fluid of patients who have IPS, TNF-alpha is increased and has been associated with poor prognosis [32]. In a series of three consecutive pediatric HSCT recipients with IPS, administration of the TNF-alpha–binding protein, etanercept, was well tolerated and was associated with clinical improvement [20].

Periengraftment respiratory distress syndrome

Definition and risk factors

In autologous bone marrow or peripheral stem cell recipients, ES has been described, characterized by fever, skin rash, generalized capillary leak, diarrhea, and pulmonary infiltrates [10,36–46]. Although the pathophysiology is poorly understood, ES has been characterized as an "autoaggression syndrome" or "cytokine storm" [10,37,41]. Lee and colleagues [41] reported median time of onset of 7 days (range, 4–22 days) after transplantation and median duration of 11 days.

Administration of granulocyte-colony stimulating factor (G-CSF) was associated with increased likelihood of ES (79%, versus 48% without G-CSF). In breast cancer patients undergoing autologous HSCT, administration of granulocyte-macrophage colony stimulating factor (GM-CSF) has been associated with a higher frequency of ES than G-CSF (24% for GM-CSF, versus 4% for G-CSF) [36]. Edenfield and colleagues [38] did not find higher risk with use of G-CSF but did correlate the frequency of ES with the dose of mononuclear cells infused during peripheral blood stem cell transplantation. In a trial of high-dose immune suppression and peripheral blood stem cell transplantation for multiple sclerosis, ES was observed in 13 of 18 patients (72%) [44]. In children receiving autologous peripheral stem cell transplants after chemotherapy for malignancy, ES has been identified as a major risk factor for early posttransplantation mortality [39]. A generalized capillary leak syndrome also occurs after allogeneic HSCT and has been associated with poor outcome [47].

Clinical features and course

Clinical features of ES overlap with those associated with acute GVHD. These features include fever, skin rash, generalized edema, weight gain, diarrhea, hypoalbuminemia, and noninfectious pulmonary infiltrates. Symptoms typically occur during the phase of neutrophil recovery after autologous stem cell transplantation. Chest radiographs often show interstitial edema and pleural effusions.

Capizzi and colleagues [10] characterized a subset of patients who developed features compatible with IPS in the setting of engraftment and termed this condition peri-engraftment respiratory distress syndrome. PERDS was identified in 19 of 416 autologous HSCT recipients (4.6%). Median time to onset was 11 days (range, 4–25 days) after transplantation, and PERDS occurred within 5 days of neutrophil recovery (defined as an absolute neutrophil count >0.5 × 10^9/L). Six patients required mechanical ventilation. BAL showed no indication of infection, but 6 of 19 patients had evidence of alveolar hemorrhage. PERDS was believed to contribute directly to death in 4 of 19 patients (21%). Of 11 patients treated with high-dose corticosteroids, 10 improved. Five of the 10 responders showed improvement in symptoms or oxygen requirement within 24 hours, suggesting a therapeutic effect. Because this syndrome has been recognized more frequently in HSCT recipients, most patients are treated with corticosteroids (eg, intravenous methylprednisolone, 1–2 mg/kg daily for 3 days, followed by a rapidly tapering schedule). Although the clinical criteria overlap with those of IPS, the subset of patients who have PERDS shows better overall outcome.

Diffuse alveolar hemorrhage

Definition

DAH represents another subset of IPS that may present in a nonspecific pattern but has been defined by specific findings. Criteria for DAH after HSCT include (1) signs and symptoms of pneumonitis, including hypoxemia and restrictive ventilatory defects, and evidence of widespread alveolar injury with radiographic infiltrates involving multiple lobes; (2) no evidence of infection; and (3) BAL showing progressively bloodier return from separate subsegmental bronchi, or more than 20% hemosiderin-laden alveolar macrophages, or blood, in at least 30% of the alveolar surfaces [9,48–50].

Incidence and risk factors

DAH occurs in approximately 5% of HSCT recipients, with a range of approximately 2% to 20% [51–55]. The reported frequency is higher in series of patients identified in the ICU or at autopsy [56]. The incidence of DAH seems to be similar among allogeneic and autologous transplant recipients. Risk factors include age greater than 40 years, intensive chemotherapy, and TBI [48,57–60]. Coagulopathy and thrombocytopenia are present in similar frequency among patients who have and do not have alveolar hemorrhage. Pretransplantation pulmonary function is not predictive of DAH after HSCT, but evidence of airway inflammation, defined as BAL neutrophils greater than 20% and any eosinophils, has been associated with subsequent DAH [61]. The timing of DAH has been correlated with the recovery of bronchial inflammatory cells after HSCT [53]. The pathogenesis may involve damage to the pulmonary endothelium, and microangiopathic changes have been observed [62].

Clinical course and prognosis

Symptoms of DAH typically include dyspnea, fever, and cough. Hemoptysis is infrequent, occurring in fewer than 20% of patients [2,63]. Chest radiographs usually show alveolar and interstitial infiltrates involving middle and lower lung zones [55]. In early phases, the radiographic changes may be subtle, unilateral, or asymmetrical. CT scanning may show ground-glass infiltrates or areas of consolidation [64]. The diagnosis is usually made or confirmed by bronchoscopy, either by the appearance of progressively bloody return during bronchoalveolar lavage or by the quantitative report of more than 20% hemosiderin-laden macrophages on iron stains of cellular preparations [49,65,66]. Fig. 1 shows BAL hemosiderin macrophages identified by Prussian-blue iron stain.

The treatment of DAH has included empiric corticosteroids. Metcalf and colleagues [53] observed

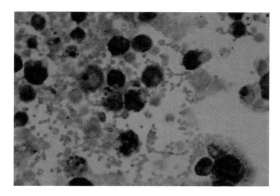

Fig. 1. Hemosiderin-laden macrophages (*darkly stained cells*) from bronchoalveolar lavage (Prussian blue staining).

that patients who received more than 30 mg of methylprednisolone daily for DAH had better outcome than those who received no steroids or a lower dose. Higher-dose steroid therapy, averaging approximately 500 mg to 1 g of methylprednisolone daily, was associated with lower mortality and lesser frequency of mechanical ventilation. Despite high-dose corticosteroid therapy, mortality of approximately 70% to 75% has been observed [52,53]. As noted in other causes of IPS, sepsis, and multiorgan failure are the most common immediate causes of death.

Afessa and colleagues [63] reviewed the outcome of 48 patients who had identified DAH among 1215 HSCT recipients. Fifty-two percent received autologous transplants, and peripheral blood was the stem cell source in 67%. DAH occurred in the first month in 28 of 48 patients (58%). Diagnostic criteria included progressively bloodier return on BAL in 88% and greater than 20% hemosiderin macrophages in only 40%. Eighty-five percent of patients were admitted to the ICU, and mechanical ventilation was required in 77%. Most patients received methylprednisolone, in a typical regimen of approximately 1 g given in four divided doses daily for 4 to 5 days, then 1 mg/kg for 3 days, and a tapering schedule over 2 to 4 weeks. The overall hospital mortality was 48% but differed by type of transplant and timing of the onset of DAH. Mortality was significantly less in autologous than in allogeneic recipients (28% versus 70%, $P < .004$). Also, DAH in the first 30 days after HSCT was associated with better survival (32% mortality versus 70% in patients who had DAH developing after 30 days, $P < .01$). The findings suggest that survival may be improving, and that early onset of DAH and autologous HSCT are favorable indicators.

Clinical approach and outcome of acute respiratory failure after hematopoietic stem cell transplantation

For the HSCT recipient who develops dyspnea and pulmonary infiltrates, the differential diagnosis includes infection, hemorrhage, edema, and IPS. The type of transplant, the timing of the onset, and the pattern of symptoms may be important but often are nonspecific. Bronchoscopy usually is performed with BAL for bacterial, viral, fungal, and mycobacterial organisms and for the diagnosis of hemorrhage. In non–HSCT-immunosuppressed patients, the yield for BAL for the diagnosis of infection is approximately 70% to 80%, but the overall diagnostic yield in HSCT patients is significantly lower [67–69]. Gruson and colleagues [67] reported an overall diagnostic yield of 49% from BAL in neutropenic patients. The subset of HSCT patients was more likely to have negative BAL findings, and those patients who did not have a specific diagnosis showed higher mortality.

There are limited data regarding the added diagnostic value of lung biopsy in HSCT recipients with pulmonary infiltrates. In most series, the majority of patients are already intubated and receiving mechanical ventilation, greatly increasing the risk of pneumothorax from transbronchoscopic lung biopsy. In many patients, coagulopathy and thrombocytopenia also increase the risks of serious bleeding. Soubani and colleagues [69], in a review of 27 bronchoscopies in patients receiving allogeneic HSCT for breast cancer, reported a specific diagnosis in 59%. BAL was diagnostic in only 22%, whereas transbronchoscopic lung biopsy yielded a diagnosis in 10 of 14 patients (71%), including drug toxicity in eight patients and metastatic breast cancer in two patients.

Surgical lung biopsy has been advocated for indeterminate pulmonary infiltrates in HSCT patients, especially to exclude infection [8]. Biopsy increases diagnostic yield, particularly for invasive pulmonary aspergillosis, for which BAL alone may be diagnostic in less than one third of HSCT patients [68]. Surgical biopsy increases morbidity, however, and there are limited data to suggest improved survival. Among 18 lung biopsies in HSCT recipients, Dunn and colleagues [70] found pneumonitis in 6, fibrosis in 6, bronchiolitis obliterans organizing pneumonia in 3, hemorrhage in 2, and infarction in 1. Overall mortality was 67%, and eight of nine patients (89%) receiving mechanical ventilation before biopsy died. Cultures were positive in six patients, but the findings did not significantly alter therapy. The investigators concluded that surgical lung biopsy was unlikely to redirect therapy and did not alter outcome [70]. Recently, Wang and colleagues [71] reported that among 35 patients in Taiwan who underwent surgical lung biopsy for diffuse pulmonary infiltrates after HSCT, idiopathic interstitial pneumonia was identified in 40%, cytomegalovirus in 20%, and miliary tuberculosis in 9%. Biopsy findings led to a change of therapy in 22 patients (63%), and clinical improvement was noted in 16 (46%). In contrast to the conclusions reached by Dunn and colleagues, Wang and colleagues suggested that lung biopsy offered additional diagnostic information and therapeutic benefit.

Outcomes of intensive care for acute respiratory failure in hematopoietic stem cell transplantation

Life-threatening complications of HSCT frequently lead to ICU admission. Early reports of the outcomes of intensive care, especially mechanical ventilation for respiratory failure, indicated mortality greater than 90% [22,72–75]. Death may be a direct result of hypoxemic respiratory failure but often is caused by late complications of sepsis and multiorgan failure. It has been suggested that invasive support be restricted to subsets of HSCT recipients who might have a better chance of recovery [76,77]. Unfortunately, accurate clinical assessment of prognosis is difficult, and physiologic scoring systems such as the Acute Physiology and Chronic Health Evaluation II have not predicted outcome accurately enough for use in individual patients [22,78].

During the past 20 years, techniques in stem cell transplantation and in ICU management have evolved, and outcomes might be expected to have changed. Recent reports do suggest that, for all HSCT recipients admitted to the ICU, survival has improved compared with previous series [22,23]. Soubani and colleagues [23] described 85 HSCT patients admitted to the ICU, representing 11.4% of transplant recipients during the study period. Fifty-one patients (60%) required mechanical ventilation, and 19 (37%) survived the ICU stay. In a series of HSCT patients requiring ICU care at the Mayo Clinic between 1982 and 1990, the authors observed overall hospital mortality of 77% [22]. In a subsequent cohort of 114 HSCT patients admitted between 1996 and 2000, the ICU, hospital, and 30-day mortality rates were 33%, 46%, and 52%, respectively. Sixty-two patients received mechanical ventilation, with 30-day mortality of 74%. Increased mortality was associated with allogeneic HSCT, the need for mechanical ventila-

tion, the use of vasopressors, sepsis, number of organ failures, and higher Acute Physiology and Chronic Health Evaluation III score [22]. Although the mortality of respiratory failure remains high, reported outcomes have improved.

Summary

Noninfectious pulmonary complications after HSCT are common and severe. IPS describes a pattern of acute, bilateral pulmonary infiltrates with associated physiologic derangement. The spectrum of IPS includes PERDS, DAH, and other idiopathic causes of acute lung injury. Overall mortality remains high but seems to have improved during the past 10 years. An aggressive approach to diagnosis and therapy is warranted, because infections may respond to specific treatment, and high-dose corticosteroid therapy seems to improve outcome in the subsets of patients who have PERDS and alveolar hemorrhage.

References

[1] Cordonnier CJ, Bernaudin F, Bierling P, et al. Pulmonary complications occurring after allogeneic bone marrow transplantation A study of 130 consecutive transplanted patients. Cancer 1986;58:1047–54.

[2] Jules-Elysee K, Stover DE, Yahalom J, et al. Pulmonary complications in lymphoma patients treated with high-dose therapy autologous bone marrow transplantation. Am Rev Respir Dis 1992;146:485–91.

[3] Robien K, Schubert MM, Bruemmer B, et al. Predictors of oral mucositis in patients receiving hematopoietic cell transplants for chronic myelogenous leukemia. J Clin Oncol 2004;22:1268–75.

[4] Sonis ST, Oster G, Fuchs H, et al. Oral mucositis and the clinical and economic outcomes of hematopoietic stem-cell transplantation. J Clin Oncol 2001;19:2201–5.

[5] Wardley AM, Jayson GC, Swindell R, et al. Prospective evaluation of oral mucositis in patients receiving myeloablative conditioning regimens and haemopoietic progenitor rescue. Br J Haematol 2000;110:292–9.

[6] Chen CI, Abraham R, Tsang R, et al. Radiation-associated pneumonitis following autologous stem cell transplantation: predictive factors, disease characteristics and treatment outcomes. Bone Marrow Transplant 2001;27:177–82.

[7] van der Wall E, Schaake-Koning CC, van Zandwijk N, et al. The toxicity of radiotherapy following high-dose chemotherapy with peripheral blood stem cell support in high-risk breast cancer: a preliminary analysis. Eur J Cancer 1996;32A:1490–7.

[8] Clark JG, Hansen JA, Hertz MI, et al. NHLBI workshop summary. Idiopathic pneumonia syndrome after bone marrow transplantation. Am Rev Respir Dis 1993;147:1601–6.

[9] Afessa BA, Tefferi MR, Litzow MJ, et al. Diffuse alveolar hemorrhage in hematopoietic stem cell transplant recipients. Am J Respir Crit Care Med 2002;166:641–5.

[10] Capizzi SA, Kumar S, Huneke NE, et al. Peri-engraftment respiratory distress syndrome during autologous hematopoietic stem cell transplantation. Bone Marrow Transplant 2001;27:1299–303.

[11] Griese M, Rampf U, Hofmann D, et al. Pulmonary complications after bone marrow transplantation in children: twenty-four years of experience in a single pediatric center. Pediatr Pulmonol 2000;30:393–401.

[12] Kantrow SP, Hackman RC, Boeckh M, et al. Idiopathic pneumonia syndrome: changing spectrum of lung injury after marrow transplantation. Transplantation 1997;63:1079–86.

[13] Chen CS, Boeckh M, Seidel K, et al. Incidence, risk factors, and mortality from pneumonia developing late after hematopoietic stem cell transplantation. Bone Marrow Transplant 2003;32:515–22.

[14] Crawford SW, Hackman RC. Clinical course of idiopathic pneumonia after bone marrow transplantation. Am Rev Respir Dis 1993;147:1393–400.

[15] Fukuda T, Hackman RC, Guthrie KA, et al. Risks and outcomes of idiopathic pneumonia syndrome after nonmyeloablative and conventional conditioning regimens for allogeneic hematopoietic stem cell transplantation. Blood 2003;102:2777–85.

[16] Wingard JR, Mellits ED, Sostrin MB, et al. Interstitial pneumonitis after allogeneic bone marrow transplantation. Nine-year experience at a single institution. Medicine (Baltimore) 1988;67:175–86.

[17] Weiner RS, Bortin MM, Gale RP, et al. Interstitial pneumonitis after bone marrow transplantation. Assessment of risk factors. Ann Intern Med 1986;104:168–75.

[18] Afessa B, Litzow MR, Tefferi A. Bronchiolitis obliterans and other late onset non-infectious pulmonary complications in hematopoietic stem cell transplantation. Bone Marrow Transplant 2001;28:425–34.

[19] Crawford SW, Longton G, Storb R. Acute graft-versus-host disease and the risks for idiopathic pneumonia after marrow transplantation for severe aplastic anemia. Bone Marrow Transplant 1993;12:225–31.

[20] Yanik G, Hellerstedt B, Custer J, et al. Etanercept (Enbrel) administration for idiopathic pneumonia syndrome after allogeneic hematopoietic stem cell transplantation. Biol Blood Marrow Transplant 2002;8:395–400.

[21] Clark JG, Madtes DK, Martin TR, et al. Idiopathic pneumonia after bone marrow transplantation: cytokine activation and lipopolysaccharide amplification in the bronchoalveolar compartment. Crit Care Med 1999;27:1800–6.

[22] Afessa B, Tefferi A, Hoagland HC, et al. Outcome of recipients of bone marrow transplants who require intensive-care unit support. Mayo Clin Proc 1992;67:117–22.

[23] Soubani AO, Kseibi E, Bander JJ, et al. Outcome and prognostic factors of hematopoietic stem cell transplantation recipients admitted to a medical ICU. Chest 2004;126:1604–11.

[24] Afessa B, Tefferi A, Dunn WF, et al. Intensive care unit support and Acute Physiology and Chronic Health Evaluation III performance in hematopoietic stem cell transplant recipients. Crit Care Med 2003;31:1715–21.

[25] Hilbert G, Gruson D, Vargas F, et al. Noninvasive ventilation in immunosuppressed patients with pulmonary infiltrates, fever, and acute respiratory failure. N Engl J Med 2001;344:481–7.

[26] Rabitsch W, Staudinger T, Brugger SA, et al. Successful management of adult respiratory distress syndrome (ARDS) after high-dose chemotherapy and peripheral blood progenitor cell rescue by non-invasive ventilatory support. Bone Marrow Transplant 1998;21:1067–9.

[27] Ognibene FP, Martin SE, Parker MM, et al. Adult respiratory distress syndrome in patients with severe neutropenia. N Engl J Med 1986;315:547–51.

[28] Gerbitz A, Nickoloff BJ, Olkiewicz K, et al. A role for tumor necrosis factor-alpha-mediated endothelial apoptosis in the development of experimental idiopathic pneumonia syndrome. Transplantation 2004;78:494–502.

[29] Hildebrandt GC, Olkiewicz KM, Corrion LA, et al. Donor-derived TNF-alpha regulates pulmonary chemokine expression and the development of idiopathic pneumonia syndrome after allogeneic bone marrow transplantation. Blood 2004;104:586–93.

[30] Hildebrandt GC, Duffner UA, Olkiewicz KM, et al. A critical role for CCR2/MCP-1 interactions in the development of idiopathic pneumonia syndrome after allogeneic bone marrow transplantation. Blood 2004;103:2417–26.

[31] Schots R, Kaufman L, Van Riet I, et al. Proinflammatory cytokines and their role in the development of major transplant-related complications in the early phase after allogeneic bone marrow transplantation. Leukemia 2003;17:1150–6.

[32] Hauber HP, Mikkila A, Erich JM, et al. TNFalpha, interleukin-10 and interleukin-18 expression in cells of the bronchoalveolar lavage in patients with pulmonary complications following bone marrow or peripheral stem cell transplantation: a preliminary study. Bone Marrow Transplant 2002;30:485–90.

[33] Hildebrandt GC, Corrion LA, Olkiewicz KM, et al. Blockade of CXCR3 receptor:ligand interactions reduces leukocyte recruitment to the lung and the severity of experimental idiopathic pneumonia syndrome. J Immunol 2004;173:2050–9.

[34] Panoskaltsis-Mortari A, Strieter RM, Hermanson JR, et al. Induction of monocyte- and T-cell-attracting chemokines in the lung during the generation of idiopathic pneumonia syndrome following allogeneic

murine bone marrow transplantation. Blood 2000;96: 834–9.

[35] Cooke KR, Hill GR, Gerbitz A, et al. Tumor necrosis factor-alpha neutralization reduces lung injury after experimental allogeneic bone marrow transplantation. Transplantation 2000;70:272–9.

[36] Akasheh M, Eastwood D, Vesole DH. Engraftment syndrome after autologous hematopoietic stem cell transplant supported by granulocyte-colony-stimulating factor (G-CSF) versus granulocyte-macrophage colony-stimulating factor (GM-CSF). Bone Marrow Transplant 2003;31:113–6.

[37] de Arriba F, Corral J, Ayala F, et al. Autoaggression syndrome resembling acute graft-versus-host disease grade IV after autologous peripheral blood stem cell transplantation for breast cancer. Bone Marrow Transplant 1999;23:621–4.

[38] Edenfield WJ, Moores LK, Goodwin G, et al. An engraftment syndrome in autologous stem cell transplantation related to mononuclear cell dose. Bone Marrow Transplant 2000;25:405–9.

[39] Foncillas MA, Diaz MA, Sevilla J, et al. Engraftment syndrome emerges as the main cause of transplant-related mortality in pediatric patients receiving autologous peripheral blood progenitor cell transplantation. J Pediatric Hematol Oncol 2004;26:492–6.

[40] Khan SA, Gaa B, Pollock BH, et al. Engraftment syndrome in breast cancer patients after stem cell transplantation is associated with poor long-term survival. Biol Blood Marrow Transplant 2001;7:433–8.

[41] Lee CK, Gingrich RD, Hohl RJ, et al. Engraftment syndrome in autologous bone marrow and peripheral stem cell transplantation. Bone Marrow Transplant 1995;16:175–82.

[42] Maiolino A, Biasoli I, Lima J, et al. Engraftment syndrome following autologous hematopoietic stem cell transplantation: definition of diagnostic criteria. Bone Marrow Transplant 2003;31:393–7.

[43] Marin D, Berrade J, Ferra C, et al. Engraftment syndrome and survival after respiratory failure post-bone marrow transplantation. Int Care Med 1998;24:732–5.

[44] Nash RA, Bowen JD, McSweeney PA, et al. High-dose immunosuppressive therapy and autologous peripheral blood stem cell transplantation for severe multiple sclerosis. Blood 2003;102:2364–72.

[45] Ravenel JG, Scalzetti EM, Zamkoff KW. Chest radiographic features of engraftment syndrome. J Thoracic Imag 2000;15:56–60.

[46] Ravoet C, Feremans W, Husson B, et al. Clinical evidence for an engraftment syndrome associated with early and steep neutrophil recovery after autologous blood stem cell transplantation. Bone Marrow Transplant 1996;18:943–7.

[47] Cahill RA, Spitzer TR, Mazumder A. Marrow engraftment and clinical manifestations of capillary leak syndrome. Bone Marrow Transplant 1996;18:177–84.

[48] Robbins RA, Linder J, Stahl MG, et al. Diffuse alveolar hemorrhage in autologous bone marrow transplant recipients. Am J Med 1989;87:511–8.

[49] De Lassence A, Fleury-Feith J, Escudier E, et al. Alveolar hemorrhage. Diagnostic criteria and results in 194 immunocompromised hosts. Am J Respir Crit Care Med 1995;151:157–63.

[50] Agusti C, Ramirez J, Picado C, et al. Diffuse alveolar hemorrhage in allogeneic bone marrow transplantation. A postmortem study. Am J Respir Crit Care Med 1995;151:1006–10.

[51] Ho VT, Weller E, Lee SJ, Alyea EP, et al. Prognostic factors for early severe pulmonary complications after hematopoietic stem cell transplantation. Biol Blood Marrow Transplant 2001;7:223–9.

[52] Lewis ID, DeFor T, Weisdorf DJ. Increasing incidence of diffuse alveolar hemorrhage following allogeneic bone marrow transplantation: cryptic etiology and uncertain therapy. Bone Marrow Transplant 2000; 26:539–43.

[53] Metcalf JP, Rennard SI, Reed EC, et al. Corticosteroids as adjunctive therapy for diffuse alveolar hemorrhage associated with bone marrow transplantation. University of Nebraska Medical Center Bone Marrow Transplant Group. Am J Med 1994;96:327–34.

[54] Nevo SV, Swan V, Enger C, et al. Acute bleeding after bone marrow transplantation (BMT)- incidence and effect on survival. A quantitative analysis in 1,402 patients. Blood 1998;91:1469–77.

[55] Witte RJ, Gurney JW, Robbins RA, et al. Diffuse pulmonary alveolar hemorrhage after bone marrow transplantation: radiographic findings in 39 patients. AJR Am J Roentgenol 1991;157:461–4.

[56] Huaringa AJ, Leyva FJ, Giralt SA, et al. Outcome of bone marrow transplantation patients requiring mechanical ventilation. Crit Care Med 2000;28:1014–7.

[57] Crilley P, Topolsky D, Styler MJ, et al. 1995. Extramedullary toxicity of a conditioning regimen containing busulphan, cyclophosphamide and etoposide in 84 patients undergoing autologous and allogenic bone marrow transplantation. Bone Marrow Transplant 1995;15:361–5.

[58] Mulder PO, Meinesz AF, de Vries EG, et al. Diffuse alveolar hemorrhage in autologous bone marrow transplant recipients. Am J Med 1991;90:278–81.

[59] Raptis A, Mavroudis D, Suffredini A, et al. High-dose corticosteroid therapy for diffuse alveolar hemorrhage in allogeneic bone marrow stem cell transplant recipients. Bone Marrow Transplant 1999;24:879–83.

[60] Wojno KJ, Vogelsang GB, Beschorner WE, et al. Pulmonary hemorrhage as a cause of death in allogeneic bone marrow recipients with severe acute graft-versus-host disease. Transplantation 1994;57:88–92.

[61] Sisson JH, Thompson AB, Anderson JR, et al. Airway inflammation predicts diffuse alveolar hemorrhage during bone marrow transplantation in patients with Hodgkin disease. Am Rev Respir Dis 1992;146: 439–43.

[62] Srivastava A, Gottlieb D, Bradstock KF. Diffuse alveolar haemorrhage associated with microangiopathy after allogeneic bone marrow transplantation. Bone Marrow Transplant 1995;15:863–7.

[63] Afessa B, Tefferi A, Litzow MR, et al. Outcome of diffuse alveolar hemorrhage in hematopoietic stem cell transplant recipients. Am J Respir Crit Care Med 2002;166:1364–8.

[64] Worthy SA, Flint JD, Muller NL. Pulmonary complications after bone marrow transplantation: high-resolution CT and pathologic findings. Radiographics 1997;17:1359–71.

[65] Huaringa AJ, Leyva FJ, Signes-Costa J, et al. Bronchoalveolar lavage in the diagnosis of pulmonary complications of bone marrow transplant patients. Bone Marrow Transplant 2000;25:975–9.

[66] Grebski E, Hess T, Hold G, et al. Diagnostic value of hemosiderin-containing macrophages in bronchoalveolar lavage. Chest 1992;102:1794–9.

[67] Gruson D, Hilbert G, Valentino R, et al. Utility of fiberoptic bronchoscopy in neutropenic patients admitted to the intensive care unit with pulmonary infiltrates. Crit Care Med 2000;28(7):2224–30.

[68] Reichenberger F, Habicht J, Matt P, et al. Diagnostic yield of bronchoscopy in histologically proven invasive pulmonary aspergillosis. Bone Marrow Transplant 1999;24(11):1195–9.

[69] Soubani AO, Qureshi MA, Baynes RD. Flexible bronchoscopy in the diagnosis of pulmonary infiltrates following autologous peripheral stem cell transplantation for advanced breast cancer. Bone Marrow Transplant 2001;28:981–5.

[70] Dunn JC, West KW, Rescorla FJ, et al. The utility of lung biopsy in recipients of stem cell transplantation. J Pediatr Surg 2001;36:1302–3.

[71] Wang J-Y, Chang Y-L, Lee L-N, et al. Diffuse pulmonary infiltrates after bone marrow transplantation: the role of open lung biopsy. Ann Thorac Surg 2004;78:267–72.

[72] Jackson SR, Tweeddale MG, Barnett MJ, et al. Admission of bone marrow transplant recipients to the intensive care unit: outcome, survival and prognostic factors. Bone Marrow Transplant 1998;21:697–704.

[73] Crawford SW, Schwartz DA, Petersen FB, et al. Mechanical ventilation after marrow transplantation. Risk factors and clinical outcome. Am Rev Respir Dis 1998;137:682–7.

[74] DeNardo SJ, Oye RK, Bellamy PE. Efficacy of intensive care for bone marrow transplant patients with respiratory failure. Crit Care Med 1989;17:4–6.

[75] Torrecilla C, Cortes JL, Chamorro C, et al. Prognostic assessment of the acute complications of bone marrow transplantation requiring intensive therapy. Intensive Care Med 1998;14:393–8.

[76] Rubenfeld GD, Crawford SW. Withdrawing life support from mechanically ventilated recipients of bone marrow transplants: a case for evidence-based guidelines. Ann Intern Med 1996;125:625–33.

[77] Faber-Langendoen K, Caplan AL, McGlave PB. Survival of adult bone marrow transplant patients receiving mechanical ventilation: a case for restricted use. Bone Marrow Transplant 1993;12:501–7.

[78] Shorr AF, Moores LK, Edenfield WJ, et al. Mechanical ventilation in hematopoietic stem cell transplantation: can we effectively predict outcomes? Chest 1999;116:1012–8.

ELSEVIER
SAUNDERS

Clin Chest Med 26 (2005) 571 – 586

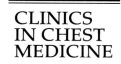

CLINICS
IN CHEST
MEDICINE

Chronic Lung Disease After Hematopoietic Stem Cell Transplantation

Bekele Afessa, MD*, Steve G. Peters, MD

*Division of Pulmonary and Critical Care Medicine, Mayo Clinic College of Medicine, 200 First Street SW,
Rochester, MN 55905, USA*

Tens of thousands of patients undergo hematopoietic stem cell transplantation (HSCT) each year, mainly for hematologic disorders [1,2]. In addition to the underlying diseases, the chemotherapy and radiation therapy that HSCT recipients receive can result in damage to multiple organ systems. Pulmonary complications develop in 30% to 60% of HSCT recipients [3–5]. With the widespread use of prophylaxis for certain infections, the spectrum of pulmonary complications after HSCT has shifted from more infectious to noninfectious complications [6]. This article reviews some of the noninfectious, chronic pulmonary complications (Box 1 and Table 1).

Pulmonary function abnormalities

Studies of pulmonary function tests in HSCT recipients have shown that restrictive and obstructive ventilatory defects and gas transfer abnormalities are frequent long-term sequelae, particularly after allogeneic transplantation [6,7]. A systematic review of 20 reports published between 1996 and 2001 found decreased carbon monoxide diffusion (DLCO) in 83%, restriction in 35%, and obstruction in 23% of allogeneic HSCT recipients [8]. A retrospective cohort study of more than 500 HSCT patients from the University of Toronto covering the period between 1980 and 1997 documented somewhat lower frequencies: impaired diffusion in 35%, restriction in 12%,

and obstruction in only 6% of long-term survivors [9]. Although the frequency of restricted and impaired diffusion seemed to be constant over time, this study suggested a declining frequency of airflow obstruction, from 15% in patients transplanted before 1987 to only 5% for those receiving transplantation after 1987. The extremely low incidence of airflow obstruction documented in this study probably reflects the stringent diagnostic criteria used by the authors. Using a more sensitive definition in a contemporary series from the Fred Hutchinson Cancer Center, Chien and colleagues [10] identified airflow obstruction in 26% of long-term survivors of allogeneic HSCT. Notably, the development of airflow obstruction serves as a marker for increased risk of mortality after transplantation [9–11].

Risk factors for the development of pulmonary function test abnormalities after HSCT include smoking history, pretransplantation pulmonary infection, and viral infection in the early posttransplantation period, older age, underlying disease, a pretransplantation chemotherapy and conditioning regimen, graft-versus-host-disease (GVHD), and human leukocyte antigen–mismatch [9,10,12–25]. Respiratory muscle weakness caused by GVHD-associated myositis has been described after allogeneic HSCT and, rarely, may be a contributing factor to restrictive pulmonary function abnormalities [26–28].

Several studies have suggested that abnormal pulmonary function may be a risk factor for the subsequent development of pulmonary complications in HSCT recipients [12,29–32]. Conflicting data exist, however. For example, a prospective study of 43 allogeneic HSCT recipients did not find a sig-

---

* Corresponding author.
E-mail address: afessa.bekele@mayo.edu (B. Afessa).

Box 1. Chronic noninfectious pulmonary
complications in hematopoietic stem cell
transplant recipients

Isolated abnormality in
    pulmonary function
Asthma
Bronchiolitis obliterans
Bronchiolitis obliterans
    organizing pneumonia
Idiopathic pneumonia syndrome
Delayed pulmonary toxicity syndrome
Pulmonary cytolytic thrombi
Pulmonary veno-occlusive disease
Progressive pulmonary fibrosis
Pulmonary hypertension
Hepatopulmonary syndrome
Pulmonary alveolar proteinosis
Eosinophilic pneumonia

limitations, the use of baseline pulmonary function tests to identify recipients at risk for pulmonary complications and to guide preventive and therapeutic interventions is of limited utility; further investigations are warranted.

Asthma

There are case reports of asthma developing after allogeneic HSCT [33–36]. Limited data suggest that the serum IgE level, of donor origin, is elevated after transplantation [37]. Allergen-specific IgE-mediated hypersensitivity can be transferred by HSCT from donor to recipient by B cells with allergen-specific memory leading to atopic dermatitis, allergic rhinitis, and asthma [33,34,37,38]. The management of asthma in HSCT recipients is similar to that in other populations.

nificant association between baseline pulmonary function values and subsequent pulmonary complications [21]. Moreover, there is considerable variability among published studies in the particular pulmonary parameters considered predictive, the posttransplantation complications that they predict, and the strength of the association. In light of these

Bronchiolitis obliterans

Chronic GVHD occurs in about 45% of allogeneic HSCT recipients who survive more than 3 months after transplantation [39]. Infectious and noninfectious pulmonary complications are common in HSCT recipients who have GVHD. The pulmonary

Table 1
Characteristics of selected pulmonary complications in hematopoietic stem cell transplant recipients

| Characteristics | Complications | | | | |
	BO	BOOP	DPTS	PCT	PVOD
Incidence	3.8% in allogeneic HSCT Rare in autologous HSCT	Low	Up to 72% of autologous HSCT for breast cancer	Rare Allogeneic	Rare
Clinical features	Dyspnea Cough Wheezing	Dyspnea Cough Fever	Dyspnea Cough Fever	Fever Cough	Dyspnea Cough Lethargy
PFT	Airway obstruction	↓ TLC ↓ DLCO	↓ TLC ↓ DLCO	Not available	↓ DLCO
Radiographic features	Air trapping Hyperinflation Normal	Consolidation Ground glass opacity Nodular opacity	Ground glass opacity Linear-nodular opacity Consolidation	Pulmonary nodules	Kerley B Prominent PA Pulmonary edema
Definite diagnosis	Surgical biopsy	Surgical biopsy Transbronchial biopsy	Clinical/PFT	Surgical biopsy	Surgical biopsy
Treatment	Immunosuppressant	Steroids	Steroids	None	None
Case fatality [reference]	High (59%) [6,16,40,43,44,46,47, 50,51,54,58,64,91]	Low (19%) [40,52,94–102,104]	0% [114,115,119,121]	0% [127,128]	High [142]

Abbreviations: BO, bronchiolitis obliterans; BOOP, bronchiolitis obliterans organizing pneumonia; DLCO, diffusion of carbon monoxide; DPTS, delayed pulmonary toxicity syndrome; PA, pulmonary artery; PCT, pulmonary cytolytic thrombi; PFT, pulmonary function test; PVOD, pulmonary veno-occlusive disease; TLC, total lung capacity.

histology of HSCT recipients who have GVHD may show diffuse alveolar damage, lymphocytic bronchitis/bronchiolitis with interstitial pneumonitis, bronchiolitis obliterans organizing pneumonia (BOOP), and bronchiolitis obliterans (BO) [40]. BO is a nonspecific inflammatory injury primarily affecting the small airways, often sparing the interstitium [41]. The term "bronchiolitis obliterans" has been used to describe a heterogeneous group of conditions [42]. In the clinical literature, it has been used to describe various conditions that result in airflow limitation. Philit and colleagues [43] have recommended the term "post-transplant obstructive lung disease" instead of "bronchiolitis obliterans" because it takes into account both the functional definition and the clinical context of the syndrome. Although BO can be idiopathic, it is often associated with connective tissue disease, inhaled toxins, infections, drugs, and chronic GVHD [41]. In the HSCT recipient, BO in most cases is considered a severe manifestation of chronic GVHD, although infection and drug toxicity may be contributing factors [44].

Incidence and risk factors

Airway disease as a complication of HSCT was first recognized in the early 1980s [45]. BO almost exclusively affects allogeneic HSCT recipients who have GVHD; there are only rare case reports of BO in autologous recipients [46]. In a recent publication from the University of Minnesota, 47 of the 1789 allogeneic HSCT recipients (2.6%) developed BO compared with none of the 1070 autologous HSCT recipients [47]. The reported incidence of BO varies among studies, related in part to patient population and to variable definitions and diagnostic criteria. Although some studies have included pathologic findings, most of the reported cases of BO were defined by the presence of airflow limitation in the appropriate clinical setting. The frequency of BO was 3.9% among 4180 allogeneic HSCT recipients reported in 13 studies [16,21,23,43,44,47–54]. A recent study employing a highly sensitive definition of airflow obstruction documented an incidence of 26% [10]. The incidence varies between 6% and 35% in long-term survivors who have GVHD [15,44, 47,49,50].

GVHD, older donor and recipient age, methotrexate use, antecedent respiratory infection, and serum immunoglobulin deficiency are risk factors for BO [10,15,16,44,47,51]. Patients who receive allogeneic HSCT after nonmyeloablative chemotherapy may have a lower incidence of pulmonary complications, including BO [55]. Although pulmonary infections are identified in many patients who have BO, it is not clear whether they are directly related to airway disease or result from immune suppression.

Pathogenesis

The pathogenesis of BO in HSCT recipients is not well understood. The strong association between BO and chronic GVHD suggests that host bronchiolar epithelial cells serve as targets for donor cytotoxic T lymphocytes [56]. Recurrent aspiration of oral material caused by esophagitis associated with GVHD, abnormal local immunoglobulin secretory function in the lungs, and unrecognized infections may also be involved [44,56]. The variations in histopathology, bronchoalveolar lavage cellular composition, and clinical course; the frequency of associated pulmonary infection; the increased risk in association with methotrexate, and the rare occurrence after autologous HSCT suggest a multifactorial pathogenesis [46,47,56,57].

Clinical findings and diagnostic evaluation

BO can occur 2 months to 9 years after transplantation [16,47,50,51,58]. Most patients present insidiously with dry cough and dyspnea, 40% develop wheezing, and 20% report antecedent "cold" symptoms; fever is notably absent [50,51]. Twenty percent of the patients who had BO had no respiratory symptoms at the time of the abnormal pulmonary function testing [51]. Because the presenting respiratory symptoms are nonspecific, a complete history, including prior medications and infections, and thorough physical examination focusing on signs of chronic GVHD should be obtained. Appropriate microbiology studies and laboratory evaluations including complete blood count with differential, blood urea nitrogen, creatinine, total bilirubin, hepatic transaminases, gamma globulin levels and subclasses, and urinalysis are recommended to exclude infection and complications of GVHD [56]. Because there is a high prevalence of sinusitis in allogeneic HSCT recipients who have GVHD, radiographic assessment of the paranasal sinuses is also recommended [56,59–62]. If gastrointestinal GVHD or aspiration is a consideration, esophageal studies should be performed [56,63].

Pulmonary function testing is the mainstay of diagnosis of BO [64]. Although normal airflow has been reported in HSCT recipients who have histologically proven BO [46], irreversible airflow obstruction is the hallmark of clinically significant disease. In lung transplant recipients, BO is classified

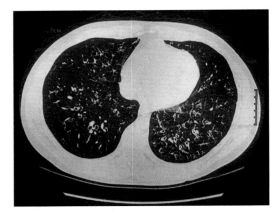

Fig. 1. CT of the chest in a patient with BO showing diffuse areas of parenchymal hypoattenuation, proximal bronchiectasis, and subsegemental bronchial dilatation. (*From* Afessa B, Litzow MR, Tefferi A. Bronchiolitis obliterans and other late onset non-infectious pulmonary complications in hematopoietic stem cell transplantation. Bone Marrow Transplant 2001;28(5):427; with permission.)

based on spirometry into stage 1 (forced expiratory volume in 1 second [FEV$_1$] 66% to 80% of peak posttransplantation baseline), stage 2 (FEV$_1$ 51% to 65% of baseline) and stage 3 (FEV$_1$<51% of baseline) [65]. This classification scheme has not been applied to the HSCT population, and its utility in defining severity or prognosis in this population remains to be established.

The chest radiograph is usually normal or may show hyperinflation [43,51,52,66]. High-resolution CT of the chest may show decreased lung attenuation, segmental or subsegmental bronchial dilatation, diminution of peripheral vascularity, centrilobular nodules, and expiratory air trapping (Fig. 1) [23,43, 52,67]. The most common finding on high-resolution CT of the chest is decreased lung attenuation. The decreased lung attenuation and bronchial dilatations are more frequent and extensive in the lower lobes [67].

Fiberoptic bronchoscopy with bronchoalveolar lavage is used in HSCT recipients suspected of having BO, mainly to exclude infection as the cause of airflow obstruction [57]. Because BO involves the respiratory and membranous bronchioles and is patchy in distribution, transbronchial lung biopsy rarely demonstrates the characteristic histologic changes and consequently is of limited utility. Furthermore, transbronchial biopsy is contraindicated in the presence of severe airways obstruction or thrombocytopenia. Bronchoalveolar lavage shows neutrophilic or lymphocytic inflammation, but this finding is nonspecific [53,57].

Video-assisted thoracoscopic lung biopsy is required to make a definitive histologic diagnosis. Lung biopsies show small airways involvement with fibrinous obliteration of the lumen with or without associated interstitial pneumonia, fibrosis, or diffuse alveolar damage (Fig. 2) [43,50,68–70]. Necrotizing bronchitis and bronchiolitis have been reported [68].

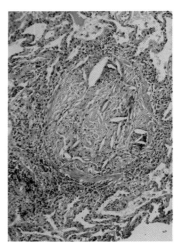 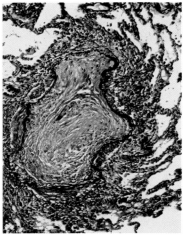

Fig. 2. Lung pathology in bronchiolitis obliterans showing bronchiolar inflammation and luminal obliteration associated with excess fibrous connective tissue. Alveoli and their ducts are spared (Hematoxylin and eosin and Verhoeff-Van Gieson elastic tissue stain). (*From* Afessa B, Litzow MR, Tefferi A. Bronchiolitis obliterans and other late onset non-infectious pulmonary complications in hematopoietic stem cell transplantation. Bone Marrow Transplant 2001;28(5):427; with permission.)

The inflammatory cellular infiltrates are usually peribronchiolar and consist of neutrophils and lymphocytes in varying proportions [54]. Surgical biopsies are rarely indicated because the diagnosis usually can be made on clinical grounds.

The diagnostic criteria for BO in HSCT recipients have not been clearly defined. Obstructive airways disease and BO may exist as distinct clinical entities in HSCT recipients. Bronchiolitis may occur without airway obstruction [56], and, conversely, airflow obstruction can occur for a number of reasons other than BO (eg, asthma, pre-existent chronic obstructive pulmonary disease, viral bronchiolitis). The diagnosis of BO is established by the presence of irreversible airflow obstruction and the exclusion of other causes of this functional abnormality. BO should be suspected in allogeneic HSCT recipients, particularly those who have chronic GVHD or who present with chronic cough, wheezing, dyspnea, or hypoxemia with a normal chest radiograph and no evidence of respiratory infection [56,71]. Similarly, the diagnosis should be considered in asymptomatic patients who have new onset of airflow obstruction on screening spirometry. Other chronic diseases, such as pulmonary veno-occlusive disease (PVOD) and early diffuse interstitial disease, can present with similar signs and symptoms. PVOD, however, is rare and unlikely to show airflow obstruction. Interstitial lung disease typically is associated with a restrictive defect on pulmonary function testing and parenchymal abnormalities on high-resolution CT of the chest.

Treatment

The treatment of BO in the HSCT recipient is empiric and typically consists of corticosteroids and augmented immunosuppression, targeting chronic GVHD. Only a minority of patients shows clinical improvement in response to treatment [6,23,43,46, 47,51,52]. Typically, prednisone in a range of 1 to 1.5 mg/kg/d is given for 4 to 6 weeks [56]. If the respiratory status remains stable, corticosteroid therapy is tapered and discontinued over 6 to 12 months. If no improvement is noted within 1 month, or if deterioration continues, cyclosporin or azathioprine can be added [56]. Antithymocyte globulin and high-dose intravenous methylprednisolone have also been used with mixed results [47].

Macrolide antibiotics are known to have anti-inflammatory properties and have been shown to improve symptoms, lung function, and mortality in patients who have panbronchiolitis [72–78]. Additionally, there are recent reports of improved lung function in lung transplant recipients who have

BO syndrome and who received macrolide therapy [79,80]. Currently, there is only one published study examining the effects of macrolides for post-HSCT BO. Khalid and colleagues [81] reported on eight HSCT patients who had BO and who were given azithromycin at an initial dose of 500 mg daily for 3 days followed by 250 mg three times weekly for 12 weeks. All patients demonstrated improvement in spirometric parameters, with a mean improvement in FEV_1 of 20.6% (range, 7.3%-42.9%). This preliminary evidence, coupled with the lack of significant adverse effects, makes macrolide therapy an attractive therapeutic option, but validation with a prospective, randomized trial is necessary before this approach can be strongly endorsed.

Although case reports have suggested beneficial response to thalidomide in HSCT recipients who have BO, a recent study showed no benefit [47,82,83]. Although hypogammaglobulinemia has been described as a risk factor for chronic GVHD, prophylaxis with intravenous immunoglobulin has not been shown to prevent BO [84]. Cyclosporin may play a protective role against BO, but its role in established BO is unproven [85]. A randomized clinical trial showed inhaled corticosteroids to be ineffective in lung transplant recipients who have BO syndrome, and there is no reason to suspect that this intervention would be any more efficacious when applied to post-HSCT BO [86].

In addition to immunosuppression and anti-inflammatory therapy, adjunctive treatments are important in the management of HSCT recipients who have BO. Prophylaxis for *Pneumocystis jiroveci* pneumonia and *Streptococcus pneumoniae* should be maintained. Bacterial infections, especially sinusitis, are common in patients who have BO and should be treated aggressively. Bronchodilator therapy is recommended, although only a minority of patients respond [51,60,68].

In selected HSCT recipients who have respiratory failure secondary to BO and who are deemed to be cured of the underlying malignancy for which HSCT was performed, lung transplantation is an option [40,87–90].

Clinical course

Serial pulmonary function tests in allogeneic HSCT recipients who have BO have shown that the rate of decline in FEV_1 is widely variable [51]. Deterioration in FEV_1 correlates with increased mortality rate [51]. The FEV_1 improves in only 8% to 20% [50,52,56,64]. The reported case fatality rates vary widely, ranging from 14% to 100%, with an average case fatality rate of 59% [6,16,40,43,44,46,47, 50,51,54,58,64,91]. In one study published 16 years ago, the 3-year mortality of 35 allogeneic HSCT recipients who had GVHD and obstructive airway disease was 65% compared with 44% for those who GVHD but did not have obstructive airway disease [51]. In a more recent study, the 5-year survival rate of 47 HSCT recipients who had BO was 10%, compared with 40% for those who did not have BO, highlighting the lack of progress in the management of BO during the last 2 decades [47].

Bronchiolitis obliterans organizing pneumonia

BOOP is an uncommon lung disease characterized by the presence of granulation tissue within the terminal and respiratory bronchioles as well as the alveolar ducts and alveoli. It was first described as a distinct clinical entity in 1985 [92]. BOOP can be either idiopathic or associated with other conditions such as infections, drugs, radiation, or connective tissue diseases [93]. The first cases of BOOP in HSCT recipients were reported in the early 1990s [94,95]. BOOP is not as common as BO in HSCT recipients.

HSCT recipients accounted for 4 of the 296 patients who had BOOP (1.4%) reported in 63 publications [96]. At Vancouver General Hospital, 5 of the 25 (20%) patients identified as having BOOP over an 8-year period were allogeneic HSCT recipients [96]. At the Mayo Clinic, the incidence of BOOP was 1.7% among 179 allogeneic HSCT recipients who survived for 3 months or longer [52]. The published medical literature on BOOP in HSCT recipients is limited to case reports with a maximum number of five patients [40,52,94–102].

Idiopathic BOOP is an inflammatory lung disease of unknown cause [93]. It occurs almost exclusively in allogeneic HSCT recipients who have GVHD, suggesting that it may represent a form of alloimmune injury to the lung by the transplanted stem cell [96]. The rare occurrence of BOOP in autologous HSCT recipients suggests that other mechanisms may be involved as well [97]. A recent case report of BOOP associated with human herpes virus-6 in a HSCT recipient suggests unrecognized infections may play role [103].

Clinical presentation and diagnostic evaluation

Onset is usually 1 month to 2 years after transplantation [52,94–96,98–102,104]. The presenting symptoms of BOOP include dry cough, dyspnea, and fever; rarely, the disease may be asymptomatic [52]. Physical examination may reveal inspiratory crackles.

BOOP should be included in the differential diagnosis of airspace disease in HSCT recipients who do not respond to antibiotics. Although the airspace disease usually is bilateral, it can be unilateral [97]. Pulmonary function tests usually show a restrictive defect, decreased DLCO, and normal flow rates [94,96,99,105]. Arterial blood gas analysis may reveal mild hypoxemia [96]. Chest radiographs and CT show patchy air space consolidation, ground-glass attenuation, and nodular opacities [94–96,99,106, 107]. The radiographic abnormalities usually have a peripheral distribution [108]. One recent study demonstrated increased exhaled nitric oxide concentration in HSCT recipients who have BOOP that decreases with response to treatment [99].

Although pulmonary function test and CT scan findings in conjunction with the clinical features may suggest the diagnosis, confirmation requires either surgical or transbronchial lung biopsy. The diagnosis of BOOP in the HSCT recipient occasionally can be made with transbronchial lung biopsy in the appropriate clinical setting, but about 85% of the patients require surgical lung biopsy [96]. Histologic confirmation of the diagnosis is warranted before the patient is subjected to long-term corticosteroid therapy. Surgical lung biopsy, usually by videoassisted thoracoscopy, is considered the criterion for the diagnosis of BOOP. The histologic hallmark of BOOP is the presence of patchy intraluminal fibrosis consisting of polypoid plugs of immature fibroblast tissue resembling granulation tissue obliterating the distal airways, alveolar ducts, and peribronchial alveolar space (Fig. 3) [42].

Treatment and prognosis

Corticosteroid therapy is the treatment of choice for symptomatic patients who have BOOP [52, 93–96,99]. About 80% of HSCT recipients who have BOOP respond favorably to treatment [52,94–96,98–101,104]. The duration and dosage of corticosteroid therapy in the HSCT recipient who has BOOP have not been clearly defined. Based on the experience from non-HSCT recipients, the initial dose of prednisone is in the range of 0.75 to 1.5 mg/kg/d, to a maximum daily dose of 100 mg, administered for 1 to 3 months, then 40 mg/d for 3 months, and then 10 to 20 mg/d or every other day for a total of 1 year [93,109]. Radiographic abnormalities usually clear within 1 to 3 months of initiating corticosteroid therapy [95,96,99,100]. Erythromycin, 10 mg/kg/d for 14 months, has been used in conjunction with

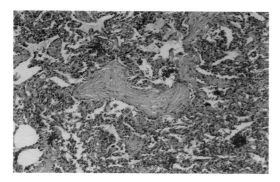

Fig. 3. Lung pathology in bronchiolitis obliterans organizing pneumonia showing the presence of intraluminal granulation tissue in bronchioli, alveolar ducts, and alveoli. There is also interstitial infiltration with mononuclear cells and foamy macrophages (Hematoxylin and eosin stain). (*From* Afessa B, Litzow MR, Tefferi A. Bronchiolitis obliterans and other late onset non-infectious pulmonary complications in hematopoietic stem cell transplantation. Bone Marrow Transplant 2001;28(5):429; with permission.)

corticosteroid to treat BOOP in one allogeneic HSCT recipient [98].

The case fatality rate of treated BOOP is 7.9% in the general population but seems to be higher in HSCT recipients [96]. Among 27 HSCT recipients who were documented in the literature as having BOOP, the overall case fatality rate was 19% [40,52, 94–102,104].

Delayed pulmonary toxicity syndrome

Chemotherapeutic agents and radiation therapy have been associated with pulmonary toxicities that manifest weeks to years later [110,111]. In the 1990s, many patients who had breast cancer were treated with a high-dose chemotherapy regimen consisting of cyclophosphamide, cisplatin, and bischloroethylinitrosurea (BCNU) followed by autologous HSCT [112]. After transplantation, a significant number of these patients developed pulmonary complications, one of the more common of which is the delayed pulmonary toxicity syndrome (DPTS) [113–120]. DPTS develops in up to 72% of autologous HSCT recipients who have received high-dose chemotherapy for breast cancer [114,115,121]. The relatively high frequency, low mortality, and good response to corticosteroid treatment distinguish DPTS from idiopathic pneumonia syndrome [114,118,119,122]. Because recent studies have not shown a survival benefit, the use of autologous HSCT after high-dose chemotherapy for breast cancer has declined [1,123].

The pathogenesis of DPTS is not known. The depletion of reduced glutathione and impaired antioxidant defenses caused by cyclophosphamide and BCNU have been implicated [118]. One study showed no significant correlation between patient age, stage of breast cancer, chemotherapy regimen, chest wall radiotherapy, tobacco use, prior lung disease, or baseline pulmonary function and the development of DPTS [121].

Clinical findings and diagnostic evaluation

Patients who have DPTS present with cough, dyspnea, and fever [115,119,121]. The onset of symptoms ranges from 2 weeks to 4 months after transplantation [119,121]. In the context of prior breast cancer treated with high-dose chemotherapy and autologous HSCT, DPTS is diagnosed by demonstration of a decline in DLCO capacity and exclusion of infectious causes [119,121]. The DLCO declines in more than 70% of patients who have breast cancer and who are treated with high-dose chemotherapy and autologous HSCT [116]. In patients who have DPTS, the median absolute DLCO decrement is 26% (range, 10%–73%), and a nadir is reached 15 to 18 weeks after transplantation [119,121]. The most common findings on CT of the chest are ground-glass opacities [119]. Other abnormalities include linear or nodular opacities and consolidation. Many patients may have a normal chest CT at the onset of DPTS [119]. Because of the typical clinical presentation and response to therapy, invasive procedures such as bronchoscopy are not usually required [114,115,119,121].

Treatment and prognosis

Corticosteroid therapy for DPTS usually results in resolution of symptoms and improvement in DLCO without long-term pulmonary sequelae [115, 119,121]. Treatment usually consists of prednisone initiated at a dose of 60 mg/d for 14 days and subsequently tapered over 5 to 7 weeks [114]. While patients are being treated with steroids, they should also receive oral trimethoprim-sulfamethoxazole or aerosolized pentamidine prophylaxis for *Pneumocystis jiroveci* pneumonia [114,121]. One case of DPTS refractory to steroid was treated successfully with interferon-gamma [124].

A study using prophylactic inhaled fluticasone propionate, 880 µg every 12 hours for 12 weeks starting from the date of high-dose chemotherapy, demonstrated a reduction in the frequency of DPTS to 35%, compared with 73% in historical controls [125].

No deaths attributable to DPTS have been reported [114,115,119,121]. The 3-year survival of stage II and III breast cancer patients who developed DPTS is 84%, which is not significantly different from that of patients who did not develop DPTS [121].

Pulmonary cytolytic thrombi

Pulmonary cytolytic thrombi (PCT) is a noninfectious pulmonary complication of unknown origin. Among HSCT recipients, PCT occurs exclusively after allogeneic procedures, typically in the setting of GVHD. PCT has also been described at autopsy in a nontransplant patient who died after hip replacement surgery [126]. All except 1 of the 16 HSCT recipients who had PCT reported in the medical literature are from a single institution [127,128]. Fifteen of the 16 patients were under age 18 years at the time of diagnosis [127,128]. Despite the seemingly rare and previously unrecognized nature of PCT, it was found in 15 of 33 (45%) HSCT recipients who underwent surgical lung biopsy for diagnosis of pulmonary nodules at the University of Minnesota [127].

Pathogenesis

The pathogenesis of PCT is not known. Although the hemorrhagic infarcts in PCT are similar to those seen in angioinvasive fungal infections, none of the lung biopsies in the reported PCT cases had evidence of infection [127,128]. The development of PCT exclusively in allogeneic HSCT recipients, and chiefly in those with GVHD, suggests that it may be a manifestation of GVHD targeting the endothelium of the lungs [127]. Demonstration of clinical and radiological improvement after increased immunosuppression also favors that GVHD as the underlying pathogenic mechanism [127,128].

Clinical findings and diagnostic evaluation

Most HSCT recipients who have PCT have active GVHD at the time of presentation [128–130]. The onset of PCT is between 8 and 343 days (median, 72 days) after transplantation [128–130]. All patients are febrile, and some have cough at presentation [128–130]. Dyspnea has not been reported at presentation.

Chest radiographs, usually performed as part of the evaluation of persistent fever, may be normal in 25% of the patients who have PCT [130]. Abnormal chest radiographic findings include nodules, interstitial prominence, and atelectasis [130]. Chest CT

shows multiple peripheral pulmonary nodules, ranging from a few mm to 4 cm in size (Fig. 4). Pleural effusion was reported in 1 of 13 patients who had undergone chest CT examination [130].

Bronchoscopy with bronchoalveolar lavage is used to exclude infection. Because of the peripheral and intravascular location of the nodules in PCT, transbronchial lung biopsy is unlikely to yield a diagnosis. Histologic demonstration of PCT requires surgical lung biopsy or necropsy [128,130]. The histologic features of PCT include occlusive vascular lesions and hemorrhagic infarcts caused by thrombi that consist of intensely basophilic, amorphous material that may extend into the adjacent tissue through the vascular wall (Fig. 5) [127]. The amorphous material suggests cellular breakdown products [129]. Immunohistochemical studies show a discontinuous endothelial cell layer.

Treatment and prognosis

Because of the unclear causes of PCT and concerns that lung nodules may have an infectious cause, patients have been treated with broad-spectrum antibiotics, antifungals, and systemic corticosteroids [130]. In one recent case report, treatment with intravenous methylprednisolone, 2 mg/kg/d, and cyclosporin, 3 mg/kg three times daily, for 1 week followed by oral prednisone, 30 mg/d, and 125 mg cyclosporin twice daily resulted in improvement [128]. Although it is unclear which of these various interventions is actually beneficial, most of the patients

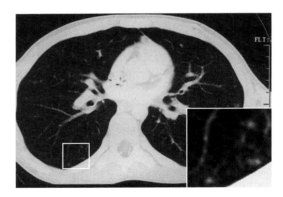

Fig. 4. CT of the chest in a patient with pulmonary cytolytic thrombi showing multiple bilateral pulmonary nodules with predominantly subpleural distribution. Inset shows magnified (×3) view of right-sided nodules. (*From* Morales IJ, Anderson PM, Tazelaar HD, et al. Pulmonary cytolytic thrombi: unusual complication of hematopoietic stem cell transplantation. J Pediatr Hematol Oncol 2003;25(1):90; with permission.)

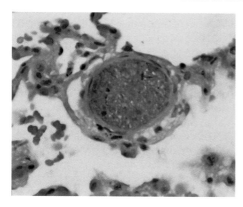

Fig. 5. Lung pathology in pulmonary cytolytic thrombi showing its granular basophilic nature. (*From* Morales IJ, Anderson PM, Tazelaar HD, et al. Pulmonary cytolytic thrombi: unusual complication of hematopoietic stem cell transplantation. J Pediatr Hematol Oncol 2003;25(1):89–92; with permission.)

who have PCT described in the literature improved clinically within 1 to 2 weeks and radiographically over weeks to months [130]. There has been no reported death attributed to PCT [127,128]. Of the 15 HSCT recipients who had PCT reported from the University of Minnesota, 10 were still alive at an average of 13 months after diagnosis; 5 died, 1 from GVHD and 4 from infectious complications [127]. The one patient reported from the Mayo Clinic died of progressive pulmonary hypertension 4 months after the diagnosis of PCT, with no evidence of PCT at autopsy [128].

Pulmonary veno-occlusive disease

PVOD is a rare cause of pulmonary hypertension that has been associated with various conditions, including HSCT. Pulmonary hypertension in PVOD results from intimal fibrosis obstructing the pulmonary veins and venules.

The incidence of PVOD in HSCT recipients is not known. Wingard and colleagues [131] reported PVOD in 19 of 154 autopsies of allogeneic HSCT recipients (12%). A recent autopsy review of 71 adult HSCT recipients (39 allogeneic) from the Mayo Clinic did not identify any case of PVOD, however [132]. PVOD affects both genders. In the published literature, there are about 28 cases of HSCT recipients who have PVOD [128,131,133–139]. The predominant underlying disease in HSCT recipients who have PVOD is hematologic malignancy, but PVOD has been found after HSCT for neuroblastoma

and aplastic anemia [128,137]. Only 2 of the 28 HSCT patients who had PVOD had received autologous grafts [135,137]. The frequency of PVOD is particularly high in allogeneic HSCT recipients who have concurrent interstitial pneumonia and hepatic veno-occlusive disease [131]. PVOD has been reported at autopsy after resolution of PCT [128].

Pathogenesis

Because the reported cases of HSCT recipients who have PVOD are limited in scope and number, its cause is not well defined. Infection, radiation, and chemotherapy are hypothesized to be contributing factors for the development of PVOD [133–135, 137,140–142]. BCNU, mitomycin C, and bleomycin are among the chemotherapeutic agents implicated as potential causes of vascular injury [140,142–145].

Clinical findings and diagnostic evaluation

Presenting symptoms are nonspecific and include dyspnea, lethargy, and chronic cough [142]. As the pulmonary hypertension worsens, orthopnea, cyanosis, chest pain, abdominal pain caused by hepatic congestion, and exertional syncope may be noted. Physical examination is also nonspecific and may reveal bibasilar crackles and inspiratory squeaks on auscultation of the lungs and findings indicative of pulmonary hypertension, including right ventricular heave, loud pulmonic heart sound, lower extremity edema, and elevated jugular venous pressure [139].

Radiographic findings include Kerley B lines, prominent central pulmonary arteries, and scattered patchy opacities [139,142]. Unlike other forms of primary pulmonary hypertension, pleural effusions are common in PVOD [142]. Echocardiogram and right heart catheterization show elevated pulmonary artery pressure. Pulmonary arteriogram may show delayed runoff and venous filling without arterial filling defects [139]. Pulmonary function testing demonstrates a decreased DLCO and restrictive ventilatory defect [139,142,146].

The triad of pulmonary arterial hypertension, radiographic evidence of pulmonary edema, and normal pulmonary artery occlusion pressure suggests PVOD. Many patients who have PVOD do not have this triad, however, and it is often difficult to get an accurate pulmonary artery occlusion pressure tracing in these patients [142].

The diagnosis cannot be made by bronchoscopy, although the finding of hemosiderosis and sclerosed venules in transbronchial lung biopsies suggests PVOD

[138]. The definitive diagnosis of PVOD requires surgical lung biopsy. In the absence of surgical lung biopsy, most cases are diagnosed at postmortem examination [131,137]. The pathologic hallmark of PVOD is the extensive and diffuse occlusion of pulmonary veins and venules by fibrous tissue [131,142,147].

Treatment and prognosis

There is no proven therapy for PVOD. Because observational trials involving patients who have primary pulmonary hypertension have suggested improved survival in those treated with anticoagulation, some advocate treating PVOD with long-term warfarin [142]. There are case reports suggesting that steroids may be beneficial in HSCT recipients who have PVOD [133,139]. The data supporting the use of steroid therapy and anticoagulation in HSCT recipients who have PVOD are limited to case reports, however [133,139]. In one report of two HSCT recipients who had PVOD, methylprednisolone, 2 mg/kg daily, resulted in improvement of arterial oxygenation and dyspnea within 1 to 2 weeks [133]. In one of these two patients, discontinuation of steroid therapy led to recurrent disease that responded to additional treatment [133]. On the other hand, there are reports of HSCT recipients who had PVOD who deteriorated and died despite treatment with steroid therapy [135]. The role of vasodilators in PVOD is unclear. Despite case reports of successful therapy with oral vasodilators or intravenous administration of prostacyclin in PVOD, these agents can dilate the arterial vessels without concomitant venodilation, leading to increased transcapillary hydrostatic pressures, acute pulmonary edema, and death [142,148]. Lung transplantation is a consideration in patients free of other comorbidities, including the underlying condition for which HSCT was performed, but there is currently no published experience on outcomes of lung transplantation in this unique setting [141,142]. In light of the limited treatment options and the generally progressive nature of the disease, it is not surprising that most patients who have PVOD die within 2 years of diagnosis [142].

Other pulmonary complications

Several cases of pulmonary arterial hypertension have been reported in HSCT recipients [136, 149–151]. The pathogenesis is not clearly defined. Normal pulmonary endothelium releases vasodilators such as prostacyclin- and endothelial-derived relaxing factors. Radiation- and chemotherapy-associated endothelial damage may be the mechanism for the development of the pulmonary hypertension [136, 149–151]. Prostacyclin infusion and calcium channel antagonists have been used for the treatment of pulmonary arterial hypertension in HSCT recipients [149–151].

Pulmonary alveolar proteinosis is characterized by excessive accumulation of surfactant lipoprotein in the alveoli leading to abnormal gas exchange [152]. The diagnosis of pulmonary alveolar proteinosis is made by the presence of periodic acid Schiff–positive proteinaceous material in bronchoalveolar fluid [153]. Cordonnier and colleagues [153] described three HSCT recipients who had pulmonary alveolar proteinosis. All three had received allogeneic HSCT for leukemia 12 to 90 days before the onset of pulmonary symptoms. Chest radiographs showed diffuse infiltrates. The clinicians had suspected infection in two patients and alveolar hemorrhage in one. Only one of the three survived.

Three cases of chronic eosinophilic pneumonia have been reported in HSCT recipients, one autologous and two allogeneic [154–156]. Despite initial response to steroid therapy, one patient had a fatal course [154].

Summary

About 50% of HSCT recipients develop pulmonary complications after transplantation. BO, BOOP, DPTS, PVOD, and PCT are among the noninfectious pulmonary complications that have been documented with varying frequency. The pathogenesis of these complications has not been defined clearly, and treatment is derived from anecdotal reports rather than from randomized clinical trials. BO affects allogeneic transplant recipients exclusively, is thought possibly to be a manifestation of chronic GVHD, and is associated with high case fatality rate because of the absence of effective therapy. Less common than BO, BOOP affects both autologous and allogeneic transplant recipients and typically responds to steroid therapy. DPTS develops in the majority of autologous HSCT recipients who have received high-dose chemotherapy for breast cancer before transplantation. It usually responds to corticosteroid treatment and has not been reported to cause death. All 16 reported HSCT recipients who had PCT had received allogeneic grafts, and most had active GVHD at the time of presentation. HSCT recipients who have PCT present with fever and pulmonary nodules. Despite the absence of specific therapy, HSCT recipients who have PCT usually improve. Most of the reported HSCT recipients who had PVOD had received allogeneic transplants. Because most cases of PVOD in HSCT recipients are diagnosed postmortem, the natural course is not known. Despite anecdotal reports of favorable response to steroid therapy, the prognosis of PVOD is poor.

References

[1] Report on state of the art in blood and marrow transplantation. International Bone Marrow Transplant Registry/Autologous Blood and Marrow Transplant Registry Newsletter 2003;10(1):7–10.

[2] Report on state of the art in blood and marrow transplantation—part II. International Bone Marrow Transplant Registry/Autologous Blood and Marrow Transplant Registry Newsletter 2004;10(2):6–9.

[3] Breuer R, Lossos IS, Berkman N, et al. Pulmonary complications of bone marrow transplantation. Respir Med 1993;87(8):571–9.

[4] Cordonnier C, Bernaudin JF, Bierling P, et al. Pulmonary complications occurring after allogeneic bone marrow transplantation. A study of 130 consecutive transplanted patients. Cancer 1986;58(5):1047–54.

[5] Jules-Elysee K, Stover DE, Yahalom J, et al. Pulmonary complications in lymphoma patients treated with high-dose therapy autologous bone marrow transplantation. Am Rev Respir Dis 1992;146(2):485–91.

[6] Griese M, Rampf U, Hofmann D, et al. Pulmonary complications after bone marrow transplantation in children: twenty-four years of experience in a single pediatric center. Pediatr Pulmonol 2000;30(5):393–401.

[7] Cerveri I, Zoia MC, Fulgoni P, et al. Late pulmonary sequelae after childhood bone marrow transplantation. Thorax 1999;54(2):131–5.

[8] Marras TK, Szalai JP, Chan CK, et al. Pulmonary function abnormalities after allogeneic marrow transplantation: a systematic review and assessment of an existing predictive instrument. Bone Marrow Transplant 2002;30(9):599–607.

[9] Marras TK, Chan CK, Lipton JH, et al. Long-term pulmonary function abnormalities and survival after allogeneic marrow transplantation. Bone Marrow Transplant 2004;33(5):509–17.

[10] Chien JW, Martin PJ, Gooley TA, et al. Airflow obstruction after myeloablative allogeneic hematopoietic stem cell transplantation. Am J Respir Crit Care Med 2003;168(2):208–14.

[11] Chien JW, Martin PJ, Flowers ME, et al. Implications of early airflow decline after myeloablative allogeneic stem cell transplantation. Bone Marrow Transplant 2004;33(7):759–64.

[12] Badier M, Guillot C, Delpierre S, et al. Pulmonary function changes 100 days and one year after bone marrow transplantation. Bone Marrow Transplant 1993;12(5):457–61.

[13] Burgart LJ, Heller MJ, Reznicek MJ, et al. Cytomegalovirus detection in bone marrow transplant patients with idiopathic pneumonitis. A clinicopathologic study of the clinical utility of the polymerase chain reaction on open lung biopsy specimen tissue. Am J Clin Pathol 1991;96(5):572–6.

[14] Chiou TJ, Tung SL, Wang WS, et al. Pulmonary function changes in long-term survivors of chronic myelogenous leukemia after allogeneic bone marrow transplantation: a Taiwan experience. Cancer Invest 2002;20(7–8):880–8.

[15] Clark JG, Schwartz DA, Flournoy N, et al. Risk factors for airflow obstruction in recipients of bone marrow transplants. Ann Intern Med 1987;107(5):648–56.

[16] Curtis DJ, Smale A, Thien F, et al. Chronic airflow obstruction in long-term survivors of allogeneic bone marrow transplantation. Bone Marrow Transplant 1995;16(1):169–73.

[17] Fanfulla F, Locatelli F, Zoia MC, et al. Pulmonary complications and respiratory function changes after bone marrow transplantation in children. Eur Respir J 1997;10(10):2301–6.

[18] Frisk P, Arvidson J, Bratteby LE, et al. Pulmonary function after autologous bone marrow transplantation in children: a long-term prospective study. Bone Marrow Transplant 2004;33(6):645–50.

[19] Gore EM, Lawton CA, Ash RC, et al. Pulmonary function changes in long-term survivors of bone marrow transplantation. Int J Radiat Oncol Biol Phys 1996;36(1):67–75.

[20] Leneveu H, Bremont F, Rubie H, et al. Respiratory function in children undergoing bone marrow transplantation. Pediatr Pulmonol 1999;28(1):31–8.

[21] Lund MB, Kongerud J, Brinch L, et al. Decreased lung function in one year survivors of allogeneic bone marrow transplantation conditioned with high-dose busulphan and cyclophosphamide. Eur Respir J 1995;8(8):1269–74.

[22] Lund MB, Brinch L, Kongerud J, et al. Lung function 5 yrs after allogeneic bone marrow transplantation conditioned with busulphan and cyclophosphamide. Eur Respir J 2004;23(6):901–5.

[23] Schultz KR, Green GJ, Wensley D, et al. Obstructive lung disease in children after allogeneic bone marrow transplantation. Blood 1994;84(9):3212–20.

[24] Schwarer AP, Hughes JM, Trotman-Dickenson B, et al. A chronic pulmonary syndrome associated with graft-versus-host disease after allogeneic marrow transplantation. Transplantation 1992;54(6):1002–8.

[25] Tait RC, Burnett AK, Robertson AG, et al. Subclinical pulmonary function defects following autologous and allogeneic bone marrow transplantation: relationship to total body irradiation and graft-versus-host disease. Int J Radiat Oncol Biol Phys 1991;20(6):1219–27.

[26] Oshima Y, Takahashi S, Nagayama H, et al. Fatal

GVHD demonstrating an involvement of respiratory muscle following donor leukocyte transfusion (DLT). Bone Marrow Transplant 1997;19(7):737–40.

[27] Oya Y, Kobayashi S, Nakamura K, et al. [Skeletal muscle pathology of chronic graft versus host disease accompanied with myositis, affecting predominantly respiratory and distal muscles, and hemosiderosis]. Rinsho Shinkeigaku 2001;41(9):612–6 [in Japanese].

[28] Stephenson AL, Mackenzie IR, Levy RD, et al. Myositis associated graft-versus-host-disease presenting as respiratory muscle weakness. Thorax 2001; 56(1):82–4.

[29] Baddley JW, Stroud TP, Salzman D, et al. Invasive mold infections in allogeneic bone marrow transplant recipients. Clin Infect Dis 2001;32(9):1319–24.

[30] Crawford SW, Fisher L. Predictive value of pulmonary function tests before marrow transplantation [see comments]. Chest 1992;101(5):1257–64.

[31] Horak DA, Schmidt GM, Zaia JA, et al. Pretransplant pulmonary function predicts cytomegalovirus-associated interstitial pneumonia following bone marrow transplantation. Chest 1992;102(5):1484–90.

[32] Milburn HJ, Prentice HG, du Bois RM. Can lung function measurements be used to predict which patients will be at risk of developing interstitial pneumonitis after bone marrow transplantation? Thorax 1992;47(6):421–5.

[33] Agosti JM, Sprenger JD, Lum LG, et al. Transfer of allergen-specific IgE-mediated hypersensitivity with allogeneic bone marrow transplantation. N Engl J Med 1988;319(25):1623–8.

[34] Hallstrand TS, Sprenger JD, Agosti JM, et al. Long-term acquisition of allergen-specific IgE and asthma following allogeneic bone marrow transplantation from allergic donors. Blood 2004;104(10):3086–90.

[35] Hirayama M, Azuma E, Kumamoto T, et al. Late-onset unilateral renal dysfunction combined with non-insulin-dependent diabetes mellitus and bronchial asthma following allogeneic bone marrow transplantation for acute lymphoblastic leukemia in a child. Bone Marrow Transplant 1998;22(9):923–6.

[36] Rietz H, Plummer AL, Gal AA. Asthma as a consequence of bone marrow transplantation. Chest 2002;122(1):369–70.

[37] Schuurman HJ, Verdonck LF, Geertzema JG, et al. Monotypic immunoglobulin E plasma cells in an allogeneic bone marrow transplant recipient. Histopathology 1986;10(9):963–9.

[38] Bellou A, Kanny G, Fremont S, et al. Transfer of atopy following bone marrow transplantation. Ann Allergy Asthma Immunol 1997;78(5):513–6.

[39] Carlens S, Ringden O, Remberger M, et al. Risk factors for chronic graft-versus-host disease after bone marrow transplantation: a retrospective single centre analysis. Bone Marrow Transplant 1998;22(8): 755–61.

[40] Yousem SA. The histological spectrum of pulmonary graft-versus-host disease in bone marrow transplant recipients. Hum Pathol 1995;26(6):668–75.

[41] King Jr TE. Overview of bronchiolitis. Clin Chest Med 1993;14(4):607–10.

[42] Myers JL, Colby TV. Pathologic manifestations of bronchiolitis, constrictive bronchiolitis, cryptogenic organizing pneumonia, and diffuse panbronchiolitis. Clin Chest Med 1993;14(4):611–22.

[43] Philit F, Wiesendanger T, Archimbaud E, et al. Post-transplant obstructive lung disease ("bronchiolitis obliterans"): a clinical comparative study of bone marrow and lung transplant patients. Eur Respir J 1995;8(4):551–8.

[44] Holland HK, Wingard JR, Beschorner WE, et al. Bronchiolitis obliterans in bone marrow transplantation and its relationship to chronic graft-v-host disease and low serum IgG. Blood 1988;72(2):621–7.

[45] Roca J, Granena A, Rodriguez-Roisin R, et al. Fatal airway disease in an adult with chronic graft-versus-host disease. Thorax 1982;37(1):77–8.

[46] Paz HL, Crilley P, Patchefsky A, et al. Bronchiolitis obliterans after autologous bone marrow transplantation. Chest 1992;101(3):775–8.

[47] Dudek AZ, Mahaseth H, DeFor TE, et al. Bronchiolitis obliterans in chronic graft-versus-host disease: analysis of risk factors and treatment outcomes. Biol Blood Marrow Transplant 2003;9(10): 657–66.

[48] Patriarca F, Skert C, Sperotto A, et al. Incidence, outcome, and risk factors of late-onset noninfectious pulmonary complications after unrelated donor stem cell transplantation. Bone Marrow Transplant 2004; 33(7):751–8.

[49] Alonso RR, Villa Jr A, Sequeiros GA, et al. [Obstructive lung disease after allogenic stem cell transplantation in children]. An Pediatr (Barc) 2004; 61(2):124–30 [in Spanish].

[50] Chan CK, Hyland RH, Hutcheon MA, et al. Small-airways disease in recipients of allogeneic bone marrow transplants. An analysis of 11 cases and a review of the literature. Medicine (Baltimore) 1987;66(5): 327–40.

[51] Clark JG, Crawford SW, Madtes DK, et al. Obstructive lung disease after allogeneic marrow transplantation. Clinical presentation and course. Ann Intern Med 1989;111(5):368–76.

[52] Palmas A, Tefferi A, Myers JL, et al. Late-onset noninfectious pulmonary complications after allogeneic bone marrow transplantation. Br J Haematol 1998;100(4):680–7.

[53] Trisolini R, Stanzani M, Agli LL, Colangelo A, et al. Delayed non-infectious lung disease in allogeneic bone marrow transplant recipients. Sarcoidosis Vasc Diffuse Lung Dis 2001;18(1):75–84.

[54] Urbanski SJ, Kossakowska AE, Curtis J, et al. Idiopathic small airways pathology in patients with graft-versus-host disease following allogeneic bone marrow transplantation. Am J Surg Pathol 1987; 11(12):965–71.

[55] Nusair S, Breuer R, Shapira MY, et al. Low incidence of pulmonary complications following nonmyelo-

ablative stem cell transplantation. Eur Respir J 2004;
23(3):440–5.

[56] Crawford SW, Clark JG. Bronchiolitis associated with
bone marrow transplantation. Clin Chest Med 1993;
14(4):741–9.

[57] St. John RC, Gadek JE, Tutschka PJ, et al. Analysis
of airflow obstruction by bronchoalveolar lavage following bone marrow transplantation. Implications for
pathogenesis and treatment. Chest 1990;98(3):600–7.

[58] Krowka MJ, Rosenow III EC, Hoagland HC. Pulmonary complications of bone marrow transplantation.
Chest 1985;87(2):237–46.

[59] Billings KR, Lowe LH, Aquino VM, et al. Screening
sinus CT scans in pediatric bone marrow transplant
patients. Int J Pediatr Otorhinolaryngol 2000;52(3):
253–60.

[60] Ralph DD, Springmeyer SC, Sullivan KM, et al.
Rapidly progressive air-flow obstruction in marrow
transplant recipients. Possible association between
obliterative bronchiolitis and chronic graft-versus-
host disease. Am Rev Respir Dis 1984;129(4):641–4.

[61] Savage DG, Taylor P, Blackwell J, et al. Paranasal
sinusitis following allogeneic bone marrow transplant. Bone Marrow Transplant 1997;19(1):55–9.

[62] Thompson AM, Couch M, Zahurak ML, et al. Risk
factors for post-stem cell transplant sinusitis. Bone
Marrow Transplant 2002;29(3):257–61.

[63] McDonald GB, Sullivan KM, Plumley TF. Radiographic features of esophageal involvement in chronic
graft-vs.-host disease. AJR Am J Roentgenol 1984;
142(3):501–6.

[64] Hyland RH, Chan CK, Hutcheon MA, et al. Early
diagnosis of obstructive airways disease after allogeneic bone marrow transplantation may improve outcome. Am Rev Respir Dis 1988;137(Suppl):111.

[65] Estenne M, Maurer JR, Boehler A, et al. Bronchiolitis obliterans syndrome 2001: an update of the diagnostic criteria. J Heart Lung Transplant 2002;21(3):
297–310.

[66] Benesch M, Kerbl R, Schwinger W, et al. Discrep-
ancy of clinical, radiographic and histopathologic
findings in two children with chronic pulmonary
graft-versus-host disease after HLA-identical sibling
stem cell transplantation. Bone Marrow Transplant
1998;22(8):809–12.

[67] Jung JI, Jung WS, Hahn ST, et al. Bronchiolitis
obliterans after allogenic bone marrow transplantation: HRCT findings. Korean J Radiol 2004;5(2):
107–13.

[68] Johnson FL, Stokes DC, Ruggiero M, et al. Chronic
obstructive airways disease after bone marrow transplantation. J Pediatr 1984;105(3):370–6.

[69] Ostrow D, Buskard N, Hill RS, et al. Bronchiolitis
obliterans complicating bone marrow transplantation.
Chest 1985;87(6):828–30.

[70] Wyatt SE, Nunn P, Hows JM, et al. Airways obstruction associated with graft versus host disease after bone marrow transplantation. Thorax 1984;39(12):
887–94.

[71] Afessa B, Litzow MR, Tefferi A. Bronchiolitis obli-
erans and other late onset non-infectious pulmonary
complications in hematopoietic stem cell transplantation. Bone Marrow Transplant 2001;28(5):
425–34.

[72] Ichikawa Y, Ninomiya H, Koga H, et al. Erythromycin reduces neutrophils and neutrophil-derived
elastolytic-like activity in the lower respiratory tract
of bronchiolitis patients [see comments]. Am Rev
Respir Dis 1992;146(1):196–203.

[73] Kudoh S, Azuma A, Yamamoto M, et al. Improvement of survival in patients with diffuse panbronchiolitis treated with low-dose erythromycin. Am J
Respir Crit Care Med 1998;157(6 Pt 1):1829–32.

[74] Kudoh S. Erythromycin treatment in diffuse panbronchiolitis. Curr Opin Pulm Med 1998;4(2):116–21.

[75] Nagai H, Shishido H, Yoneda R, et al. Long-term
low-dose administration of erythromycin to patients
with diffuse panbronchiolitis. Respiration (Herrlisheim) 1991;58(3–4):145–9.

[76] Oda H, Kadota J, Kohno S, et al. Erythromycin inhibits
neutrophil chemotaxis in bronchoalveoli of diffuse
panbronchiolitis. Chest 1994;106(4):1116–23.

[77] Kanazawa S, Nomura S, Muramatsu M, et al.
Azithromycin and bronchiolitis obliterans. Am J
Respir Crit Care Med 2004;169(5):654–5.

[78] Culic O, Erakovic V, Parnham MJ. Anti-inflammatory
effects of macrolide antibiotics. Eur J Pharmacol
2001;429(1–3):209–29.

[79] Verleden GM, Dupont LJ. Azithromycin therapy for
patients with bronchiolitis obliterans syndrome after lung transplantation. Transplantation 2004;77(9):
1465–7.

[80] Gerhardt SG, McDyer JF, Girgis RE, et al. Maintenance azithromycin therapy for bronchiolitis obliterans syndrome: results of a pilot study. Am J Respir
Crit Care Med 2003;168(1):121–5.

[81] Khalid M, Al Saghir A, Saleemi S, et al. Azithromycin in bronchiolitis obliterans complicating bone
marrow transplantation: a preliminary study. Eur
Respir J 2005;25(3):490–3.

[82] Browne PV, Weisdorf DJ, DeFor T, et al. Response
to thalidomide therapy in refractory chronic graft-
versus-host disease. Bone Marrow Transplant 2000;
26(8):865–9.

[83] Forsyth CJ, Cremer PD, Torzillo P, et al. Thalidomide
responsive chronic pulmonary GVHD. Bone Marrow
Transplant 1996;17(2):291–3.

[84] Sullivan KM, Storek J, Kopecky KJ, et al. A controlled trial of long-term administration of intravenous immunoglobulin to prevent late infection and
chronic graft-vs.-host disease after marrow transplantation: clinical outcome and effect on subsequent
immune recovery. Biol Blood Marrow Transplant
1996;2(1):44–53.

[85] Payne L, Chan CK, Fyles G, et al. Cyclosporine as
possible prophylaxis for obstructive airways disease
after allogeneic bone marrow transplantation. Chest
1993;104(1):114–8.

[86] Whitford H, Walters EH, Levvey B, et al. Addition of inhaled corticosteroids to systemic immunosuppression after lung transplantation: a double-blind, placebo-controlled trial. Transplantation 2002;73(11): 1793–9.

[87] Boas SR, Noyes BE, Kurland G, et al. Pediatric lung transplantation for graft-versus-host disease following bone marrow transplantation. Chest 1994;105(5): 1584–6.

[88] Favaloro R, Bertolotti A, Gomez C, et al. Lung transplant at the Favaloro Foundation: a 13-year experience. Transplant Proc 2004;36(6):1689–91.

[89] Pechet TV, de le Morena M, Mendeloff EN, et al. Lung transplantation in children following treatment for malignancy. J Heart Lung Transplant 2003;22(2): 154–60.

[90] Rabitsch W, Deviatko E, Keil F, et al. Successful lung transplantation for bronchiolitis obliterans after allogeneic marrow transplantation. Transplantation 2001; 71(9):1341–3.

[91] Paz HL, Crilley P, Topolsky DL, et al. Bronchiolitis obliterans after bone marrow transplantation: the effect of preconditioning. Respiration (Herrlisheim) 1993;60(2):109–14.

[92] Epler GR, Colby TV, McLoud TC, et al. Bronchiolitis obliterans organizing pneumonia. N Engl J Med 1985;312(3):152–8.

[93] Epler GR. Bronchiolitis obliterans organizing pneumonia. Arch Intern Med 2001;161(2):158–64.

[94] Thirman MJ, Devine SM, O'Toole K, et al. Bronchiolitis obliterans organizing pneumonia as a complication of allogeneic bone marrow transplantation [see comments]. Bone Marrow Transplant 1992; 10(3):307–11.

[95] Mathew P, Bozeman P, Krance RA, et al. Bronchiolitis obliterans organizing pneumonia (BOOP) in children after allogeneic bone marrow transplantation. Bone Marrow Transplant 1994;13(2):221–3.

[96] Alasaly K, Muller N, Ostrow DN, et al. Cryptogenic organizing pneumonia. A report of 25 cases and a review of the literature. Medicine (Baltimore) 1995; 74(4):201–11.

[97] Hayes-Jordan A, Benaim E, Richardson S, et al. Open lung biopsy in pediatric bone marrow transplant patients. J Pediatr Surg 2002;37(3):446–52.

[98] Ishii T, Manabe A, Ebihara Y, et al. Improvement in bronchiolitis obliterans organizing pneumonia in a child after allogeneic bone marrow transplantation by a combination of oral prednisolone and low dose erythromycin. Bone Marrow Transplant 2000; 26(8):907–10.

[99] Kanamori H, Fujisawa S, Tsuburai T, et al. Increased exhaled nitric oxide in bronchiolitis obliterans organizing pneumonia after allogeneic bone marrow transplantation. Transplantation 2002;74(9): 1356–8.

[100] Kanda Y, Takahashi T, Imai Y, et al. Bronchiolitis obliterans organizing pneumonia after syngeneic bone marrow transplantation for acute lymphoblastic leukemia. Bone Marrow Transplant 1997;19(12): 1251–3.

[101] Kleinau I, Perez-Canto A, Schmid HJ, et al. Bronchiolitis obliterans organizing pneumonia and chronic graft-versus-host disease in a child after allogeneic bone marrow transplantation. Bone Marrow Transplant 1997;19(8):841–4.

[102] Przepiorka D, Abu-Elmagd K, Huaringa A, et al. Bronchiolitis obliterans organizing pneumonia in a BMT patient receiving FK506 [letter; comment]. Bone Marrow Transplant 1993;11(6):502.

[103] Yata K, Nakajima M, Takemoto Y, et al. [Pneumonitis with a bronchiolitis obliterans organizing pneumonia-like shadow in a patient with human herpes virus-6 viremia after allogeneic bone marrow transplantation]. Kansenshogaku Zasshi 2002;76(5): 385–90 [in Japanese].

[104] Baron FA, Hermanne JP, Dowlati A, et al. Bronchiolitis obliterans organizing pneumonia and ulcerative colitis after allogeneic bone marrow transplantation. Bone Marrow Transplant 1998;21(9):951–4.

[105] Epler GR. Bronchiolitis obliterans organizing pneumonia. Semin Respir Infect 1995;10(2):65–77.

[106] Muller NL, Staples CA, Miller RR. Bronchiolitis obliterans organizing pneumonia: CT features in 14 patients. AJR Am J Roentgenol 1990;154(5):983–7.

[107] Worthy SA, Flint JD, Muller NL. Pulmonary complications after bone marrow transplantation: high-resolution CT and pathologic findings. Radiographics 1997;17(6):1359–71.

[108] Graham NJ, Muller NL, Miller RR, et al. Intrathoracic complications following allogeneic bone marrow transplantation: CT findings. Radiology 1991; 181(1):153–6.

[109] Cordier JF. Organising pneumonia. Thorax 2000; 55(4):318–28.

[110] Abratt RP, Morgan GW, Silvestri G, et al. Pulmonary complications of radiation therapy. Clin Chest Med 2004;25(1):167–77.

[111] Limper AH. Chemotherapy-induced lung disease. Clin Chest Med 2004;25(1):53–64.

[112] Pedrazzoli P, Ferrante P, Kulekci A, et al. Autologous hematopoietic stem cell transplantation for breast cancer in Europe: critical evaluation of data from the European Group for Blood and Marrow Transplantation (EBMT) Registry 1990–1999. Bone Marrow Transplant 2003;32(5):489–94.

[113] Bearman SI, Overmoyer BA, Bolwell BJ, et al. High-dose chemotherapy with autologous peripheral blood progenitor cell support for primary breast cancer in patients with 4–9 involved axillary lymph nodes. Bone Marrow Transplant 1997;20(11):931–7.

[114] Bhalla KS, Wilczynski SW, Abushamaa AM, et al. Pulmonary toxicity of induction chemotherapy prior to standard or high-dose chemotherapy with autologous hematopoietic support. Am J Respir Crit Care Med 2000;161(1):17–25.

[115] Chap L, Shpiner R, Levine M, et al. Pulmonary toxicity of high-dose chemotherapy for breast can-

cer: a non-invasive approach to diagnosis and treatment. Bone Marrow Transplant 1997;20(12):1063–7.

[116] Fanfulla F, Pedrazzoli P, Da Prada GA, et al. Pulmonary function and complications following chemotherapy and stem cell support in breast cancer. Eur Respir J 2000;15(1):56–61.

[117] Jones RB, Matthes S, Shpall EJ, et al. Acute lung injury following treatment with high-dose cyclophosphamide, cisplatin, and carmustine: pharmacodynamic evaluation of carmustine. J Natl Cancer Inst 1993;85(8):640–7.

[118] Todd NW, Peters WP, Ost AH, et al. Pulmonary drug toxicity in patients with primary breast cancer treated with high-dose combination chemotherapy and autologous bone marrow transplantation. Am Rev Respir Dis 1993;147(5):1264–70.

[119] Wilczynski SW, Erasmus JJ, Petros WP, et al. Delayed pulmonary toxicity syndrome following high-dose chemotherapy and bone marrow transplantation for breast cancer. Am J Respir Crit Care Med 1998;157(2):565–73.

[120] Wong R, Rondon G, Saliba RM, et al. Idiopathic pneumonia syndrome after high-dose chemotherapy and autologous hematopoietic stem cell transplantation for high-risk breast cancer. Bone Marrow Transplant 2003;31(12):1157–63.

[121] Cao TM, Negrin RS, Stockerl-Goldstein KE, et al. Pulmonary toxicity syndrome in breast cancer patients undergoing BCNU-containing high-dose chemotherapy and autologous hematopoietic cell transplantation. Biol Blood Marrow Transplant 2000; 6(4):387–94.

[122] Peters WP, Ross M, Vredenburgh JJ, et al. High-dose chemotherapy and autologous bone marrow support as consolidation after standard-dose adjuvant therapy for high-risk primary breast cancer. J Clin Oncol 1993;11(6):1132–43.

[123] Stadtmauer EA, O'Neill A, Goldstein LJ, et al. Conventional-dose chemotherapy compared with high-dose chemotherapy plus autologous hematopoietic stem-cell transplantation for metastatic breast cancer. Philadelphia Bone Marrow Transplant Group. N Engl J Med 2000;342(15):1069–76.

[124] Suratt BT, Lynch DA, Cool CD, et al. Interferon-gamma for delayed pulmonary toxicity syndrome resistant to steroids. Bone Marrow Transplant 2003; 31(10):939–41.

[125] McGaughey DS, Nikcevich DA, Long GD, et al. Inhaled steroids as prophylaxis for delayed pulmonary toxicity syndrome in breast cancer patients undergoing high-dose chemotherapy and autologous stem cell transplantation. Biol Blood Marrow Transplant 2001;7(5):274–8.

[126] Castellano-Sanchez AA, Poppiti RJ. Pulmonary cytolytic thrombi (PCT). A previously unrecognized complication of bone marrow transplantation (BMT). Am J Surg Pathol 2001;25(6):829–31.

[127] Gulbahce HE, Pambuccian SE, Jessurun J, et al. Pulmonary nodular lesions in bone marrow transplant recipients: impact of histologic diagnosis on patient management and prognosis. Am J Clin Pathol 2004;121(2):205–10.

[128] Morales IJ, Anderson PM, Tazelaar HD, et al. Pulmonary cytolytic thrombi: unusual complication of hematopoietic stem cell transplantation. J Pediatr Hematol Oncol 2003;25(1):89–92.

[129] Gulbahce HE, Manivel JC, Jessurun J. Pulmonary cytolytic thrombi: a previously unrecognized complication of bone marrow transplantation. Am J Surg Pathol 2000;24(8):1147–52.

[130] Woodard JP, Gulbahce E, Shreve M, et al. Pulmonary cytolytic thrombi: a newly recognized complication of stem cell transplantation. Bone Marrow Transplant 2000;25(3):293–300.

[131] Wingard JR, Mellits ED, Jones RJ, et al. Association of hepatic veno-occlusive disease with interstitial pneumonitis in bone marrow transplant recipients. Bone Marrow Transplant 1989;4(6):685–9.

[132] Sharma S, Nadrous HF, Peters SG, et al. Pulmonary complications in adult blood and marrow transplant recipients: autopsy findings. Chest, in press.

[133] Hackman RC, Madtes DK, Petersen FB, et al. Pulmonary venoocclusive disease following bone marrow transplantation. Transplantation 1989;47(6):989–92.

[134] Kuga T, Kohda K, Hirayama Y, et al. Pulmonary veno-occlusive disease accompanied by microangiopathic hemolytic anemia 1 year after a second bone marrow transplantation for acute lymphoblastic leukemia. Int J Hematol 1996;64(2):143–50.

[135] Salzman D, Adkins DR, Craig F, et al. Malignancy-associated pulmonary veno-occlusive disease: report of a case following autologous bone marrow transplantation and review. Bone Marrow Transplant 1996; 18(4):755–60.

[136] Seguchi M, Hirabayashi N, Fujii Y, et al. Pulmonary hypertension associated with pulmonary occlusive vasculopathy after allogeneic bone marrow transplantation. Transplantation 2000;69(1):177–9.

[137] Trobaugh-Lotrario AD, Greffe B, Deterding R, et al. Pulmonary veno-occlusive disease after autologous bone marrow transplant in a child with stage IV neuroblastoma: case report and literature review. J Pediatr Hematol Oncol 2003;25(5):405–9.

[138] Troussard X, Bernaudin JF, Cordonnier C, et al. Pulmonary veno-occlusive disease after bone marrow transplantation. Thorax 1984;39(12):956–7.

[139] Williams LM, Fussell S, Veith RW, et al. Pulmonary veno-occlusive disease in an adult following bone marrow transplantation. Case report and review of the literature. Chest 1996;109(5):1388–91.

[140] Kotloff RM, Ahya VN, Crawford SW. Pulmonary complications of solid organ and hematopoietic stem cell transplantation. Am J Respir Crit Care Med 2004;170(1):22–48.

[141] Kramer MR, Estenne M, Berkman N, et al. Radiation-induced pulmonary veno-occlusive disease. Chest 1993;104(4):1282–4.

[142] Mandel J, Mark EJ, Hales CA. Pulmonary veno-

occlusive disease. Am J Respir Crit Care Med 2000; 162(5):1964–73.

[143] Doll DC, Yarbro JW. Vascular toxicity associated with antineoplastic agents. Semin Oncol 1992;19(5): 580–96.

[144] Doll DC, Yarbro JW. Vascular toxicity associated with chemotherapy and hormonotherapy. Curr Opin Oncol 1994;6(4):345–50.

[145] Gagnadoux F, Capron F, Lebeau B. Pulmonary veno-occlusive disease after neoadjuvant mitomycin chemotherapy and surgery for lung carcinoma. Lung Cancer 2002;36(2):213–5.

[146] Elliott CG, Colby TV, Hill T, et al. Pulmonary veno-occlusive disease associated with severe reduction of single-breath carbon monoxide diffusing capacity. Respiration (Herrlisheim) 1988;53(4):262–6.

[147] Wagenvoort CA, Wagenvoort N, Takahashi T. Pulmonary veno-occlusive disease: involvement of pulmonary arteries and review of the literature. Hum Pathol 1985;16(10):1033–41.

[148] Palmer SM, Robinson LJ, Wang A, et al. Massive pulmonary edema and death after prostacyclin infusion in a patient with pulmonary veno-occlusive disease. Chest 1998;113(1):237–40.

[149] Shankar S, Choi JK, Dermody TS, et al. Pulmonary hypertension complicating bone marrow transplantation for idiopathic myelofibrosis. J Pediatr Hematol Oncol 2004;26(6):393–7.

[150] Vaksmann G, Nelken B, Deshildre A, et al. Pulmonary arterial occlusive disease following chemotherapy and bone marrow transplantation for leukaemia. Eur J Pediatr 2002;161(5):247–9.

[151] Bruckmann C, Lindner W, Roos R, et al. Severe pulmonary vascular occlusive disease following bone marrow transplantation in Omenn syndrome. Eur J Pediatr 1991;150(4):242–5.

[152] Presneill JJ, Nakata K, Inoue Y, et al. Pulmonary alveolar proteinosis. Clin Chest Med 2004;25(3): 593–613 [viii.].

[153] Cordonnier C, Fleury-Feith J, Escudier E, et al. Secondary alveolar proteinosis is a reversible cause of respiratory failure in leukemic patients. Am J Respir Crit Care Med 1994;149(3 Pt 1):788–94.

[154] Gross TG, Hoge FJ, Jackson JD, et al. Fatal eosinophilic disease following autologous bone marrow transplantation. Bone Marrow Transplant 1994;14(2): 333–7.

[155] Brunet S, Muniz-Diaz E, Baiget M. [Chronic eosinophilic pneumonia in a patient treated with allogeneic bone marrow transplantation]. Med Clin (Barc) 1994; 103(17):677 [in Spanish].

[156] Richard C, Calavia J, Loyola I, et al. [Chronic eosinophilic pneumonia in a patient treated with allogenic bone marrow transplantation]. Med Clin (Barc) 1994; 102(12):462–4 [in Spanish].

ELSEVIER
SAUNDERS

Clin Chest Med 26 (2005) 587–597

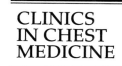

CLINICS
IN CHEST
MEDICINE

Hepatopulmonary Syndrome and Portopulmonary Hypertension: Implications for Liver Transplantation

Michael J. Krowka, MD

*Divisions of Pulmonary & Critical Care Medicine and Gastroenterology & Hepatology, Mayo Clinic College of Medicine,
200 First Street SW, Rochester, MN 55905, USA*

The success of orthotopic liver transplantation (OLT) has heightened the awareness of the two major pulmonary vascular complications of advanced liver disease, namely, hepatopulmonary syndrome (HPS) and portopulmonary hypertension (POPH) [1,2]. Survival after OLT is affected by the presence before pretransplantation of either of these distinct syndromes [2–4]. Hence, it is important to understand current diagnostic criteria, optimal screening approaches, natural history, special pretransplantation considerations, and perioperative management issues and dilemmas for the patients meeting listing criteria for liver transplantation from cadaveric or living donor sources. Key reviews are documented to guide the reader to references published before 2000. This update reflects the significant initial OLT-related contributions and emphasizes published data spanning the last 5 years.

Hepatopulmonary syndrome

Clinical presentation

HPS is characterized by the triad of liver disease complicated by arterial hypoxemia caused by pulmonary vascular dilatations [1,2]. Although arterial hypoxemia is relatively common in the setting of advanced liver disease, the frequency of hypoxemia caused by HPS is low, ranging from 5% to 20% depending upon which diagnostic criteria for hypox-

emia have been followed [2]. Severe hypoxemia should strongly suggest the existence of HPS in both the pediatric and adult age groups. No particular relationship exists between HPS and the primary cause of liver disease. Disagreement exists whether HPS is related to the severity of liver dysfunction. Although most commonly associated with hepatic cirrhosis and portal hypertension, HPS in the setting of noncirrhotic portal hypertension is well documented.

Diagnostic criteria

HPS diagnostic criteria have evolved as investigators have struggled with both the appropriate cutoff values to define hypoxemia and methods to document the presence of pulmonary vascular dilatations [2,5,6]. A recent international effort initiated by the European Respiratory Society and European Association for the Study of Liver Disease brought pulmonologists, hepatologists, anesthesiologists, and liver transplant surgeons together to address the pulmonary vascular syndromes that complicate liver disease [2]. To facilitate basic science and clinical investigation, that group put forth a working consensus of specific diagnostic criteria for HPS (Box 1). In the setting of advanced liver disease, the patient must have hypoxemia caused by pulmonary vascular dilatations as documented by either contrast-enhanced (CE) transthoracic echocardiography or brain uptake after technetium-99m macroaggregated albumen ($^{99m\text{Tc}}$MAA) lung perfusion scanning [2,7]. The exact criteria used for the determination of hypoxemia caused by HPS is an interesting issue and

E-mail address: krowka@mayo.edu

Box 1. Diagnostic criteria for
hepatopulmonary syndrome

1. Portal hypertension with or without
   cirrhotic liver disease
2. Arterial hypoxemia
      Alveolar-arterial oxygen gradient
      less than 15 mm Hg
3. Pulmonary vascular dilatation demonstrated by
      Delayed "positive" CE trans-
         thoracic echocardiography or
      Abnormal brain uptake (>6%)
         after ^{99mTc}MAA lung perfu-
         sion scanning

has raised at least three concerns [2,6]. First, what is considered an abnormal PaO_2? Second, what threshold should be used to define an increased alveolar-arterial oxygen gradient? Third, how can adjustments be made for altitude effects on oxygenation at the point of testing? These issues have been addressed recently by several authors and merit further study.

The methods used to detect pulmonary vascular dilatation are twofold: CE echocardiography and ^{99mTc}MAA brain uptake. The technical aspects of these diagnostic studies are summarized in the European Respiratory Society Task Force Report [2]. CE echocardiography involves the peripheral intravenous administration of hand-agitated saline (using a three-way stop cock). Because the normal capillary diameter is only about 8 microns, and the microbubbles average 10 to 20 microns in diameter, first-pass clearance (absorption within alveoli) of all microbubbles occurs in normal individuals. In contradistinction, the diffuse dilatations or discrete arteriovenous dilatations and communications of HPS allow passage of such microbubbles through the pulmonary circulation. CE echocardiography suggests pulmonary vascular dilatation if left atrial microbubble opacification occurs within three to six cardiac cycles after the visualization of microbubbles in the right heart. Appearance of microbubbles in the left atrium within three cardiac cycles suggests a right-to-left intracardiac shunt. The use of transesophageal echocardiography can distinguish further between intracardiac and intrapulmonary shunting by the direct visualization of microbubbles entering the left atrium from any of the pulmonary veins [2].

Use of radionuclide perfusion lung scanning, with demonstration of abnormal uptake over the brain after

a peripheral injection of ^{99mTc}MAA, follows the same logic. These aggregates are anywhere from 20 to 90 microns in size and will not traverse the normal pulmonary vascular bed but are permitted to enter the systemic circulation in the presence of dilated pulmonary vascular channels. Unlike CE and transesophageal echocardiography, the ^{99mTc}MAA method provides no clues to permit distinction between an intracardiac versus an intrapulmonary right-to-left shunt. CE echocardiography is more sensitive than ^{99mTc}MAA in detecting vascular dilatation within the lung, and, frequently, a weakly positive CE echo in patients who have advanced liver disease is reported in association with normal arterial oxygenation (ie, normal PaO_2 and alveolar-arterial oxygen gradient) [2,7]. The clinical importance of that finding remains to be determined, but preliminary data suggest that approximately 30% of patients develop hypoxemia ($PaO_2 < 70$ mm Hg) with 24 months (K.L. Swanson, Mayo Clinic, personal communication, 2005).

Pulmonary angiography as a means to demonstrate pulmonary vascular dilatations is advised only in the setting of severe hypoxemia if discrete arteriovenous communications are suspected by chest CT imaging and if poor response to inspired 100% oxygen ($PaO_2 < 300$ mm Hg) exists. The purpose of angiography in such rare patients is to conduct coil embolotherapy to obliterate discrete lesions and improve hypoxemia [7].

Screening

Pulse oximetry is a logical screening assessment for hypoxemia in the setting of liver disease [2,5]. Arterial blood gas measurement, however, remains the appropriate test of choice to establish the HPS diagnosis. Comparisons between pulse oximetry and hemoglobin saturations determined by arterial blood gases have shown that the former frequently exceeds the latter by an average of 4% [5]. Radial artery puncture, as well as cannulation, can be conducted safely in most patients despite the tendency of coagulopathy and thrombocytopenia to complicate liver disease [7].

There seems to be no consistent relationship between the severity of liver disease and the degree of arterial hypoxemia caused by HPS. It is important to note that 20% to 30% of patients who have HPS have additional pulmonary abnormalities that might affect oxygenation [7–9]. In those patients the use of ^{99mTc}MAA lung perfusion scans with brain uptake can clarify the contribution of pulmonary vascular dilatation to the finding of hypoxemia when patients present with chronic obstructive pulmonary disease, asthma, hepatic hydrothorax, and lung fibrosis [2,7].

Natural history

The 5-year survival of patients who have HPS in the absence of OLT is approximately 20% [2,8]. Causes of death usually are related to complications of liver disease and to comorbidities such as coronary disease, renal dysfunction, and neoplasm, as opposed to simply progressive hypoxemia. Nonetheless, the severity of hypoxemia documented by arterial blood gas predicts long-term survival, with significantly poorer survival associated with a room air PO_2 of less than 50 to 60 mm Hg [8].

Pathophysiology

The precise pathophysiology of HPS remains speculative. Aside from possible genetic predisposition, the vasodilating effects of nitric oxide and the role of an imbalance between pulmonary vascular endothelin receptors for vasoconstriction and vasodilatation are current areas of investigation [10,11]. The role of bacterial translocation and treatment with antibiotics is of recent interest [2].

Treatment and monitoring before transplantation

No pharmacologic therapy has been documented to improve the hypoxemia associated with HPS consistently [2]. Administration of supplemental oxygen can ameliorate some of the symptoms of hypoxemia. Such oxygen therapy should be considered during sleep and with any type of exercise. The beneficial effect of arterial hypoxemia on hepatic function seems logical but is unproven at this time. The provision of oxygen should include assessment of requirements at rest, exercise, and sleep.

Arterial oxygenation can decline in patients awaiting OLT. Limited experience suggests a mean decline of approximately 5 mm Hg/12 months in patients awaiting OLT; no correlation with hepatic change could be found (Fig. 1) [8].

Special considerations before transplantation

The priority assigned a candidate for OLT is influenced by the degree of arterial hypoxemia associated with HPS. At this time, priority for OLT is

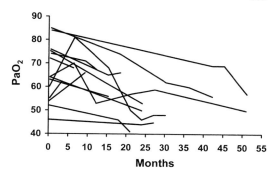

Fig. 1. Change in PaO_2 values in patients awaiting OLT (N = 14). (*From* Swanson KL, Wiesner RH, Krowka MJ. Natural history of hepatopulmonary syndrome: impact of liver transplantation. Hepatology 2005;41:1122–9; with permission.)

based on a numerical score derived from three variables (total bilirubin, serum creatinine, and international normalized ratio) as determined using the Model for End Stage Liver Disease (MELD) score [12]. The United Network for Organ Sharing, the organization that controls allocation of organs in the United States, has approved a nationwide policy by which the MELD score for a liver transplant candidate can be increased if, because of HPS, the resting PaO_2 is less than 60 mm Hg in the sitting position, thus increasing the patient's priority for OLT. The magnitude of increase varies from region to region. Even with the extensive liver transplantation experience that has evolved, approximately 20% of patients who have HPS have been denied liver transplantation because of comorbidities such as cardiac disease, age, neoplasms, and coexistence of pulmonary problems for which hypoxemia (nonvascular in origin) is not expected to improve after transplantation [4].

Factors existing before transplantation that are predictive of an increased risk of death after OLT in patients who have HPS have been identified. A retrospective study of 81 patients who had HPS reported 30% mortality within 90 days of OLT for patients who had a pretransplantation room air PaO_2 less than 50 mm Hg [13]. A recent prospective study of 24 patients who had HPS found that the combination of room air PaO_2 of 50 mm Hg or less and brain uptake of 20% or less on ^{99mTc}MAA lung perfusion scanning had a 75% positive predictive value and a 94% negative predictive value for mortality after OLT [14]. The PaO_2 response to 100% inspired oxygen does not seem to be an independent factor to predict risk for OLT [7].

Intraoperative concerns

No intraoperative deaths directly attributable to HPS have been reported in the three largest published series describing post-OLT outcomes among 136 patients who had HPS [4,13,15]. Immediate post-OLT oxygenation may worsen acutely because of superimposed problems with volume overload, noncardiogenic pulmonary edema, and infection. Prolonged mechanical ventilatory support and extended stays in the ICU may be necessary [3,13]. The use of inhaled nitric oxide, intravenous methylene blue, and Trendelenberg's positioning have been documented in single case reports as successfully improving arterial oxygenation in the period immediately after transplantation [16–19].

Clinical course and survival after orthotopic liver transplantation

Beginning with the landmark observation in 1990 [20], numerous case reports and small series detailing outcomes after OLT for patients who had HPS have been published and reviewed in recent publications [13,21–24]. Resolution of HPS is expected after OLT, although it may take several months for the normalization of arterial oxygenation, lung perfusion and brain scan imaging, and CE echocardiography [2,3]. Improvement in oxygenation precedes changes in the imaging modalities. Only one case of recurrent HPS after successful OLT has been reported. This case was attributable to the development of cirrhosis and portal hypertension after recurrence of nonalcoholic steatohepatitis 18 months after transplantation [25].

Despite overall success, in-hospital mortality after OLT remains significant. Combining the largest literature review to date and experiences from Japan and France, a 12-month post-OLT mortality in the range of 16% to 38% has been documented [8,13, 15,23]. Causes of death usually were multifactorial, with infection and sepsis representing the main causes; refractory hypoxemia per se was not a primary cause of death in most cases. Outcomes associated with the use of living-donor livers seem to be similar to those associated with cadaveric livers [23,26].

Information on long-term survival after OLT in the setting of HPS has been reported in a case-control study of 61 patients from the Mayo Clinic in which 24 patients underwent OLT and 37 patients had usual medical care (Fig. 2) [8]. Several points can be drawn from that experience. First, the 5-year survival of patients who had HPS and who underwent OLT was

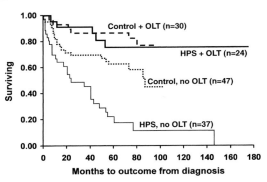

Fig. 2. Survival in 61 Mayo Clinic patients who had HPS. Survival curves from the time of HPS diagnosis or time from PaO_2 determination in age- and disease severity–matched controls are shown. Survival was significantly better in patients who had HPS and who received OLT than in patients who had HPS and did not receive OLT ($P < .001$). Survival in patients who had HPS and did not receive OLT was significantly worse than in controls ($P < .001$). No difference in the severity of hypoxemia was noted at baseline within the HPS subgroups. (*From* Swanson KL, Wiesner RH, Krowka MJ. Natural history of hepatopulmonary syndrome: impact of liver transplantation. Hepatology 2005; 41:1122–9; with permission.)

similar to that of patients undergoing transplantation who did not have HPS, with a 5-year survival of approximately 76%. Second, the long-term survival of patients who had HPS and who did not undergo OLT was only 23%, far inferior to the survival rate achieved after OLT (although one cannot assume that the groups were comparable with respect to severity of illness). Third, the 5-year post-OLT survival of patients who had HPS and who had severe hypoxemia at presentation ($PaO_2 < 50$ mm Hg) was only 55%. Such data bolster the argument that, to optimize outcomes, a higher priority for OLT should be given to patients who have HPS before they develop severe hypoxemia. Fourth, survival both with and without OLT was associated with the baseline room air PaO_2 (Fig. 3).

In short, many clinicians in the transplant community believe that, for both the pediatric and adult age groups, the presence of HPS should be an indication to proceed to OLT as a definitive therapy for the advanced liver disease and hypoxemia caused by HPS. It has been proposed that priority should be given to patients who have HPS and who have PaO_2 less than 60 mm Hg. The degree of OLT priority that should be given to such patients who have HPS and who otherwise are acceptable candidates for OLT remains a debatable issue. The dual observations that even severe hypoxemia associated with HPS resolves

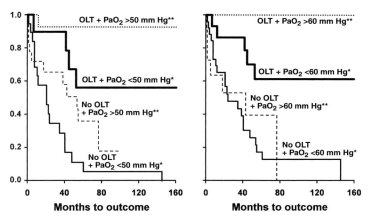

Fig. 3. Survival associated with HPS based on baseline PaO_2 cutoffs of 50 mm Hg and 60 mm Hg. Regardless of whether OLT was accomplished, patients who had HPS and had $PaO_2 < 50$ or 60 mm Hg at baseline had worse survival ($P < .001$). (*From* Swanson KL, Wiesner RH, Krowka MJ. Natural history of hepatopulmonary syndrome: impact of liver transplantation. Hepatology 2005;41:1122–9; with permission.)

after OLT and that long-term survival is attainable are major contributions to the field of liver transplantation.

Finally, although HPS may completely resolve after successful OLT, the development of pulmonary hypertension months to years later has been observed [27–29]. It has been hypothesized that pulmonary vascular dilation and pulmonary vascular obstruction might coexist (having evolved in different time periods). The clinical and hemodynamic picture of pulmonary hypertension appears after OLT and elimination of factors causing pulmonary vascular dilatation.

Portopulmonary hypertension

Definition and clinical presentation

POPH is characterized by the development of pulmonary arterial hypertension in association with portal hypertension, with or without hepatic disease [2]. Although POPH is uncommon (4%–17% frequency noted at major liver transplant centers), the clinical implications are significant [1,2].

POPH can produce many nonspecific symptoms: exertional dyspnea, dyspnea at rest, chest pain, chest pressure, palpitations, and near-syncope or syncope [1,2]. Abnormalities found on physical examination include an accentuated and split second heart sound, right ventricular heave, right-sided S3 gallop, neck vein distention, ascites, and lower leg edema [2]. Physical signs may be absent in mild POPH, except for what appears to be a hyperdynamic circulatory state.

On the other hand, severe POPH may mimic advanced liver disease, with ascites and lower extremity edema. Hence, to make the diagnosis of POPH a high degree of clinical suspicion must exist, and appropriate screening and diagnostic studies should follow.

Diagnostic criteria

The diagnosis of POPH rests on pulmonary hemodynamic measurements and calculations determined by right heart catheterization [1,2]. Transthoracic Doppler echocardiography is a reasonable screening tool (as discussed later), but abnormalities involving the right heart and estimated pulmonary artery pressures are neither sufficient nor accurate to make this diagnosis [30,31]. A key feature of POPH is the obstruction to pulmonary artery flow caused by vasoconstriction, proliferation of the endothelium and smooth muscle constituents of the vascular wall, and in situ thrombosis. Hence, an increase in calculated pulmonary vascular resistance (PVR) is necessary as part of the definition [2].

Box 2. Diagnostic criteria for portopulmonary hypertension

1. Presence of portal hypertension (clinical diagnosis)
2. MPAP greater than 25 mm Hg
3. PAOP less than 15 mm Hg
4. PVR greater than 240 dyne/sec/cm^{-5}

Table 1
Mayo Clinic classification of pulmonary hypertension in the setting of portal hypertension

	Type	MPAP	PAOP	CO	PVR
I.	Pulmonary artery high-flow state	↑	n or ↓	↑↑	↓
II.	Excess pulmonary venous volume	↑	↑	↑	↓
III.	Portopulmonary hypertension				
	a) pulmonary vascular obstruction; normal volume	↑↑↑	n or ↓	↑	↑↑↑
	b) pulmonary vascular obstruction; excess volume	↑↑	↑	↑	↑

Based upon right heart catheterization measurements (MPAP, CO, PAOP) and calculations (PVR).
Abbreviations: CO, cardiac output; MPAP, mean pulmonary artery pressure; PAOP, pulmonary artery occlusion pressure; PVR, pulmonary vascular resistance.

The diagnostic criteria for POPH are summarized in Box 2: (1) increased mean pulmonary artery pressure (MPAP); (2) increased PVR; and (3) normal pulmonary artery occlusion pressure (PAOP). The hyperdynamic (high-flow) circulatory state associated with advanced liver disease may lead to an increased pulmonary artery systolic pressure by Doppler echocardiography and elevated MPAP by right heart catheterization, in the absence of intrinsic pulmonary vascular disease. The key finding in this situation is a normal calculated PVR [2]. Likewise, increased central volume, as reflected by an increased PAOP, can result in an increase in MPAP, but PVR should be normal. Such scenarios are summarized in Table 1. On the other hand, a marked increase in volume, left heart dysfunction, or the concomitant existence of true POPH with excess volume may confound interpretation of hemodynamic patterns. The presence of an increase in the transpulmonary gradient (MPAP − PAOP > 10 mm Hg) suggests an increased resistance to pulmonary flow and merits close follow-up.

The cutoff of abnormal PVR associated with POPH has evolved over time. Initially, many investigators used the value greater than 120 dyne/sec/cm^{-5}; recently that cutoff has been raised to more than 240 dyne/sec/cm^{-5}. There is little disagreement that a value greater than 240 dyne/sec/cm^{-5} is abnormal; monitoring patients who have a PVR in the range of 120 to 240 dyne/sec/cm^{-5} is advised, because the severity of POPH can evolve over several months [2].

Screening

Transthoracic Doppler echocardiography is the screening procedure of choice for POPH [30,31]. By measuring the tricuspid systolic peak velocity (TR) and using a modified Bernoulli equation, a pressure gradient between the right atrium and ventricle can be determined. With an echo estimate of the size of the inferior vena cava, a pressure estimate of the right atrium is selected, and the right ventricular systolic pressure (RVsys) is reported:

$$\Delta \text{ gradient} = 4 \times \left(\text{TR peak velocity}^2 \right)$$

$$\text{RVsys} = \text{RA pressure} + \Delta \text{ gradient}$$

For example, a TR of 4.0 m/sec (normal usually < 2.5) and a right atrium estimate of 14 mm based upon a distended inferior vena cava results in an abnormal RVsys of 78 mm Hg (normal may be center specific but should be 30–35 mm Hg maximum). The estimated RVsys, in turn, accurately mirrors the pulmonary artery systolic pressure in the absence of pulmonic valve abnormalities. Qualitative assessment of right ventricular size and function can be made even if the TR cannot be measured, as happens in 10% to 20% of cases.

The Mayo Clinic experience with Doppler echocardiography as a screening tool for POPH suggests that an estimated RVsys pressure (ie, pulmonary artery systolic pressure) in excess of 50 mm should prompt performance of a right heart catheterization. Based on 958 patients screened (100 had RVsys > 50 mm Hg), the author and colleagues found that 86% of patients exceeding this echo pressure estimate had a PVR greater than 120 dyne/sec/cm^{-5}, and 64% had a PVR greater than 240 dyne/sec/cm^{-5} on subsequent catheterization. Cotton and colleagues [31] from the University of Chicago found that an estimated pulmonary artery pressure of greater than 50 mm by echocardiography had a positive predictive value of 38% and a negative predictive value of 92% in detecting pulmonary hypertension of this magnitude by catheterization. Thus, an estimated RVsys pressure (pulmonary artery systolic pressure) greater than 50 mm Hg by echocardiography seems to be the optimal cutoff for subjecting patients to right heart catheterization, although this finding may be center specific.

Chest radiographs and ECG are poor screening methods for POPH. Abnormalities in the chest ra-

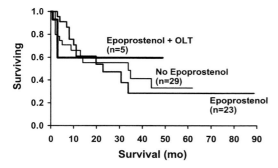

Fig. 4. Survival in 57 Mayo Clinic patients who had POPH, with and without the use of intravenous epoprostenol (P = not significant). Severity of POPH was similar in the subgroups. Patients who underwent OLT had a nonsignificant trend toward better survival.

diograph (enlarged central pulmonary arteries, cardiomegaly) and ECG (right axis, right bundle branch block, t-wave inversion in the anterior leads) are late findings that suggest the existence of significant and quite possibly severe pulmonary artery hypertension [32]. Measurement of plasma B-type natriuretic peptide levels, which may reflect right ventricular stress and strain caused by pressure and volume overload, seems to be a reasonable surrogate marker of the degree of pulmonary hemodynamic abnormality in idiopathic pulmonary artery hypertension [33], but currently there are no data to suggest a screening role for plasma B-type natriuretic peptide in POPH.

Natural history

In the pre–liver transplant era, the median and mean survival times of patients who had POPH were 6 and 15 months, respectively. Death within 12 months of diagnosis was the expectation [34]. With the advent of better patient selection for OLT, prostacyclins (epoprostenol, treprostinil, and iloprost), endothelin antagonists, and phosphodiesterase inhibitors, it is hoped that the natural history will be modified [2]. Although no large series have been published to date, preliminary data from the Mayo Clinic suggest a 5-year survival of 30% regardless of whether a prostacyclin is used (Fig. 4) [35]. Causes of mortality seemed to be distributed equally between right heart failure and consequences of advanced liver disease.

Pathophysiology

Specific mediators responsible for the development of POPH have not been identified, but ge-

netic susceptibility and elevated circulating levels of endothelin-1 seem to be associated with the presence of POPH [2,36]. Despite pathologic similarities between POPH and idiopathic pulmonary arterial hypertension, the hemodynamic profile is distinctive because of the splanchnic vasodilatation and high cardiac output that can occur in POPH despite marked increases in pulmonary resistance [1,2].

Pretransplantation issues

Three practical concerns related to liver transplant candidacy exist when the diagnosis of POPH has been established. First, does the degree of pulmonary hemodynamic severity warrant therapy before OLT is attempted? Second, what therapy should be selected? Third, what pulmonary hemodynamic goals will facilitate safe OLT (Fig. 5)? Limited data suggest an increased risk of death after OLT in patients who have POPH if the MPAP exceeds 35 mm Hg; therefore, it seems prudent to consider that value as an indication for vasomodulating therapy before OLT [37–39]. This recommendation parallels the value commonly cited for starting therapy in patients who have idiopathic pulmonary arterial hypertension.

No studies have addressed the question of which medications are most efficacious and safe in patients who have POPH. To date, the greatest experience is with intravenous epoprostenol, although a concern regarding the development of progressive thrombocytopenia with splenomegaly (out of proportion to liver disease) has been posed [2,40–44]. Other prostacyclin analogues, bosentan, and sildenafil have shown promise in the setting of POPH [45–48]. A preference for a particular drug or combination of drugs depends upon investigator experience, drug availability, and safety considerations, but clinical trials are needed before definitive recommendations can be made.

Retrospective analyses suggest that successful reduction in MPAP to below 35 mm Hg and in PVR below 250 dyne/sec/cm^{-5} minimize the post-OLT risk for mortality and therefore define a suitable candidate for OLT [39]. Patients receiving vasomodulating therapy who continue to have a MPAP between 35 and 50 mm Hg and a PVR between 240 and 400 dyne/sec/cm^{-5} are at increased risk, with a perioperative mortality approximating 50% [2]; the decision to proceed with OLT is center dependent. Patients who have a MPAP in excess of 50 mm Hg despite therapy are at highest risk and would be excluded from consideration for OLT at most major transplant centers [39,40]. Nonetheless, there are reports of successful OLT even in this exceptionally

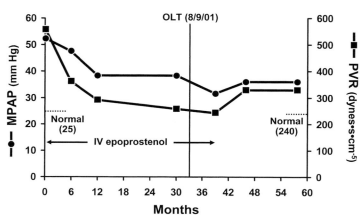

Fig. 5. Pulmonary hemodynamics in a 48-year-old woman who had cryptogenic cirrhosis and severe POPH. Treatment with 24-hour continuous infusion of epoprostenol for 30 months preceded successful OLT. Treatment with epoprostenol was discontinued 6 months after OLT, and treatment with amlodipine was started. MPAP, mean pulmonary artery pressure; PVR, pulmonary vascular resistance.

high-risk group [49] Regardless of the hemodynamic numbers, right ventricle function is a key issue that is difficult to assess in a manner that simulates the rigors of the liver transplantation procedure. Rarely, multiorgan transplantation (heart-lung-liver or lung-liver) can be attempted in patients unresponsive to current therapies [50].

Finally, it should be understood that POPH can evolve quickly over months. A patient on the OLT waiting list should have repeated Doppler echocardiography annually to ensure that a major change in hemodynamics has not occurred.

Intraoperative concerns

A literature review of the early experience in dealing with pulmonary hypertension and OLT revealed that the initial diagnosis of POPH was made in the operating room at the time of OLT in 28 of 43 cases reviewed (65%) [39]. That statistic was unacceptable, given the subsequent intraoperative deaths (two patients) and deaths that occurred within 30 months of OLT (12 patients) directly caused by cardiopulmonary dysfunction. After publication of this review, it was hoped that screening Doppler echocardiography and careful patient selection would improve OLT outcomes in the setting of POPH. Unfortunately, intraoperative mortality has remained a vexing problem, as evidenced by a mortality rate of 14% documented in the most recent multicenter database report of 36 patients who had POPH and who underwent OLT [4].

Clinical course after orthotopic liver transplantation

Aside from case reports and limited case series, the understanding of the clinical course after OLT is rudimentary. It is likely that poor outcomes have been underreported in the literature [2]. Long-term follow-up has yet to be studied systematically. In the setting of POPH, denial for OLT, intraoperative death, and death before and after hospital discharge have been reported (Table 2). On the other hand, partial or complete normalization of pulmonary hemodynamics, as well as long-term survival, have been

Table 2
Orthotopic liver transplantation dispositions and outcomes in the setting of portopulmonary hypertension

Disposition and outcome	References
Denied OLT because of severity of POPH	[4]
OLT attempted; intraoperative death	[4,40,41]
OLT; death during hospitalization for transplantation	[4,37,40,41, 51,52]
Death after hospitalization for transplantation	[40,41,53]
Long-term survival after OLT	
Resolution of POPH after OLT	[38,40,41,43–45, 49,50]
Improvement of POPH after OLT	[39–42,47–49, 51,54]
Progression of POPH after OLT	[40,41]

Abbreviations: OLT, orthotopic liver transplantation; POPH, portopulmonary hypertension.

Table 3

Mean pre-orthotopic liver transplantation pulmonary hemodynamics in patients with portopulmonary hypertension

Parameter	All PortoPH (N=66)	Denied OLT (N=30)	Transplanted	
			Survivors (N=23)	Nonsurvivors (N=13)
MPAP	48 ± 11	53 ± 11[a]	45 ± 14[3]	44 ± 8
PVR	462 ± 202	614 ± 288[b]	341 ± 181[3]	322 ± 139
CO	7.3 + 3.1	6.2 ± 3.3	8.2 ± 2.7[3]	8.6 ± 4.3
RA	10 ± 6	11 ± 7	8 ± 3	7 ± 3
PCWP	11 ± 6	10 ± 6	11 ± 5	14 ± 6

Abbreviations: CO, cardiac output (L/min); MPAP, mean pulmonary artery pressure (mm Hg); PCWP, pulmonary capillary wedge pressure (mm Hg); PVR, pulmonary vascular resistance (dyne/sec/cm^{-5}); RA, mean right atrial pressure (mm Hg).
  [a] $P < .015$.
  [b] $P < .005$.

Adapted from Krowka MJ, Mandell RS, Ramsay MAE, et al. Hepatopulmonary syndrome and portopulmonary hypertension: a report of the multicenter liver transplant database. Liver Transpl 2004;10:174–82; with permission.

documented [39,40,49,51]. Unlike HPS, POPH has been considered a relative contraindication to OLT because of the increased mortality and unpredictable outcomes.

The incomplete picture provided by previously published case reports set the stage for a prospective, multicenter effort to describe better the pre-OLT characteristics and post-OLT course of patients who have POPH (Table 3). In this multicenter study from 10 liver transplant centers, 30 of the 66 patients were excluded from OLT because of the severity of POPH. Despite this seemingly stringent selection of candidates, post-OLT in-hospital mortality occurred in 13 of 36 cases (36%). Twelve of 13 deaths were caused by right heart failure in the setting of variable approaches to managing POPH before and after OLT [4].

The role of living-donor OLT for patients who have mild to moderate POPH is an area of active consideration but carries a similar risk of an unpredictable outcome regarding pulmonary hemodynamics and mortality after transplantation [52–54].

Summary

HPS and POPH are uncommon but potentially serious pulmonary consequences of advanced liver disease. The major considerations for liver transplantation posed by these disorders are summarized in Table 4. Remarkably, HPS may completely resolve after OLT; the post-OLT outcome of POPH is less predictable. Both syndromes, under certain conditions, may represent high-risk situations for OLT. The unique opportunity to reverse serious dysfunction in one organ (the lungs) by the successful transplantation of another organ (the liver) is worthy of further clinical investigations.

Table 4

Summary of liver transplant considerations for hepatopulmonary syndrome and portopulmonary hypertension

	Hepatopulmonary syndrome	Portopulmonary hypertension
High risk for OLT (↑mortality)	PaO$_2$ < 50 mm Hg ^{99mTc}MAA brain uptake > 20%	MPAP > 35 mm Hg
UNOS indication for OLT	Yes	No
Higher priority for OLT	Yes, if PaO$_2$ < 60 mm Hg	No
Syndrome deterioration awaiting OLT	Yes	Yes
Sudden death due to syndrome	No	25%
5-Year survival without OLT	23%	30%
Pharmacologic treatment before OLT helpful	Not proven	Strongly suggested
Intraoperative death	Not reported	Yes
Transplant hospitalization mortality	16%	35%
Syndrome resolution after OLT	Common	Extremely variable

Abbreviations: MPAP, mean pulmonary arterial pressure; OLT, orthotopic liver transplantation; ^{99mTc}MAA, tecnetium-99m macroaggregated albumin; UNOS, United Network for Organ Sharing.

References

[1] Krowka MJ. Hepatopulmonary syndrome and porto-pulmonary hypertension: distinctions and dilemmas. Hepatology 1997;25:1282–4.

[2] Rodriguez-Roisin R, Krowka MJ, Herve P, et al. Pulmonary-hepatic vascular disorders: a task force report. Eur Respir J 2004;24:861–80.

[3] Mazzeo AT, Lucanto T, Santamaria LB. Hepatopulmonary syndrome: a concern for the anesthetist? Preoperative evaluation of hypoxemic patients with liver disease. Acta Anesthesiol Scand 2004;48:178–86.

[4] Krowka MJ, Mandell MS, Ramsay MAE, et al. Hepatopulmonary syndrome and portopulmonary hypertension: a report of the multicenter liver transplant database. Liver Transpl 2004;10:174–82.

[5] Abrams GA, Sanders MK, Fallon MB. Utility of pulse oximetry in the detection of arterial hypoxemia in liver transplant candidates. Liver Transpl 2002;8:391–6.

[6] Schenk P, Fuhrmann V, Madl C, et al. Hepatopulmonary syndrome: prevalence and predictive value of cutoffs for arterial oxygenation and their clinical consequences. Gut 2002;51:853–9.

[7] Krowka MJ, Wiseman GA, Burnett OL, et al. Hepatopulmonary syndrome: a prospective study of relationships between severity of liver disease, PaO_2 response to 100% oxygen, and brain uptake after [99m] TcMAA lung scanning. Chest 2000;118:615–24.

[8] Swanson KL, Wiesner RH, Krowka MJ. Natural history of hepatopulmonary syndrome: impact of liver transplantation. Hepatology 2005;41(5):1122–9.

[9] Martinez G, Barbera JA, Navasa M, et al. Hepatopulmonary syndrome associated with cardiorespiratory disease. J Hepatol 1999;30:882–9.

[10] Rolla G, Brussino L, Colagrande P. Exhaled nitric oxide and impaired oxygenation in cirrhotic patients before and after liver transplantation. Ann Intern Med 1998;129:375–8.

[11] Ling Y, Zhang J, Luo B, et al. The role of endothelin-1 and endothelin B receptor in the pathogenesis of hepatopulmonary syndrome in the rat. Hepatology 2004; 39:1593–602.

[12] Wiesner RH, Edwards E, Freeman R, et al. Model for end-stage liver disease (MELD) and allocation of liver donors. Gastroenterology 2003;124:91–6.

[13] Krowka MJ, Porayko MK, Plevak DJ, et al. Hepatopulmonary syndrome with progressive hypoxemia as an indication for liver transplantation. Mayo Clin Proc 1997;72:44–53.

[14] Arguedas M, Abrams GA, Krowka MJ, et al. Prospective evaluation of outcomes and predictors of mortality in patients with hepatopulmonary syndrome undergoing liver transplantation. Hepatology 2003;37: 192–7.

[15] Taille C, Cadranel J, Bellocq A, et al. Liver transplantation for hepatopulmonary syndrome: a ten-year experience in Paris, France. Transplantation 2003;75: 1446–7.

[16] Meyers C, Low L, Kaufman L, et al. Trendelenburg positioning and continuous lateral rotation improves oxygenation in hepatopulmonary syndrome following liver transplantation. Liver Transpl Surg 1998;4: 510–2.

[17] Durand P, Baujard C, Grosse AL, et al. Reversal of hypoxemia by inhaled nitric oxide in children with severe hepatopulmonary syndrome type I during and after liver transplantation. Transplantation 1998;65: 437–9.

[18] Alexander J, Greenough A, Baker A, et al. Nitric oxide treatment of severe hypoxemia after liver transplantation in hepatopulmonary syndrome. Liver Transpl Surg 1997;3:54–5.

[19] Schenk P, Madl C, Rezale-Majd S, et al. Methylene blue improves hepatopulmonary syndrome. Ann Intern Med 2000;133:701–6.

[20] Stoller JK, Moodie D, Schiavone WA, et al. Reduction in intrapulmonary shunt and resolution of digital clubbing associated with primary biliary cirrhosis after liver transplantation. Hepatology 1990;11:54–8.

[21] Laberge JM, Brandt ML, Lebecque P. Reversal of cirrhosis-related pulmonary shunting in two children by orthotopic liver transplantation. Transplantation 1992;53:1135–45.

[22] Krowka MJ. Hepatopulmonary syndrome: recent literature (up to 1999) and implications for liver transplantation. Liver Transpl 2000;6(4 Suppl 1):S31–5.

[23] Uemoto S, Inomata Y, Egawa H. Effects of hypoxemia on early postoperative course of liver transplantation in pediatric patients with intrapulmonary shunting. Transplantation 1997;63:407–14.

[24] Collison EA, Nourmand H, Fraiman MH, et al. Retrospective analysis of the results of liver transplantation for adults with severe hepatopulmonary syndrome. Liver Transpl 2002;8:925–31.

[25] Krowka MJ, Wiseman GA, Steers JL, et al. Late recurrence and rapid evolution of severe hepatopulmonary syndrome after liver transplantation. Liver Transpl 1999;5:451–3.

[26] Carey EJ, Douglas DD, Bala V, et al. Hepatopulmonary syndrome after living donor liver transplantation and deceased donor liver transplantation: a single center experience. Liver Transpl 2004;10:529–33.

[27] Avendano CE, Flume PA, Baliga P, et al. Hepatopulmonary syndrome occurring after orthotopic liver transplantation. Liver Transpl 2001;7:1081–4.

[28] Kaspar MD, Ramsay MA, Shuey CB, et al. Severe pulmonary hypertension and amelioration of hepatopulmonary syndrome after liver transplantation. Liver Transpl Surg 1998;4:177–9.

[29] Martinez-Pauli G, Barbera JA, Taura P, et al. Severe portopulmonary hypertension after liver transplantation in a patient with preexisting hepatopulmonary syndrome. J Hepatol 1999;31:1075–9.

[30] Kim WR, Krowka MJ, Plevak DJ, et al. Accuracy of Doppler echocardiography in the assessment of portopulmonary hypertension in liver transplant candidates. Liver Transpl 2000;6:453–8.

[31] Cotton CL, Gandhi S, Vaitkus PT, et al. Role of

echocardiography in detecting portopulmonary hypertension in liver transplant candidates. Liver Transpl 2002;8:1051–4.

[32] Pilatis ND, Jacobs LE, Rekpattanappipat P, et al. Clinical predictors of pulmonary hypertension in patients undergoing liver transplantation. Liver Transpl 2000;6:85–91.

[33] Henriksen JH, Gotz JP, Fuglsang S, et al. Increased circulating pro-brain natriuretic peptide (proBNP) and brain natriuretic peptide (BNP) in patients with cirrhosis: relation to cardiovascular dysfunction and severity of disease. Gut 2003;52:1511–7.

[34] Robalino BD, Moodie DS. Association between primary pulmonary hypertension and portal hypertension: analysis of its pathophysiology and clinical, laboratory and hemodynamic manifestations. J Am Coll Cardiol 1991;17:492–8.

[35] Swanson KL, McGoon MD, Krowka MJ. Survival in portopulmonary hypertension with the use of intravenous epoprostenol [abstract]. Am J Respir Crit Care Med 2003;167:A683.

[36] Benjaminov FS, Prentice M, Sniderman KW, et al. Portopulmonary hypertension in decompensated cirrhosis and refractory ascites. Gut 2003;52:1355–62.

[37] DeWolf AM, Gasior T, Kang Y. Pulmonary hypertension in a patient undergoing liver transplantation. Transplant Proc 1991;23:2000–1.

[38] Castro M, Krowka MJ, Schroeder DR, et al. Frequency and clinical implications of increased pulmonary artery pressures in liver transplant patients. Mayo Clin Proc 1996;71:543–51.

[39] Krowka MJ, Plevak DJ, Findlay JY, et al. Pulmonary hemodynamics and perioperative cardiopulmonary mortality in patients with portopulmonary hypertension undergoing liver transplantation. Liver Transpl 2000;6: 443–50.

[40] Ramsay MAE, Simpson BR, Nguyen AT, et al. Severe pulmonary hypertension in liver transplant candidates. Liver Transpl Surg 1997;3:494–500.

[41] Krowka MJ, Frantz RP, McGoon MD, et al. Improvement in pulmonary hemodynamics during intravenous epoprostenol (prostacyclin): a study of 15 patients with moderate to severe portopulmonary hypertension. Hepatology 1999;30:641–8.

[42] Plotkin JS, Kuo PC, Rubin LJ, et al. Successful use of chronic epoprostenol as a bridge to liver transplantation in severe portopulmonary hypertension. Transplantation 1998;65:457–9.

[43] Tan HP, Markowitz JS, Montgomery RA, et al. Liver transplantation in patients with severe portopulmonary hypertension treated with preoperative chronic intravenous epoprostenol. Liver Transpl 2001;7:745–9.

[44] Kett DH, Acost RC, Campos MA, et al. Recurrent portopulmonary hypertension after liver transplantation: management with epoprostenol and resolution after retransplantation. Liver Transpl 2001;7:645–8.

[45] Minder S, Fishler M, Muelihaupt B, et al. Intravenous iloprost bridging to orthotopic liver transplantation in portopulmonary hypertension. Eur Respir J 2004;24: 703–7.

[46] Hoeper MM, Halank M, Marx C, et al. Bosentan for the treatment of portopulmonary hypertension. Eur Respir J 2005;25:502–8.

[47] Clift PF, Bramhill S, Isaac JL. Successful treatment of severe portopulmonary hypertension after liver transplantation by bosentan. Transplantation 2004;77: 1774–6.

[48] Makisalo H, Koivusalo A, Vakkuri A, et al. Sidenafil for portopulmonary hypertension in a patient undergoing liver transplantation. Liver Transpl 2004;10: 945–50.

[49] Starkel P, Vera A, Gunson B, et al. Outcome of liver transplantation for patients with pulmonary hypertension. Liver Transpl 2002;8:383–8.

[50] Pirenne J, Verlede G, Nevens F, et al. Combined liver and heart-lung transplantation in liver transplant candidates with refractory portopulmonary hypertension. Transplantation 2002;73:140–2.

[51] Schott R, Chaouat A, Launoy A, et al. Improvement of pulmonary hypertension after liver transplantation. Chest 1999;115:1748–9.

[52] Urashima Y, Tojimbara T, Nakajima I, et al. Living related liver transplantation for biliary atresia with portopulmonary hypertension. Transplant Proc 2004; 36:2237–8.

[53] Kikuchi H, Ohkoohchi N, Orli T, et al. Living-related liver transplantation in patients with pulmonary vascular disease. Transplant Proc 2000;32:2177–8.

[54] Sulica R, Emre S, Poon M. Medical management of portopulmonary hypertension and right heart failure prior to living-related liver transplantation. Congestive Heart Failure 2004;10:192–4.

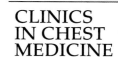

Clin Chest Med 26 (2005) 599 – 612

Allograft Rejection After Lung Transplantation

Timothy P.M. Whelan, MD*, Marshall I. Hertz, MD

*Division of Pulmonary, Allergy, and Critical Care Medicine, University of Minnesota, 420 Delaware Street SE,
Minneapolis, MN 55455, USA*

James Hardy at the University of Mississippi performed the first human lung transplantation in 1963 [1]. The patient survived 18 days and ultimately died of multiorgan failure. Over the next 20 years, there were approximately 40 attempts at human lung transplantation with a maximum posttransplant survival of 10 months [2–4]. Early immunosuppressive therapy consisted primarily of corticosteroids, sometimes in combination with azathioprine. Although episodes of rejection could be identified and then treated with augmented corticosteroid therapy, treatment led to increased risk of infection and bronchial anastomosis dehiscence, which were the major limitations to successful lung transplantation. In 1981, the introduction of cyclosporine led to the first successful heart-lung transplantation and opened the era to subsequent successful single-lung transplantation in 1983 [5].

Today, lung transplantation has become an accepted therapy for treatment of selected patients who have advanced lung disease. More than 100 centers worldwide performed more than 1600 lung transplantations in 2002 [6]. As is the case for all organ transplantations, suppression of the alloimmune response is necessary for the transplanted lung to remain functional. Acute rejection remains a common occurrence in lung transplantation but rarely leads directly to mortality in the transplant recipient. Bronchiolitis obliterans syndrome (BOS) or chronic rejection, on the other hand, accounts for more than 30% of late deaths after transplantation [6].

The immune system is a complex array of mechanisms that developed to help identify "self"

from "nonself." This ability allows the organism to identify foreign bacterial, viral, fungal, and parasitic organisms and defend itself against infection. This defense often is referred to as innate immunity, because it is active innately in all members of a species without prior antigen exposure. Major components of this same system allow organ transplant recipients to recognize transplanted organs as "nonself," leading to multiple host responses identified as rejection. These mechanisms are known as the adaptive immune system. The major histocompatibility complex is a region of highly polymorphic genes that produce glycoprotein cell-surface antigens found in all cells. In humans, these antigens are the human leukocyte antigens (HLA). The primary role of HLA is to allow the immune system to mount a response against an invading infection without destroying the "self" cells identified by the unique HLA component. Identical twins have the same HLA; therefore, an organ transplanted from one identical twin to another is accepted without the need for immunosuppression. Except in this unusual situation, the recipient's unique HLA allows his immune system to identify a donor allograft as foreign; the result is rejection.

This article covers three broad areas related to immune reactivity against the transplanted lung: hyperacute rejection, acute rejection, and bronchiolitis obliterans (often referred to as chronic rejection).

Hyperacute rejection

Hyperacute rejection is a well-known cause of immediate graft dysfunction in kidney transplantation [7,8]. It is a predominantly antibody-mediated

---

* Corresponding author.
E-mail address: whela011@umn.edu (T.P.M. Whelan).

0272-5231/05/$ – see front matter © 2005 Elsevier Inc. All rights reserved.
doi:10.1016/j.ccm.2005.06.008

chestmed.theclinics.com

response that occurs immediately upon revascularization of the graft. Preformed recipient antibodies bind to donor antigens resulting in complement activation and a cascade of events ultimately leading to thrombosis of the organ within minutes to hours after transplantation. Pre-existing antibodies to HLA or ABO blood type antigens are the classic mediators of this response.

Frost and colleagues [9–11] reported the first well-documented case of hyperacute rejection after lung transplantation in 1996; there have been at least two other case reports since then. The clinical presentation of hyperacute rejection is consistent among these reports. The transplant recipient develops sudden onset of respiratory failure within minutes to several hours after allograft reperfusion. The respiratory failure is heralded by a marked increase in mean pulmonary artery pressure and an increase in measured airway pressures, signaling a fall in lung compliance. This reduced compliance results in a dramatic drop in arterial oxygenation and blood pressure. On bronchoscopic examination, large amounts of frothy, blood-tinged fluid can be seen pouring from the airways of the transplanted lung. Chest radiographs reveal dense infiltrates throughout the transplanted lung. Several nonimmunologic complications can lead to a similar presentation early after transplantation; these complications include obstruction of the pulmonary veins, acute left ventricular failure, infection with acute respiratory distress syndrome, and development of nonimmunologic primary graft dysfunction.

Once other potential causes are excluded, the diagnosis is corroborated by the identification of a donor-specific IgG antibody in recipient serum. Confirmation of the diagnosis from pathologic specimens is challenging at acute presentation, because the severity of illness often precludes adequate tissue sampling. In the confirmed case reports, however, the pathologic specimens were consistent with those of other organs undergoing hyperacute rejection. Specifically, marked interstitial neutrophilic infiltration with platelet and fibrin thrombi in small arterioles is apparent. Accumulation of edema fluid and neutrophils within alveolar airspaces is also characteristic. Immunohistochemical staining reveals deposition of antibodies on the endothelial surface and within the vascular walls [9,10]. In single-lung transplantation, these findings are limited to the allograft.

Treatment options for hyperacute rejection are directed at removing the preformed antibodies from the recipient's serum by plasmapheresis and preventing the production of further antibody by adjunctive immunosuppression with cyclophosphamide and anti-thymocyte globulin. With this treatment, at least one successful outcome has been documented, with recovery of graft function, discontinuation of mechanical ventilation on the sixth postoperative day, and prolonged survival [11].

Although a successful recovery has been reported, mortality from hyperacute rejection remains exceedingly high, and prevention remains the best therapy. One study has confirmed that patients who have elevated preformed antibodies to both class I and class II HLA, even at low levels, have an increased risk of acute graft dysfunction [12]. In addition, the International Society for Heart and Lung Transplantation (ISHLT) Registry shows that elevation of panel-reactive antibodies (which indicates the presence of preformed antibodies to class I or class II HLA molecules) is a risk factor for 1-year mortality after transplantation [6]. As a result, it is recommended that potential lung transplant recipients undergo screening to detect antibodies to common HLA antigens. A history of pregnancy, blood transfusion, prior transplantation, or connective tissue disease increases the risk for development of these antibodies. For patients who have high levels of antibody, a donor-specific lymphocytotoxic crossmatching should be performed before transplantation of the organ to ensure there is no significant reactivity and the patient is not at risk for hyperacute rejection. In addition, all patients who have low-titer anti-HLA antibodies should undergo concomitant or retrospective flow cytometry crossmatching whenever possible [13]. Prospective crossmatching should reduce the risk of hyperacute rejection, and concomitant or retrospective crossmatching ensures early identification and treatment of cases of hyperacute rejection.

Immunopathogenesis of acute rejection

Acute rejection is a T-cell–mediated response directed against "nonself" antigens. These allograft antigens include HLA proteins, but other non-HLA proteins can also fuel the rejection response. Class I HLA antigens (HLA A, B, and C) are located on all nucleated cells. These antigens are recognized by $CD8^+$ cytotoxic T lymphocytes. Once activated, the $CD8^+$ T cells lyse the antigen-bearing target cell. Class II HLA antigens (HLA DP, DQ, and DR) are found on endothelial cells, antigen-presenting cells, activated T lymphocytes, and some epithelial cells. These antigens are recognized by $CD4^+$ T lymphocytes. Once activated, $CD4^+$ T lymphocytes release a number of chemokines and cytokines that result in further proliferation and activation of T cells, amplifying the rejection process [14,15].

Acute rejection remains one of the most common complications after lung transplantation. Two large series indicate that only between 24% and 40% of recipients remain free from acute rejection at 1 year after transplantation [16,17]. Several factors may play a role in this exceedingly high rate of rejection. The lung is a highly vascular organ, it is constantly exposed to the environment, and it has a large lymphocyte network. Most initial episodes of acute rejection reverse with augmented immunosuppression. For a smaller subset of patients, multiple episodes of acute rejection occur. Morbidity results not only from the loss of lung function but also from complications related to increased immunosuppression (ie, increased infection, weakness, and metabolic complications). Furthermore, repeated episodes of acute rejection have been implicated consistently in the later development of BOS [18–24].

For these reasons, prevention of the development of acute rejection is a major goal of therapy. Acute rejection is a T-cell–mediated response to "nonself" antigens. To activate a T cell, three signals are required: (1) interaction of the T-cell receptor with an intact foreign HLA antigen (direct allorecognition) or with a foreign peptide presented by the recipient's own antigen-presenting cell (indirect allorecognition); (2) a costimulatory signal from the antigen-presenting cell to the T cell; and (3) an autocrine interaction of interleukin (IL)-2, from activated T cells, with increased expression of IL-2 receptors on their cell surfaces. Interference with these three mechanisms should result in decreased acute rejection [25]. IL-2 is clearly one of the most important factors in the cascade. Altering these interactions forms the basis for immunosuppression regimens in the lung transplant recipient.

Induction immunosuppression

In 2002, approximately 40% of transplant centers used augmented immunosuppression in the early posttransplantation period (induction therapy) [6]. There are several potential benefits to induction therapy. First, it is hoped that additional immunosuppression may decrease episodes of early acute rejection. In addition, induction therapy allows the transplant team more flexibility in calcineurin inhibitor dosing in the early postoperative course. This flexibility is particularly helpful in recipients who develop early renal insufficiency that may be exacerbated by full-dose calcineurin inhibitors [26].

Induction therapy typically is composed of a polyclonal anti–T-cell antibody, a monoclonal antibody, or an IL-2 receptor antagonist (eg, basiliximab, daclizumab) added to the patient's maintenance regimen. Table 1 lists the major induction agents, their mechanisms of action, and major side effects. Polyclonal and monoclonal anti–T-cell antibodies bind to T-cells and cause cell lysis, resulting in profound and prolonged T-cell depletion. There has been one single-center prospective, randomized trial comparing a noncommercial rabbit anti-thymocyte globulin (ATG) preparation versus conventional therapy without induction in 44 patients [27]. In the patients who received ATG, there was a 23% prevalence of acute rejection (grade A2 or higher) in the first year, compared with 55% in those who did not receive ATG ($P < .05$). There was a nonsignificant decrease in the development of BOS, and rates of infection and malignancy were similar in the two groups. Muromonab-CD3 has not been evaluated in a prospective, randomized clinical trial versus conventional therapy. It has, however, been compared with ATG and daclizumab induction by Brock and colleagues [28]. In a protocol initially intended to compare ATG versus muromonab-CD3, there were no differences in freedom from acute rejection or the development of BOS. Higher rates of infection were noted in the muromonab-CD3 group, but this difference only developed 2 months after transplantation. There were no differences in survival between the muromonab-CD3 and ATG groups.

IL-2 receptor antagonists are the newest class of induction agents available. IL-2 binds to a receptor on T lymphocytes, CD-25, which activates the cells. Once activated, T cells increase the production of CD-25, making T lymphocytes highly responsive to IL-2. IL-2 receptor antagonists selectively block activated T cells. As mentioned previously, Brock and colleagues [28] included daclizumab in their study of induction agents. Although the follow-up period was significantly shorter than for ATG and muromonab-CD3, there was no difference in the incidence of acute rejection. In addition, there seemed to be fewer infections than in the other arms of the study. A retrospective analysis by Bhorade and colleagues [29] suggested that daclizumab significantly decreased acute rejection rates by univariate analysis. Once adjustments were made for diagnosis of cystic fibrosis and age, however, the differences between groups were no longer statistically significant. This study also found no difference in infection rates between the groups that received daclizumab and those that did not.

At present, there are some theoretical advantages to induction therapy for lung transplant re-

Table 1
Common immunosuppression agents used in lung transplantation

Drug	Mechanism of action	Side effects
Induction agents		
Muromonab-CD3	Murine monoclonal antibody against CD3; binds CD3 causing initial activation and cytokine release then blockade of function and cell lysis	First-dose reaction: fever, rigors, nausea, vomiting, diarrhea, chest pain, dyspnea, wheezing, hypotension Pulmonary edema: risk greater for patients with fluid overload
Polyclonal anti-thymocyte globulin	Polyclonal IgG from horse or rabbit serum blocking T-cell membrane proteins; alters T-cell function, causes lysis and T-cell depletion	Fevers, chills, pruritus, rash, gastrointestinal intolerance, arthralgias, back pain, headache, thrombocytopenia, leukopenia, anaphylaxis, and serum sickness
Basiliximab or daclizumab	IL-2 receptor antagonist	Hypersensitivity reactions (uncommon)
Maintenance agents		
Cyclosporine[a]	Inhibits calcineurin	Hirsutism, hypertension, tremor, headache, nephrotoxicity, diabetes mellitus, hyperlipidemia, gum hyperplasia
Tacrolimus[a]	Inhibits calcineurin	Similar to cyclosporine except lower incidence of hypertension, hirsutism, and gum hyperplasia; higher incidence diabetes mellitus and neurotoxicity
Azathioprine	Inhibits purine synthesis	Nausea, vomiting, hepatotoxicity, leukopenia, thrombocytopenia, pancreatitis
Mycophenolate mofetil	Inhibits de novo purine synthesis	Hypertension, peripheral edema, gastrointestinal intolerance, gastrointestinal bleeding
Corticosteroids	Block cytokine transcription; lyse T cells	Hyperglycemia, hypertension, mood changes, insomnia, myopathy, cataracts, osteoporosis
Sirolimus[a]	Inhibits T-cell activation (non–calcineurin dependent)	Hyperlipidemia, thrombocytopenia, pneumonitis, delayed wound healing, peripheral edema, increased toxicity of calcineurin inhibitors

[a] Metabolized by cytochrome P-450 system. Azole antifungals, diltiazem, and macrolide antibiotics increase levels; rifampin, phenobarbital, and phenytoin decrease levels.

cipients. In addition, there is suggestive evidence that induction therapy decreases rates of acute rejection in the first year after transplantation. To date, however, there is no clear evidence that induction therapy decreases rates of BOS. If induction therapy is used, ATG or an IL-2 receptor antagonist seems to be a reasonable choice. Muromonab-CD3 is being used much less frequently because of its less favorable side-effect profile [6].

Maintenance immunosuppression

Beyond the early postoperative phase, almost all patients are maintained using three major drug classes: a calcineurin inhibitor, a purine synthesis inhibitor, and corticosteroids. Although most regimens taper corticosteroids to low doses by the end of the first year after transplantation, patients generally take all three drug classes throughout their lives [6]. In terms of specific agents in these categories, the optimal immunosuppression regimen remains unclear [17]. Keenan and colleagues [30] randomly assigned 133 patients to treatment with cyclosporine versus tacrolimus with azathioprine and steroids. A trend toward fewer acute rejection episodes was noted at 6 and 12 months in the tacrolimus group. A statistically significant decrease in the frequency of BOS was observed in the tacrolimus group as well [30]. More recently, a trial of tacrolimus versus cyclosporine with mycophenolate mofetil and corticosteroids found no significant differences in episodes of acute rejection, development of BOS, or survival [17]. Similarly, two large, prospective, randomized studies (one short term, one long term) indicate no clear advantage of either mycophenolate mofetil or azathioprine over the other [31,32]. Based on data from the ISHLT registry, there is a trend toward increased use of tacrolimus with mycophenolate mofetil and prednisone. All of the following immunosuppressants are commonly prescribed for lung transplant recipients, however. A brief description of these agents is provided here and is summarized in Table 1; an excellent review by Knoop and colleagues [33] provides more extensive information.

Cyclosporine A is a cyclic polypeptide that is a metabolite of the species *Tolypocladium inflatum Gams*. Cyclosporine A is highly lipophilic and enters the cell easily. It binds to cyclophilin and inhibits T lymphocytes by decreasing production of cytokines, including IL-2 and gamma interferon. In addition, production of the receptor site for interleukin-2 on T lymphocytes is inhibited by cyclosporine.

Tacrolimus, a macrolide antibiotic produced by the soil fungus *Streptomyces tsukubaensis*, similarly inhibits secretion of cytokines (including IL-2 and gamma interferon). Tacrolimus binds to an intracellular protein, FK Binding Protein-12 (FKBP-12), which inhibits calcineurin but is distinct from cyclophilin. This inhibition decreases gene transcription for lymphokines and results in inhibition of T-lymphocyte activation.

Both cyclosporine and tacrolimus are monitored with serum trough levels. Target drug levels depend on the assay used but typically are maintained at higher levels in the early posttransplantation period because of the greater risk of acute rejection. Although cyclosporine traditionally has been monitored with the C0 level or trough level, it was reported in heart transplant recipients that levels 2 hours after dosing (C2 levels) correlate better than C0 levels with area under the curve measurements [34]. There are also several reports that C2 levels correlate with risk of rejection in renal transplant recipients, whereas C0 levels do not [35]. There is only one published report of C2 monitoring in lung transplantation [36]. In 18 patients followed with C2 monitoring, the rates of acute rejection, lung function, and survival at 3 months were similar to those in 18 patients followed with traditional C0 monitoring. There was, however, a significant difference in the change in creatinine level over 3 months, with C0 monitoring seemingly more nephrotoxic. At this point, there are insufficient data to recommend C2 monitoring over traditional trough measurement of cyclosporine; however, the preliminary evidence

suggests that C2 monitoring may be the recommended assay in the future.

Both cyclosporine and tacrolimus are metabolized by the cytochrome P-450 system. As a result, commonly prescribed medications may have dramatic effects on the patient's serum level of these medications. Azole antifungals, some calcium-channel blockers (ie, diltiazem), and macrolide antibiotics can increase drug levels. Rifampin, phenytoin, and phenobarbital have the opposite effect, dramatically decreasing cyclosporine or tacrolimus levels in serum. Therefore, when a patient's medication regimen is altered, possible drug interactions should always be considered, and drug levels should be re-evaluated as necessary.

Azathioprine is a purine analogue that is cleaved in vivo to 6-mercaptopurine. By affecting purine nucleotide synthesis, azathioprine alters RNA and DNA synthesis and function. The drug suppresses T-cell more so than B-cell activity and has potent anti-inflammatory properties. Mycophenolate mofetil, a macrolide antibiotic isolated from *Penicillium* species, also affects purine synthesis. It blocks de novo synthesis of guanosine nucleotides. Because lymphocytes depend on the de novo pathway for purine synthesis, the result is selective inhibition of the proliferative response of T and B cells.

Corticosteroids have broad effects on the immune response. These effects include blocking cytokine gene transcription and secretion from mononuclear lymphocytes as well as a direct effect of lysing T cells.

In addition to the three major classes of immunosuppressive medications discussed thus far, sirolimus and its derivative, everolimus, are used in approximately 10% of lung transplant recipients 1 and 5 years after transplantation [6]. Sirolimus is a macrocyclic triene antibiotic (structurally related to tacrolimus) produced by fermentation of *Streptomyces hygroscopicus*. Similar to tacrolimus, sirolimus binds to FKBP-12; however, the complex does not affect calcineurin activity. Instead, it inhibits a key regulatory kinase, mammalian target of rapamycin (mTOR) resulting in decrease cytokine production and inhibition of T-cell proliferation. It typically is used to treat BOS (as an additional immunosuppressant) or to replace either tacrolimus or cyclosporine to spare the kidney from the nephrotoxicity of these agents.

Acute rejection

As noted previously, despite triple-drug immunosuppression after lung transplantation, acute rejection remains common. The greatest risk for the development of acute rejection is during the first several months after transplantation [16,37,38]. Mild rejection may be entirely asymptomatic. With higher grades of rejection, the clinical presentation is similar to that of acute respiratory infection. Patients often present with symptoms of fever, cough, fatigue, dyspnea, a decrease in oxygenation, or evidence of an infiltrate on chest radiograph. Chest radiographs are nonspecific and cannot distinguish between rejection and infection. Radiographic abnormalities are more likely to be present in the early posttransplantation period than beyond 1 month after transplantation [39,40].

Several studies show the utility of following patients with pulmonary function tests [41–44]. Once acute rejection develops, the forced expiratory volume in one second (FEV_1) and the mean forced expiratory flow during the middle half of the forced vital capacity ($FEF_{25\%-75\%}$) often decline from the patient's baseline. Unfortunately, pulmonary function testing cannot distinguish acute rejection from infection or nonimmunologic causes of respiratory dysfunction such as airway stenosis. Transplant centers typically follow both the FEV_1 and $FEF_{25\%-75\%}$ and use this information in conjunction with the patient's symptoms to determine appropriate further diagnostic strategies. A drop in FEV_1 of more than 10% is considered a significant change that warrants clinical evaluation.

Once infection has been ruled out, empiric treatment for acute rejection may be instituted when histologic confirmation cannot be obtained. The diagnosis is confirmed by a rapid improvement with high-dose corticosteroid therapy. This approach has limitations, because the treatment for rejection usually is diametrically opposed to the treatment of the principle alternative diagnosis (ie, infection). Because noninvasive measures cannot distinguish between infection and rejection, the bronchoscopy with transbronchial biopsy has been used extensively in patients after lung transplantation [16,45].

The reported sensitivity of bronchoscopy to detect abnormalities is variable. In animal models in which known acute rejection is present, the sensitivity of bronchoscopy has been noted to be as high as 94% when adequate tissue is obtained [46]. Sensitivity decreases in the human lung transplant population, however [47]. For patients who have clinical symptoms, the sensitivity of bronchoscopy to diagnose infection or rejection is greater than 80% [16,45,48]. For asymptomatic patients undergoing routine surveillance bronchoscopy, acute rejection or infection is found in approximately 20% of cases [16,45]. In addition to clinical presentation, the confidence of the di-

agnosis obtained with bronchoscopy depends on the number of biopsy specimens obtained. The consensus reached from the Lung Rejection Study Group (LRSG) is that at least five pieces of alveolated tissue, each containing bronchioles and more than 100 air sacs, are necessary to grade acute rejection confidently [49]. To obtain this quantity of tissue, the bronchoscopist usually must perform more than five biopsies. In a recent study in which the protocol called for 10 to 12 biopsy specimens at each bronchoscopy, 98% of the procedures achieved the criteria outlined by the LRSG for interpretable biopsies [16].

In 1995 the LRSG further clarified the histologic grading system for acute rejection (Table 2) [49]. The goal of this grading system was to ensure accurate comparisons of data from independent institutions. This grading system has been readily accepted within the transplant community and is used routinely when evaluating the significance of pathologic

Table 2
Histologic grading system for acute rejection

Grade	Description of pathology
A0 (no AR)	Normal pulmonary parenchyma
A1 (minimal AR)	Scattered, infrequent perivascular mononuclear infiltrates in alveolated lung parenchyma that are not obvious on low magnification
A2 (mild AR)	Frequent perivascular mononuclear infiltrates surrounding venules and arterioles easily seen at low magnification
A3 (moderate AR)	Readily recognizable cuffing of venules and arterioles by dense perivascular mononuclear infiltrates with extension of the inflammatory cell infiltrate into perivascular and peribronchiolar alveolar septae and air spaces
A4 (severe AR)	Diffuse perivascular, interstitial, and air space mononuclear infiltrates and prominent alveolar pneumocyte damage usually associated with intra-alveolar necrotic cells, macrophages, hyaline membranes, hemorrhage, and neutrophils

Abbreviation: AR, acute rejection.
Data from Yousem SA, Berry GJ, Cagle PT, et al. Revision of the 1990 working formulation for the classification of pulmonary allograft rejection: lung rejection study group. J Heart Lung Transplant 1996;15:1–15.

specimens obtained by transbronchial biopsy. Acute rejection is characterized by perivascular and subendothelial mononuclear infiltrates and by lymphocytic bronchitis and bronchiolitis. Although acute rejection is a continuum of inflammation, for the purposes of diagnosis of acute rejection by the grading system, acute rejection is based solely on the presence of perivascular and interstitial mononuclear infiltrates (Fig. 1).

Perivascular infiltrates are identified clearly in patients who have acute rejection. These findings, however, must be interpreted cautiously in a patient who has infection. The differential diagnosis includes viral infection (including Cytomegalovirus pneumonitis), Pneumocystis jeroveci pneumonia, posttransplantation lymphoproliferative disease, bronchial-associated lymphoid tissue, previous biopsy sites, recurrent primary disease (eg, sarcoidosis), and, in the early posttransplantation period, ischemia-reperfusion injury [49].

Airway inflammation or lymphocytic bronchiolitis often is associated with infection. The varying numbers of bronchioles present on transbronchial biopsy specimens often limit the ability to comment on this aspect of the pathology in the lung transplant recipient. Based on the recommendations of the LRSG, airway inflammation should be documented, but its presence alone does not signify acute rejection. The presence of lymphocytic bronchiolitis, however, has been clearly associated with the development of BOS and is discussed later in this article [20,23,50].

Once transbronchial biopsy material is obtained, which patients should be treated for histologically evident acute rejection? It is clear that patients who

have had at least mild acute rejection (grade $\geq$ A2) should have augmented immunosuppression, regardless of symptoms. For patients who have clinical symptoms (eg, drop in FEV_1, fatigue, shortness of breath), minimal acute rejection (A1) should be treated. For patients who have minimal rejection on biopsies but no clinical symptoms, the consensus is less clear. Treatment of these asymptomatic patients must also weigh the risks of high-dose corticosteroids, including infection, with the potential benefits of treatment. Two early studies reported that a subset of patients who have asymptomatic minimal or mild acute rejection demonstrate resolution without treatment [51,52]. A recent study from Australia, where asymptomatic A1 rejection was not treated, found that 25% of patients go on to develop A2 rejection or greater within 3 months. For patients who did not progress to higher grade rejection but had persistent asymptomatic A1 rejection, there was a statistically significant higher risk of the development of BOS compared with patients who had one or fewer episodes of A1 rejection on biopsy [53]. It remains to be seen if treatment of asymptomatic minimal rejection will have any impact on the development of BOS.

High-dose corticosteroids are often used to treat acute rejection. The standard dosing regimen is approximately 15 mg/kg of intravenous methylprednisolone each day for 3 consecutive days. The physician should review the maintenance immunosuppression regimen and, if agents have been tapered, consider a return to pretaper dosages. In terms of corticosteroid therapy after the bolus, if the main-

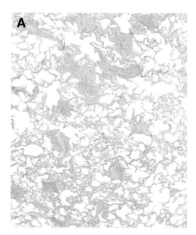
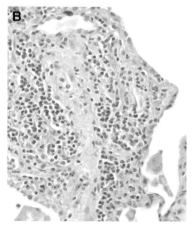

Fig. 1. Acute rejection. (A) Low-power view showing numerous perivascular lymphocytic infiltrates. (B) Dense perivascular infiltrates compress and focally infiltrate the wall of the vessel (hematoxylin and eosin stain). (Courtesy of Jose Jessurun, MD, Minneapolis, Minnesota.)

tenance prednisone has been tapered, increasing the prednisone to 1 mg/kg/d and tapering over the next 10 days may be helpful [54]. Early episodes of acute rejection typically respond rapidly to treatment with improvement in spirometry, radiographic abnormalities and in clinical symptoms [52]. A significant percentage of patients who have histologically proven acute rejection more than 6 months after transplantation have a progressive decline in FEV_1 despite corticosteroid therapy [55]. Unfortunately, this decline may be the precursor to the development of BOS. This finding and previous reports of persistent acute rejection histology after treatment despite apparent clinical resolution [38,45,52] highlight the need for transbronchial biopsy sampling after treatment to ensure resolution of acute rejection.

A small subset of patients have refractory or recurrent acute rejection despite adequate maintenance immunosuppression and repeated boluses of intravenous corticosteroids. This finding is the main risk factor for the development of BOS [56]. Therefore, consideration of additional immunosuppression strategies is warranted for these patients. One option is to convert cyclosporine to tacrolimus. Several small studies and one large retrospective study suggest that a switch from cyclosporine to tacrolimus decreases the rate of subsequent acute rejection in patients who have refractory or recurrent acute rejection [57–60]. Patients often are treated with multiple modalities in addition to a conversion in calcineurin therapy. These modalities include the addition of methotrexate [61], muromonab-CD3 monoclonal antibody [62], antithymocyte globulin, total lymphoid irradiation [63], extracorporeal photochemotherapy (photopheresis) [64,65], and aerosolized cyclosporine [66]. More recently, a case report with the use of alemtuzumab has also been published [67].

At this time, the best treatment combination for patients who have refractory or recurrent acute rejection is unknown. It seems a reasonable strategy to convert patients to a tacrolimus-based regimen (if not already receiving such) and to consider augmented immunosuppression with one of the adjunctive modalities described previously. It remains unknown if preventing further episodes of acute rejection in this patient population will prevent the development of BOS.

Bronchiolitis obliterans syndrome

The histologic presence of bronchiolitis obliterans in a lung allograft was first described in 1984 in heart-lung recipients who developed progressive airflow obstruction on pulmonary function testing [68]. Lung biopsy of these patients revealed intraluminal polyps of fibromyxoid granulation tissue and plaques of dense submucosal eosinophilic scar (Fig. 2). The development of bronchiolitis remains a major limitation to long-term survival in lung transplantation today. It accounts for approximately 30% of all mortality after 1 year of survival after transplantation and is the largest single cause of late posttransplantation mortality [6].

Bronchiolitis obliterans is a histologic diagnosis. Unfortunately, transbronchial biopsy often provides inadequate tissue samples to identify this lesion. As a result, the ISHLT defined the term "bronchiolitis obliterans syndrome" to identify patients by decline in pulmonary function rather than by histology [69]. The system proposed staging based on FEV_1. Patients with stable lung function are defined as BOS 0; progressive declines in FEV_1 correlate with BOS stages 1 through 3. More recently, the ISHLT updated the diagnostic criteria because of concerns that the system was not sensitive enough to detect early, small, but potentially important changes in pulmo-

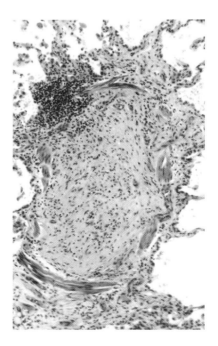

Fig. 2. Obliterative bronchiolitis. Complete fibrous obliteration of the bronchiolar lumen. Smooth muscle fibers corresponding to the bronchiolar wall surround the fibrous scar. Notice the presence of residual lymphocytic inflammation (hematoxylin and eosin stain). (Courtesy of Jose Jessurun, MD, Minneapolis, Minnesota.)

nary function. Earlier detection of BOS may allow earlier interventions that may alter the grim prognosis of this disease. As a result, the addition of mid-expiratory flow rates and a more subtle decrease in FEV_1 have been added to the diagnostic criteria (Table 3) [70].

BOS should be diagnosed only after confounding diagnoses have been ruled out. These confounding diagnoses include infection, acute rejection, anastomotic complications, disease recurrence, and aging. For single-lung transplant recipients, native lung hyperinflation (in patients who have underlying emphysema) and disease progression in the native lung should be excluded also. When pulmonary function tests reveal reduced vital capacity and FEV_1 with a normal FEV_1/forced vital capacity ratio, restrictive causes must be ruled before the patient is given the diagnosis of BOS. These restrictive causes include pleural effusion, increased body mass index, and neuromuscular weakness [70].

There are clear data to attest to the potential utility of $FEF_{25\%-75\%}$ measurements in early detection of BOS in heart-lung and bilateral-lung transplant recipients [71–74]. On the other hand, the utility of this grading system was not validated in single-lung transplant recipients at the time of its publication. Subsequently, Nathan and colleagues [75] evaluated a decrease in $FEF_{25\%-75\%}$ to less than 75% of the baseline value for its sensitivity and specificity in predicting development of BOS grade 1 in single-lung transplant recipients. The decline in $FEF_{25\%-75\%}$ was 92% sensitive and 69% specific for the future development of BOS grade 1 in patients who had chronic obstructive pulmonary disease. In patients who had

idiopathic pulmonary fibrosis, decline in $FEF_{25\%-75\%}$ was 63% sensitive and 100% specific for the development of BOS grade 1. This study was limited by its small size, and further studies are needed to validate the utility of BOS 0p in single-lung transplant recipients.

Several factors confer an increased risk for the development of BOS. These factors can be separated into two broad categories, alloimmune dependent and alloimmune independent [76]. The most widely accepted risk factor for the development of BOS is acute rejection [18–24]. The risk seems to increase for patients who have severe or persistent acute rejection despite augmentation of immunosuppression [18,56,70]. A recent report, however, suggests that asymptomatic patients who have grade A1 (minimal) rejection more than once on surveillance bronchoscopy are also at increased risk for the development of BOS [53]. Nonetheless, patients who never have documented acute rejection do go on to develop BOS, suggesting a complex relationship between these two factors.

Alloreactivity toward HLA antigens has been implicated in the development of BOS, but its relationship is less clear. Several studies found no relationship with mismatches to HLA A, B, and DR [20,23,77], whereas others have found an association between mismatches at the A locus or total mismatch at A, B, and DR loci and development of BOS [24,50,78,79]. Despite this suggestive evidence that HLA alloreactivity may be a factor in the development of BOS, the largest of these studies (>3000 patients from the United Network for Organ Sharing/ISHLT registry) found a minimally increased risk of death for HLA mismatch 1, 3, and 5 years after transplantation. This finding suggests that the effect of HLA mismatch on outcomes is quite small [77].

Distinct from HLA mismatch, several studies have found the development of anti-HLA antibodies to both class I and class II HLA is associated with the development of BOS [80–83]. A potential mechanism for the development of BOS is the binding of these HLA antibodies to class I molecules, inducing proliferation of airway epithelial cells [84]. In addition, many tissues in the lung, including vascular endothelium and bronchial epithelium, can be induced to express class II antigens by cytokines such as IL-2 and gamma interferon [85]. Therefore, direct binding of class II anti-HLA antibodies to airway epithelium may also induce epithelial injury that leads to the development of BOS [82].

Alloimmune-independent mechanisms for the development of BOS include viral infection. Cytomegalovirus pneumonitis has been associated with the

Table 3
Bronchiolitis obliterans classification system

Grade	Pulmonary function
BOS 0	$FEV_1 > 90\%$ of baseline and $FEF_{25\%-75\%} > 75\%$ of baseline
BOS 0p	FEV_1 81%–90% of baseline and/or $FEF_{25\%-75\%} \leq 75\%$ of baseline
BOS 1	FEV_1 66%–80% of baseline
BOS 2	FEV_1 51%–65% of baseline
BOS 3	$FEV_1 \leq 50\%$ of baseline

Abbreviations: BOS, bronchiolitis obliterans syndrome; $FEF_{25\%-75\%}$, mid-expiratory flow rate; FEV_1, forced expiratory volume in 1 second.
Adapted from Estenne M, Maurer JR, Boehler A, et al. Bronchiolitis obliterans syndrome 2001: an update of the diagnostic criteria. J Heart Lung Transplant 2002;21:297–310; with permission.

development of BOS in several series [18,24,79,86]. Prophylaxis with ganciclovir or immunoglobulin may help reduce the development of BOS; but this benefit must be confirmed by further study. Community-acquired respiratory viruses such as respiratory syncytial virus, parainfluenza, and influenza have been associated with the development of BOS [87,88]. There is precedent for this observation, because community-acquired respiratory viruses are known to be associated with chronic airflow obstruction (albeit rarely) in the nontransplant population.

Other factors have been implicated in the pathogenesis of BOS. It has been suggested that airway ischemia may play a role in development of BOS [76]. In addition, donor age and allograft ischemic time have been associated with BOS [89]. Non-immune primary graft dysfunction has also been suggested as a potential cause for the development of BOS [90]. Gastroesophageal reflux disease is common in the pretransplant population, particularly in patients who have cystic fibrosis and idiopathic pulmonary fibrosis [91,92]. Lung transplant surgery may increase the risk of esophageal and upper gastrointestinal dysmotility that may, along with a denervated lung, predispose the lung transplant recipient to increased risk of injury secondary to aspiration. Supportive evidence for gastrointestinal dysmotility as a contributor to the development of BOS is derived from retrospective analyses in which gastric fundoplication was associated with a decreased risk of BOS. In addition, in some cases, gastric fundoplication after BOS developed was associated with improvement in pulmonary function [93,94].

Once BOS develops, the course of the disease is variable. Some patients experience rapid loss of lung function that is relentless. Others have slowly progressive or stepwise progression of disease over a longer period [70]. Currently, treatment consists primarily of augmentation of immunosuppression. As with refractory acute rejection, a switch from cyclosporine to tacrolimus may be beneficial [60,95]. Unfortunately, these series suggest a stabilization of disease and not improvement of FEV_1 for the average patient.

Multiple other medication and immunomodulating therapies have been used in attempts to modify the course of disease. These measures include methotrexate [96], cyclophosphamide [97], total lymphoid irradiation [98,99], antilymphocyte antibody formulations [100,101], and extracorporeal photochemotherapy [65,102,103]. Although each study reports a small series of patients, their outcomes provide hope that the natural course of this disease can be inhibited through immunomodulation. Un-

fortunately, these regimens also increase the risk of toxicity to the patient, and this cumulative toxicity may outweigh the gains from stabilization of the BOS in some cases.

Potential nonimmunosuppressant therapies for the treatment of BOS include 3-hydroxy-3-methylglutaryl coenzyme A reductase inhibitors (statins). In a retrospective analysis comparing patients who received statins for treatment of hypercholesterolemia versus those who were not exposed to statins, the investigators found a significant survival advantage at 6 years in those treated with statins [104]. In addition, for patients who received statins, there was a trend toward decreased BOS ($P = .06$). The authors hypothesized that statins may be better in preventing BOS than in treating disease once it develops. Patients who received statin therapy soon after transplantation were at significantly less risk of developing BOS than patients who never received statin therapy.

Azithromycin is another agent that has been reported recently as treatment for BOS. In a small pilot study, six patients with BOS grades 1 through 3 were treated with 250 mg azithromycin daily for 5 days followed by 250 mg three times per week. Five of the six patients had improvement in FEV_1 with the treatment [105]. Similar results were found recently in another small series of patients [106]. The mechanism of action for this response is not clear. Reports have suggested azithromycin may possess anti-inflammatory properties [107,108] or nonbactericidal antimicrobial effects on *Pseudomonas* [109–111]. Alternatively, azithromycin may treat atypical infections such as mycoplasma or *Chlamydia pneumoniae* or prevent gastroesophageal reflux through its promotility actions. These promising results are limited, given the small numbers of patients and the lack of a control group. Therefore, azithromycin should be studied further.

BOS remains the major limitation to long-term success in lung transplantation. Further studies are necessary to identify the causes of this complication. Preventative strategies are likely to be more successful because, once this complication develops, treatment options are limited.

References

[1] Hardy JD, Webb WR, Dalton Jr ML, et al. Lung homotransplantation in man. JAMA 1963;186: 1065–74.
[2] Wildevuur CR, Benfield JR. A review of 23 human lung transplantations by 20 surgeons. Ann Thorac Surg 1970;9:489–515.

[3] Veith FJ. Lung transplantation. Surg Clin North Am 1978;58:357–64.

[4] Derom F, Barbier F, Ringoir S, et al. Ten-month survival after lung homotransplantation in man. J Thorac Cardiovasc Surg 1971;61:835–46.

[5] Unilateral lung transplantation for pulmonary fibrosis. Toronto Lung Transplant Group. N Engl J Med 1986;314:1140–5.

[6] Trulock EP, Edwards LB, Taylor DO, et al. The registry of the International Society for Heart and Lung Transplantation: twenty-first official adult heart transplant report–2004. J Heart Lung Transplant 2004;23:804–15.

[7] Williams GM, Hume DM, Hudson Jr RP, et al. "Hyperacute" renal-homograft rejection in man. N Engl J Med 1968;279:611–8.

[8] Kissmeyer-Nielsen F, Olsen S, Petersen VP, et al. Hyperacute rejection of kidney allografts, associated with pre-existing humoral antibodies against donor cells. Lancet 1966;2:662–5.

[9] Frost AE, Jammal CT, Cagle PT. Hyperacute rejection following lung transplantation. Chest 1996;110: 559–62.

[10] Choi JK, Kearns J, Palevsky HI, et al. Hyperacute rejection of a pulmonary allograft. Immediate clinical and pathologic findings. Am J Respir Crit Care Med 1999;160:1015–8.

[11] Bittner HB, Dunitz J, Hertz M, et al. Hyperacute rejection in single lung transplantation–case report of successful management by means of plasmapheresis and antithymocyte globulin treatment. Transplantation 2001;71:649–51.

[12] Scornik JC, Zander DS, Baz MA, et al. Susceptibility of lung transplants to preformed donor-specific HLA antibodies as detected by flow cytometry. Transplantation 1999;68:1542–6.

[13] Reinsmoen NL, Nelson K, Zeevi A. Anti-HLA antibody analysis and crossmatching in heart and lung transplantation. Transpl Immunol 2004;13:63–71.

[14] Rogers NJ, Lechler RI. Allorecognition. Am J Transplant 2001;1:97–102.

[15] Denton MD, Magee CC, Sayegh MH. Immunosuppressive strategies in transplantation. Lancet 1999; 353:1083–91.

[16] Hopkins PM, Aboyoun CL, Chhajed PN, et al. Prospective analysis of 1,235 transbronchial lung biopsies in lung transplant recipients. J Heart Lung Transplant 2002;21:1062–7.

[17] Zuckermann A, Reichenspurner H, Birsan T, et al. Cyclosporine A versus tacrolimus in combination with mycophenolate mofetil and steroids as primary immunosuppression after lung transplantation: one-year results of a 2-center prospective randomized trial. J Thorac Cardiovasc Surg 2003;125:891–900.

[18] Bando K, Paradis IL, Similo S, et al. Obliterative bronchiolitis after lung and heart-lung transplantation. an analysis of risk factors and management. J Thorac Cardiovasc Surg 1995;110:4–13 [discussion: 13–4].

[19] Whitehead B, Rees P, Sorensen K, et al. Incidence of obliterative bronchiolitis after heart-lung transplantation in children. J Heart Lung Transplant 1993;12: 903–8.

[20] Girgis RE, Tu I, Berry GJ, et al. Risk factors for the development of obliterative bronchiolitis after lung transplantation. J Heart Lung Transplant 1996;15: 1200–8.

[21] Scott JP, Higenbottam TW, Sharples L, et al. Risk factors for obliterative bronchiolitis in heart-lung transplant recipients. Transplantation 1991;51:813–7.

[22] Sharples LD, Tamm M, McNeil K, et al. Development of bronchiolitis obliterans syndrome in recipients of heart-lung transplantation–early risk factors. Transplantation 1996;61:560–6.

[23] Husain AN, Siddiqui MT, Holmes EW, et al. Analysis of risk factors for the development of bronchiolitis obliterans syndrome. Am J Respir Crit Care Med 1999;159:829–33.

[24] Kroshus TJ, Kshettry VR, Savik K, et al. Risk factors for the development of bronchiolitis obliterans syndrome after lung transplantation. J Thorac Cardiovasc Surg 1997;114:195–202.

[25] Halloran PF. Immunosuppressive drugs for kidney transplantation. N Engl J Med 2004;351:2715–29.

[26] Meyers BF, Lynch J, Trulock EP, et al. Lung transplantation: a decade of experience. Ann Surg 1999; 230:362–70 [discussion 370–1].

[27] Palmer SM, Miralles AP, Lawrence CM, et al. Rabbit antithymocyte globulin decreases acute rejection after lung transplantation: results of a randomized, prospective study. Chest 1999;116:127–33.

[28] Brock MV, Borja MC, Ferber L, et al. Induction therapy in lung transplantation: a prospective, controlled clinical trial comparing OKT3, anti-thymocyte globulin, and daclizumab. J Heart Lung Transplant 2001;20:1282–90.

[29] Bhorade SM, Jordan A, Villanueva J, et al. Comparison of three tacrolimus-based immunosuppressive regimens in lung transplantation. Am J Transplant 2003;3:1570–5.

[30] Keenan RJ, Konishi H, Kawai A, et al. Clinical trial of tacrolimus versus cyclosporine in lung transplantation. Ann Thorac Surg 1995;60:580–4 [discussion: 584–5].

[31] Palmer SM, Baz MA, Sanders L, et al. Results of a randomized, prospective, multicenter trial of mycophenolate mofetil versus azathioprine in the prevention of acute lung allograft rejection. Transplantation 2001;71:1772–6.

[32] Glanville AR, Corris PA, McNeil KD, et al. Mycophenolate mofetil (MMF) vs azathioprine (AZA) in lung transplantation for the prevention of bronchiolitis obliterans syndrome (BOS): results of a 3 year international randomised trial. J Heart Lung Transplant 2003;22:S207. Available from: http://www.science direct.com/science/article/B6VSG-47T8W48-H3/2/ fa92ba8c68e2b73b3fd286aa1c68c642. Accessed February 1, 2005.

[33] Knoop C, Haverich A, Fischer S. Immunosuppres-

sive therapy after human lung transplantation. Eur Respir J 2004;23:159–71.

[34] Cantarovich M, Besner JG, Barkun JS, et al. Two-hour cyclosporine level determination is the appropriate tool to monitor neoral therapy. Clin Transplant 1998; 12:243–9.

[35] Levy G, Thervet E, Lake J, et al. Consensus on Neoral C(2): Expert Review in Transplantation (CONCERT) Group. Patient management by neoral C(2) monitoring: an international consensus statement. Transplantation 2002;73:S12–8.

[36] Morton JM, Aboyoun CL, Malouf MA, et al. Enhanced clinical utility of de novo cyclosporine C2 monitoring after lung transplantation. J Heart Lung Transplant 2004;23:1035–9.

[37] Baz MA, Layish DT, Govert JA, et al. Diagnostic yield of bronchoscopies after isolated lung transplantation. Chest 1996;110:84–8.

[38] Trulock EP, Ettinger NA, Brunt EM, et al. The role of transbronchial lung biopsy in the treatment of lung transplant recipients. an analysis of 200 consecutive procedures. Chest 1992;102:1049–54.

[39] Millet B, Higenbottam TW, Flower CD, et al. The radiographic appearances of infection and acute rejection of the lung after heart-lung transplantation. Am Rev Respir Dis 1989;140:62–7.

[40] Kundu S, Herman SJ, Larhs A, et al. Correlation of chest radiographic findings with biopsy-proven acute lung rejection. J Thorac Imaging 1999;14: 178–84.

[41] Otulana BA, Higenbottam T, Ferrari L, et al. The use of home spirometry in detecting acute lung rejection and infection following heart-lung transplantation. Chest 1990;97:353–7.

[42] Van Muylem A, Melot C, Antoine M, et al. Role of pulmonary function in the detection of allograft dysfunction after heart-lung transplantation. Thorax 1997;52:643–7.

[43] Becker FS, Martinez FJ, Brunsting LA, et al. Limitations of spirometry in detecting rejection after single-lung transplantation. Am J Respir Crit Care Med 1994;150:159–66.

[44] Morlion B, Knoop C, Paiva M, et al. Internet-based home monitoring of pulmonary function after lung transplantation. Am J Respir Crit Care Med 2002; 165:694–7.

[45] Guilinger RA, Paradis IL, Dauber JH, et al. The importance of bronchoscopy with transbronchial biopsy and bronchoalveolar lavage in the management of lung transplant recipients. Am J Respir Crit Care Med 1995;152:2037–43.

[46] Tazelaar HD, Nilsson FN, Rinaldi M, et al. The sensitivity of transbronchial biopsy for the diagnosis of acute lung rejection. J Thorac Cardiovasc Surg 1993;105:674–8.

[47] Trulock EP, Ettinger NA, Brunt EM, et al. The role of transbronchial lung biopsy in the treatment of lung transplant recipients. An analysis of 200 consecutive procedures. Chest 1992;102:1049–54.

[48] De Hoyos A, Chamberlain D, Schvartzman R, et al. Prospective assessment of a standardized pathologic grading system for acute rejection in lung transplantation. Chest 1993;103:1813–8.

[49] Yousem SA, Berry GJ, Cagle PT, et al. Revision of the 1990 working formulation for the classification of pulmonary allograft rejection: lung rejection study group. J Heart Lung Transplant 1996;15: 1–15.

[50] El-Gamel A, Sim E, Hasleton P, et al. Transforming growth factor beta (TGF-beta) and obliterative bronchiolitis following pulmonary transplantation. J Heart Lung Transplant 1999;18:828–37.

[51] Yousem SA. Significance of clinically silent untreated mild acute cellular rejection in lung allograft recipients. Hum Pathol 1996;27:269–73.

[52] Sibley RK, Berry GJ, Tazelaar HD, et al. The role of transbronchial biopsies in the management of lung transplant recipients. J Heart Lung Transplant 1993; 12:308–24.

[53] Hopkins PM, Aboyoun CL, Chhajed PN, et al. Association of minimal rejection in lung transplant recipients with obliterative bronchiolitis. Am J Respir Crit Care Med 2004;170:1022–6.

[54] Hertz MI, Bolman RM. University of Minnesota. Physicians Transplant Program, Fairview Health Services manual of lung transplant medical care. 2nd edition. Minneapolis (MN): Fairview Publications; 2001.

[55] Kesten S, Maidenberg A, Winton T, et al. Treatment of presumed and proven acute rejection following six months of lung transplant survival. Am J Respir Crit Care Med 1995;152:1321–4.

[56] Sharples LD, McNeil K, Stewart S, et al. Risk factors for bronchiolitis obliterans: a systematic review of recent publications. J Heart Lung Transplant 2002; 21:271–81.

[57] Vitulo P, Oggionni T, Cascina A, et al. Efficacy of tacrolimus rescue therapy in refractory acute rejection after lung transplantation. J Heart Lung Transplant 2002;21:435–9.

[58] Horning NR, Lynch JP, Sundaresan SR, et al. Tacrolimus therapy for persistent or recurrent acute rejection after lung transplantation. J Heart Lung Transplant 1998;17:761–7.

[59] Onsager DR, Canver CC, Jahania MS, et al. Efficacy of tacrolimus in the treatment of refractory rejection in heart and lung transplant recipients. J Heart Lung Transplant 1999;18:448–55.

[60] Sarahrudi K, Estenne M, Corris P, et al. International experience with conversion from cyclosporine to tacrolimus for acute and chronic lung allograft rejection. J Thorac Cardiovasc Surg 2004;127: 1126–32.

[61] Cahill BC, O'Rourke MK, Strasburg KA, et al. Methotrexate for lung transplant recipients with steroid-resistant acute rejection. J Heart Lung Transplant 1996;15:1130–7.

[62] Shennib H, Massard G, Reynaud M, et al. Efficacy

of OKT3 therapy for acute rejection in isolated lung transplantation. J Heart Lung Transplant 1994;13: 514–9.

[63] Valentine VG, Robbins RC, Wehner JH, et al. Total lymphoid irradiation for refractory acute rejection in heart-lung and lung allografts. Chest 1996;109: 1184–9.

[64] Andreu G, Achkar A, Couetil JP, et al. Extracorporeal photochemotherapy treatment for acute lung rejection episode. J Heart Lung Transplant 1995;14: 793–6.

[65] Villanueva J, Bhorade SM, Robinson JA, et al. Extracorporeal photopheresis for the treatment of lung allograft rejection. Ann Transplant 2000;5:44–7.

[66] Keenan RJ, Iacono A, Dauber JH, et al. Treatment of refractory acute allograft rejection with aerosolized cyclosporine in lung transplant recipients. J Thorac Cardiovasc Surg 1997;113:335–40 [discussion 340–1].

[67] Reams BD, Davis RD, Curl J, et al. Treatment of refractory acute rejection in a lung transplant recipient with Campath 1H. Transplantation 2002;74:903–4.

[68] Burke CM, Theodore J, Dawkins KD, et al. Posttransplant obliterative bronchiolitis and other late lung sequelae in human heart-lung transplantation. Chest 1984;86:824–9.

[69] Cooper JD, Billingham M, Egan T, et al. A working formulation for the standardization of nomenclature and for clinical staging of chronic dysfunction in lung allografts. International Society for Heart and Lung Yransplantation. J Heart Lung Transplant 1993;12: 713–6.

[70] Estenne M, Maurer JR, Boehler A, et al. Bronchiolitis obliterans syndrome 2001: an update of the diagnostic criteria. J Heart Lung Transplant 2002;21: 297–310.

[71] Estenne M, Van Muylem A, Knoop C, et al. Detection of obliterative bronchiolitis after lung transplantation by indexes of ventilation distribution. Am J Respir Crit Care Med 2000;162:1047–51.

[72] Patterson GM, Wilson S, Whang JL, et al. Physiologic definitions of obliterative bronchiolitis in heartlung and double lung transplantation: a comparison of the forced expiratory flow between 25% and 75% of the forced vital capacity and forced expiratory volume in one second. J Heart Lung Transplant 1996; 15:175–81.

[73] Reynaud-Gaubert M, Thomas P, Badier M, et al. Early detection of airway involvement in obliterative bronchiolitis after lung transplantation. Functional and bronchoalveolar lavage cell findings. Am J Respir Crit Care Med 2000;161:1924–9.

[74] Finkelstein SM, Snyder M, Stibbe CE, et al. Staging of bronchiolitis obliterans syndrome using home spirometry. Chest 1999;116:120–6.

[75] Nathan SD, Barnett SD, Wohlrab J, et al. Bronchiolitis obliterans syndrome: utility of the new guidelines in single lung transplant recipients. J Heart Lung Transplant 2003;22:427–32.

[76] Estenne M, Hertz MI. Bronchiolitis obliterans after

human lung transplantation. Am J Respir Crit Care Med 2002;166:440–4.

[77] Quantz MA, Bennett LE, Meyer DM, et al. Does human leukocyte antigen matching influence the outcome of lung transplantation? An analysis of 3,549 lung transplantations. J Heart Lung Transplant 2000;19:473–9.

[78] Sundaresan S, Mohanakumar T, Smith MA, et al. HLA-A locus mismatches and development of antibodies to HLA after lung transplantation correlate with the development of bronchiolitis obliterans syndrome. Transplantation 1998;65:648–53.

[79] Heng D, Sharples LD, McNeil K, et al. Bronchiolitis obliterans syndrome: incidence, natural history, prognosis, and risk factors. J Heart Lung Transplant 1998; 17:1255–63.

[80] Jaramillo A, Smith MA, Phelan D, et al. Development of ELISA-detected anti-HLA antibodies precedes the development of bronchiolitis obliterans syndrome and correlates with progressive decline in pulmonary function after lung transplantation. Transplantation 1999;67:1155–61.

[81] Lau CL, Palmer SM, Posther KE, et al. Influence of panel-reactive antibodies on posttransplant outcomes in lung transplant recipients. Ann Thorac Surg 2000;69:1520–4.

[82] Palmer SM, Davis RD, Hadjiliadis D, et al. Development of an antibody specific to major histocompatibility antigens detectable by flow cytometry after lung transplant is associated with bronchiolitis obliterans syndrome. Transplantation 2002;74:799–804.

[83] Girnita AL, Duquesnoy R, Yousem SA, et al. HLA-specific antibodies are risk factors for lymphocytic bronchiolitis and chronic lung allograft dysfunction. Am J Transplant 2005;5:131–8.

[84] Reznik SI, Jaramillo A, Zhang L, et al. Anti-HLA antibody binding to HLA class I molecules induces proliferation of airway epithelial cells: a potential mechanism for bronchiolitis obliterans syndrome. J Thorac Cardiovasc Surg 2000;119:39–45.

[85] Zissel G, Ernst M, Rabe K, et al. Human alveolar epithelial cells type II are capable of regulating T-cell activity. J Invest Med 2000;48:66–75.

[86] Keller CA, Cagle PT, Brown RW, et al. Bronchiolitis obliterans in recipients of single, double, and heartlung transplantation. Chest 1995;107:973–80.

[87] Billings JL, Hertz MI, Savik K, et al. Respiratory viruses and chronic rejection in lung transplant recipients. J Heart Lung Transplant 2002;21:559–66.

[88] Khalifah AP, Hachem RR, Chakinala MM, et al. Respiratory viral infections are a distinct risk for bronchiolitis obliterans syndrome and death. Am J Respir Crit Care Med 2004;170:181–7.

[89] Hosenpud JD, Bennett LE, Keck BM, et al. The registry of the International Society for Heart and Lung Transplantation: seventeenth official report—2000. J Heart Lung Transplant 2000;19:909–31.

[90] Fiser SM, Tribble CG, Long SM, et al. Ischemia-reperfusion injury after lung transplantation increases

risk of late bronchiolitis obliterans syndrome. Ann Thorac Surg 2002;73:1041–7 [discussion 1047–8].

[91] Feigelson J, Girault F, Pecau Y. Gastro-oesophageal reflux and esophagitis in cystic fibrosis. Acta Paediatr Scand 1987;76:989–90.

[92] Tobin RW, Pope II CE, Pellegrini CA, et al. Increased prevalence of gastroesophageal reflux in patients with idiopathic pulmonary fibrosis. Am J Respir Crit Care Med 1998;158:1804–8.

[93] Davis Jr RD, Lau CL, Eubanks S, et al. Improved lung allograft function after fundoplication in patients with gastroesophageal reflux disease undergoing lung transplantation. J Thorac Cardiovasc Surg 2003; 125:533–42.

[94] Cantu III E, Appel III JZ, Hartwig MG, et al. Early fundoplication prevents chronic allograft dysfunction in patients with gastroesophageal reflux disease. Ann Thorac Surg 2004;78:1142–51 [discussion 1142–51].

[95] Verleden GM, Dupont LJ, Van Raemdonck D, et al. Effect of switching from cyclosporine to tacrolimus on exhaled nitric oxide and pulmonary function in patients with chronic rejection after lung transplantation. J Heart Lung Transplant 2003;22:908–13.

[96] Dusmet M, Maurer J, Winton T, et al. Methotrexate can halt the progression of bronchiolitis obliterans syndrome in lung transplant recipients. J Heart Lung Transplant 1996;15:948–54.

[97] Verleden GM, Buyse B, Delcroix M, et al. Cyclophosphamide rescue therapy for chronic rejection after lung transplantation. J Heart Lung Transplant 1999;18:1139–42.

[98] Fisher AJ, Rutherford RM, Bozzino J, et al. The safety and efficacy of total lymphoid irradiation in progressive bronchiolitis obliterans syndrome after lung transplantation. Am J Transplant 2005;5:537–43.

[99] Diamond DA, Michalski JM, Lynch JP, et al. Efficacy of total lymphoid irradiation for chronic allograft rejection following bilateral lung transplantation. Int J Radiat Oncol Biol Phys 1998;41:795–800.

[100] Snell GI, Esmore DS, Williams TJ. Cytolytic therapy for the bronchiolitis obliterans syndrome complicating lung transplantation. Chest 1996;109:874–8.

[101] Kesten S, Rajagopalan N, Maurer J. Cytolytic therapy for the treatment of bronchiolitis obliterans syndrome following lung transplantation. Transplantation 1996; 61:427–30.

[102] O'Hagan AR, Stillwell PC, Arroliga A, et al. Photopheresis in the treatment of refractory bronchiolitis obliterans complicating lung transplantation. Chest 1999;115:1459–62.

[103] Salerno CT, Park SJ, Kreykes NS, et al. Adjuvant treatment of refractory lung transplant rejection with extracorporeal photopheresis. J Thorac Cardiovasc Surg 1999;117:1063–9.

[104] Johnson BA, Iacono AT, Zeevi A, et al. Statin use is associated with improved function and survival of lung allografts. Am J Respir Crit Care Med 2003;167: 1271–8.

[105] Gerhardt SG, McDyer JF, Girgis RE, et al. Maintenance azithromycin therapy for bronchiolitis obliterans syndrome: results of a pilot study. Am J Respir Crit Care Med 2003;168:121–5.

[106] Verleden GM, Dupont LJ. Azithromycin therapy for patients with bronchiolitis obliterans syndrome after lung transplantation. Transplantation 2004;77:1465–7.

[107] Suzuki H, Asada Y, Ikeda K, et al. Inhibitory effect of erythromycin on interleukin-8 secretion from exudative cells in the nasal discharge of patients with chronic sinusitis. Laryngoscope 1999;109:407–10.

[108] Culic O, Erakovic V, Cepelak I, et al. Azithromycin modulates neutrophil function and circulating inflammatory mediators in healthy human subjects. Eur J Pharmacol 2002;450:277–89.

[109] Nagino K, Kobayashi H. Influence of macrolides on mucoid alginate biosynthetic enzyme from pseudomonas aeruginosa. Clin Microbiol Infect 1997;3: 432–9.

[110] Ichimiya T, Takeoka K, Hiramatsu K, et al. The influence of azithromycin on the biofilm formation of pseudomonas aeruginosa in vitro. Chemotherapy 1996;42:186–91.

[111] Yamasaki T, Ichimiya T, Hirai K, et al. Effect of antimicrobial agents on the piliation of Pseudomonas aeruginosa and adherence to mouse tracheal epithelium. J Chemother 1997;9:32–7.

ELSEVIER
SAUNDERS

Clin Chest Med 26 (2005) 613 – 622

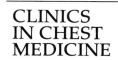

CLINICS
IN CHEST
MEDICINE

Noninfectious Pulmonary Complications After Lung Transplantation

Vivek N. Ahya, MD[a],*, Steven M. Kawut, MD, MS[b]

[a]Pulmonary, Allergy, and Critical Care Division, University of Pennsylvania School of Medicine, 832 West Gates,
3600 Spruce Street, Philadelphia, PA 19104, USA
[b]Division of Pulmonary, Allergy, and Critical Care Medicine and the Department of Epidemiology,
Columbia University College of Physicians and Surgeons, 622 West 168th Street, New York, NY 10032, USA

Lung transplantation has become an important therapeutic option for select patients who have advanced lung disease. For these patients, transplantation offers the potential for improved quality of life and long-term survival. Unfortunately, the lung transplant recipient is at risk for developing numerous complications that threaten these objectives. This article reviews several important noninfectious pulmonary complications that may occur. The absence of major posttransplantation complications, however, does not necessarily predict normal functional status and exercise capacity. The final section discusses potential mechanisms of persistent exercise limitation despite successful lung transplantation.

Primary graft dysfunction

Primary graft dysfunction (PGD) (also known as primary graft failure, severe ischemia-reperfusion injury, or reimplantation response) is a severe, acute lung injury syndrome after lung transplantation that is characterized by diffuse radiographic infiltrates in the allograft and increased alveolar–arterial oxygen gradient (Fig. 1) [1]. PGD is a diagnosis of exclusion; therefore, other causes of early graft failure such as pneumonia, pulmonary venous outflow obstruction, increased left-sided cardiac pressures, and hyperacute rejection must first be ruled out [2].

Although its pathogenesis has not been fully elucidated, recent studies suggest that PGD probably represents the result of multiple insults to the allograft resulting in increased pulmonary microvascular permeability and diffuse alveolar damage. Lung injury is initiated at the time of donor injury (thoracic trauma, aspiration, mechanical ventilation) and brain death and is amplified by a sequence of events that occur during organ retrieval, preservation, hypothermic storage, and reperfusion of the ischemic donor lung. Although most lung transplant recipients manifest some degree of ischemia-reperfusion injury, PGD identifies the subset of patients who experience the severest form of lung injury [3].

The timing of PGD is remarkably consistent across studies (within 2–3 days of transplantation). The varying incidence estimates in the literature are probably attributable to inconsistency in definition, temporal trends, and differences in surgical technique and recipient and donor characteristics. To standardize future research of PGD, the International Society for Heart and Lung Transplantation has established a severity grading system, derived from the acute respiratory distress syndrome literature and based on the ratio of arterial partial pressure of oxygen to the fraction of inspired oxygen (P/F ratio) (Table 1) [1]. A P/F ratio less than 200 within the first 48 to 72 hours after transplantation (PGD grade III) discriminates those patients who have dramatically inferior functional outcomes and survival from those who have a more favorable prognosis [4,5]. This cutoff corresponds to an incidence of approximately 15%, a rate consistent with other studies using a strict

---

* Corresponding author.
E-mail address: ahyav@uphs.upenn.edu (V.N. Ahya).

0272-5231/05/$ – see front matter © 2005 Elsevier Inc. All rights reserved.
doi:10.1016/j.ccm.2005.06.006

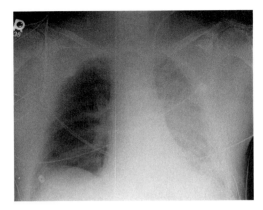

Fig. 1. Chest radiograph obtained 48 hours after left single-lung transplantation. Interstitial and alveolar infiltrates in the allograft are consistent with the diagnosis of PGD. Note that the emphysematous native lung is clear.

definition for early graft failure [6]. Less stringent oxygenation definitions have resulted in estimates approaching 50% for PGD in some transplant cohorts [7].

Certain risk factors for the development of PGD have been described. One study identified donor female sex, African American donor ethnicity, donor age of less than 21 years or more than 45 years, and a recipient diagnosis of idiopathic pulmonary arterial hypertension as risk factors for PGD [6]. Studies on the impact of prolonged graft ischemic times have yielded conflicting results [7–10]. Most recently, a large retrospective multicenter analysis has reported an increased risk of early (90-day) mortality in patients who have graft ischemic time greater than 330 minutes [10]. These findings confirm similar observations reported in the International Society for Heart and Lung Transplantation registry and suggest that, because PGD is the primary cause of early mortality after transplantation, lung ischemic times above a certain threshold may increase the risk of PGD [11,12].

There is no specific treatment for PGD that has proven efficacious. Several principles underlying the supportive care of patients who have acute respiratory distress syndrome may be helpful, however. The "leakiness" of the alveolar–pulmonary capillary barrier allows fluid translocation into the alveolar space, a problem compounded by inadequate lymphatic drainage in the new allograft. The judicious use of diuretics to maintain negative fluid balance and to reduce pulmonary venous pressure and the use of

vasopressors as needed to support organ perfusion seem prudent [13].

Conventional mechanical ventilation using low-tidal-volume strategies to reduce the risk of ventilator-induced lung injury is recommended. Independent lung ventilation may be considered in patients who have severe chronic obstructive lung disease who have developed PGD after unilateral transplantation to optimize ventilation to lungs with marked compliance differences [14]. Although inhaled nitric oxide or prostacyclin may improve oxygenation transiently, studies have not shown clinically significant benefits. A recent randomized clinical trial has shown that prophylactic administration of inhaled nitric oxide to all lung transplant recipients at the time of reperfusion neither prevents the occurrence of PGD nor improves outcomes in terms of P/F ratio, time to extubation, or length of ICU or hospital stay [15]. Additional studies will be required to determine if there is a benefit of nitric oxide when specifically targeted at patients who have evidence of graft dysfunction.

Patients who have severe PGD unresponsive to conventional therapy may benefit from early initiation (within 24–48 hours of transplantation) of extracorporeal life support; however, later use has been associated with dismal outcome [16,17]. Emergent retransplantation in the setting of ventilator-dependent respiratory failure is also associated with poor outcome [18].

PGD is a major cause of perioperative death, with studies reporting mortality rates over 60%. These patients require prolonged duration of mechanical ventilation and extended hospital stay. In addition, patients who have PGD who recover from respiratory failure and survive beyond the first transplant year continue to be at higher risk for death and on average have poorer functional outcomes than patients who do not have PGD [19,20]. Nonetheless, complete recovery is possible.

Table 1
International Society for Heart and Lung Transplantation grades of primary graft dysfunction severity

Grade	PaO$_2$/FiO$_2$	Radiographic infiltrates consistent with pulmonary edema
0	>300	Absent
1	>300	Present
2	200–300	Present
3	<200	Present

Abbreviations: FiO$_2$, fraction of inspired oxygen; PaO$_2$, arterial partial pressure of oxygen.

Native lung hyperinflation

The modern era of lung transplantation was introduced by the landmark report in 1986 from the Toronto Lung Transplant Group in which two patients who had idiopathic pulmonary fibrosis successfully underwent single-lung transplantation and achieved intermediate-term survival [21]. Patients who had pulmonary fibrosis were considered ideal candidates for single-lung transplantation because the reduced lung compliance and increased pulmonary vascular resistance of the native fibrotic lung led to preferential perfusion and ventilation of the allograft. On the other hand, patients who had emphysema were viewed as suboptimal candidates for single-lung transplantation because of concerns about preferential ventilation to the more compliant native lung. Investigators feared that profound ventilation/perfusion disparity and severe native lung hyperinflation would lead to mediastinal shift and crowding of the lung allograft, resulting in respiratory and hemodynamic compromise. These fears seemed to be substantiated in initial attempts to perform single-lung transplantation in this population [22].

Subsequent reports showed that single-lung transplantation could be performed safely in patients who have emphysema with concomitant increases in ventilation and perfusion to the allograft [23–25]. Later studies demonstrating similar short-term and intermediate-term survival between single- and double-lung recipients and excellent functional outcomes in both groups have further supported the notion that single-lung transplantation is an acceptable procedure for patients who have advanced emphysema and is perhaps a more judicious use of limited available organs [26]. Nevertheless, complications associated with native lung hyperinflation are common. These complications may be divided into two categories: acute native lung hyperinflation (ANLH) and chronic native lung hyperinflation.

ANLH is defined as early postoperative mediastinal shift and ipsilateral diaphragmatic flattening on chest radiography [27,28]. Data on the incidence and clinical significance of ANLH are somewhat conflicting. One center reported that 12 of 27 (44%) consecutive single-lung transplant recipients who had chronic obstructive pulmonary disease (COPD) developed ANLH, which was associated with increased early mortality and worse long-term pulmonary function [27]. In contrast, a review of 51 consecutive recipients at another center revealed that 16 (31%) patients developed ANLH, but only 8 (16%) were symptomatic (developed respiratory or hemodynamic instability). Although symptomatic patients had a prolonged duration of mechanical ventilation and hospital stay, 30-day mortality, forced expiratory volume in 1 second, and 6-minute walk distances were not different 1, 2, and 3 years after transplantation when compared with COPD recipients without ANLH [28].

Possible risk factors for ANLH include early graft dysfunction (magnifying the compliance differential between the allograft and native lung), prolonged positive-pressure ventilation, and severe bullous emphysema in the native lung [23,27–29]. Additionally, theoretical concerns that the right lung is more likely to cause ANLH because hepatic restriction of downward right hemidiaphragmatic movement could result in expansion into the contralateral (left) thoracic cavity have not been validated in larger case series [27,28].

Several strategies have evolved to prevent and treat ANLH. Early extubation or ventilatory strategies that permit prolonged expiration are usually adequate to prevent symptomatic ANLH. If ANLH is associated with severe gas-exchange or hemodynamic abnormalities, initiation of independent lung ventilation often leads to rapid clinical improvement. Typically, the allograft is ventilated with higher respiratory rates and positive end-expiratory pressure to promote oxygenation while the native lung receives lower respiratory rates and tidal volumes to allow emptying [30]. The requirement for a double-lumen endotracheal tube and asynchronous ventilation for independent lung ventilation is not without risk; decreased clearance of pulmonary secretions, malposition of the endotracheal tube, and the need for neuromuscular blocking agents and higher levels of sedation complicate this approach [28,30,31]. Although prophylactic lung-volume reduction surgery or bullectomy may reduce the risk of ANLH, the low incidence of symptomatic ANLH refractory to medical/ventilatory management precludes routine recommendation of this potentially risky preventative strategy [28,32].

Chronic native lung hyperinflation presents with slowly progressive dyspnea that develops months to years after single-lung transplantation for COPD. This syndrome is associated with decreasing spirometric measurements and radiographic evidence of marked mediastinal shift and allograft compression (Fig. 2). Although surgical volume reduction or lobectomy performed on the native lung have led to clinical improvement in select patients, it is important to recognize that radiographic evidence of native lung hyperinflation is quite common and usually is not clinically significant [33–37]. Thus, it is essential to consider alternative explanations for declining lung

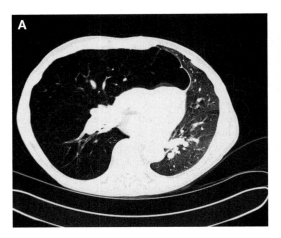
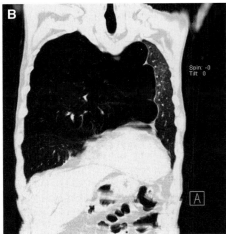

Fig. 2. (*A*) Axial and (*B*) coronal chest CT scan images obtained from a patient 4 years after left single-lung transplantation for COPD demonstrate severe chronic native lung hyperinflation. Spirometry showed a decline in both forced expiratory volume in 1 second and forced vital capacity consistent with allograft restriction by the hyperinflated native lung.

function and dyspnea such as chronic rejection, anastomotic narrowing, and infection [28,38]. Bronchoscopy with transbronchial biopsy and high-resolution CT scan of the chest may be helpful in identifying potential causes. Performance of lung-volume reduction surgery on the native lung of a recipient with a structurally abnormal allograft is unlikely to result in a clinically meaningful benefit [39].

Anastomotic complications

Lung transplantation involves completion of three anastomoses: pulmonary arterial, left atrial (encompassing the pulmonary veins), and bronchial. The airway is the most common location for anastomotic complications after lung transplantation, probably because of the disruption of the systemic blood supply. Major dehiscence of the bronchial anastomosis was once a major cause of perioperative mortality. Fortunately, refinements in surgical technique, tissue preservation, and immunosuppression have significantly reduced the risk of this life-threatening complication. Focal dehiscence is seen more commonly (in 1%–6% of cases) [40,41]. Focal dehiscence must be suspected in a transplant recipient who has a new or increasing pneumothorax and should be evaluated by performing a bronchoscopy to inspect the bronchial anastomosis directly. Focal dehiscences typically heal without surgical intervention, and reduction in corticosteroid administration is a reasonable but

unproven approach. Tube thoracostomy may be required to evacuate a persistent or large pneumothorax [14].

Narrowing of the bronchial anastomosis caused by excessive granulation tissue, fibrous stricture, or malacia is seen in 5% to 14% of patients [40,42–44]. Suspected risk factors include ischemic airway injury, telescoped rather than a modified or end-to-end bronchial anastomosis, and endobronchial infection [41,43–46]. Anastomotic narrowing may develop within several weeks of transplantation. Clues to its presence include declining spirometry, increasing sputum production, and auscultation of a focal wheeze over the anastomosis on the affected side. Direct visualization of the anastomosis during bronchoscopy is required for the diagnosis [14]. Balloon dilatation of the stenotic segment, electrocautery or laser debridement of excessive granulation tissue, and placement of an endobronchial stent are useful treatment approaches. In cases with multiple recurrences caused by granulation tissue, endobronchial brachytherapy may be attempted [47,48].

Complications of the vascular anastomoses are seen less frequently but may have devastating effects. For example, thrombus formation at the left atrial/pulmonary venous anastomotic suture line increases the risk of systemic embolization and cerebrovascular accident. Thrombi may also obstruct pulmonary venous outflow and cause severe pulmonary edema refractory to medical management [49,50]. One prospective cohort study evaluated the incidence of pulmonary venous thrombosis in 87 consecutive lung transplant recipients with transesophageal echocardiography within 48 hours of the transplant procedure. Thirteen (15%) had evidence of pulmonary venous/left atrial clot. This subset of patients had a significantly increased risk of death (90-day mortality rate of 38%). Larger thrombus size and resultant increased acceleration of flow through the narrowed pulmonary vein was associated with the poorest clinical outcome [50]. Allograft failure, multiorgan system failure, and hemorrhage caused by systemic anticoagulation were the main causes of early death. At present, there is no standardized approach to managing these patients. Patients who have symptomatic thrombi may benefit from systemic anticoagulation. Refractory hypoxemia or hemodynamic instability may require emergent surgical thrombectomy, but outcomes are usually poor [51,52].

Pulmonary artery stenosis has also been reported early and late after lung transplantation. Symptoms such as shortness of breath and signs of pulmonary hypertension and right heart failure should suggest this diagnosis. Echocardiographic evidence of increased right ventricular pressure or right ventricular dysfunction may be present [53]. Quantitative ventilation/perfusion scanning shows blood flow that is distributed unequally between lungs after bilateral transplantation or disproportionate flow to the native lung after single-lung transplantation. Pulmonary angiography usually is necessary to confirm the diagnosis of pulmonary artery anastomotic stenosis and allows therapeutic measures such as balloon dilatation and stent placement [53,54]. Surgical reconstruction is the final option for stenosis not amenable to other interventions [55].

Phrenic nerve injury

Phrenic nerve injury is relatively common after cardiac surgery. Mechanical injury from intraoperative retraction of the sternum, manipulation of the pericardium, and mediastinal dissection and hypothermic injury incurred by the use of cold topical cardioplegia have been implicated in the pathogenesis of phrenic nerve dysfunction. These risk factors are often present during the lung transplantation procedure. Thus, it is not surprising that two prospective studies of lung transplant recipients have reported phrenic nerve injury in 7% and 30%, respectively, of the study cohorts [56,57]. The significantly higher frequency found in the latter study probably reflects the use of phrenic nerve electrophysiologic testing, a sensitive method of detecting nerve injury. Phrenic nerve dysfunction has been associated with increased

morbidity, increased length of stay in the ICU, prolonged mechanical ventilation, and greater need for tracheostomy. A negative impact on long-term outcome has not been clearly established, however [56–59].

Phrenic nerve injury should be suspected in patients who are difficult to wean from mechanical ventilation, demonstrate paradoxical diaphragmatic movement on examination, and have unexplained persistent atelectasis or an elevated hemidiaphragm on radiographic studies. Patients may also report symptoms of dyspnea and orthopnea [58]. Several methods are available to evaluate for the presence of phrenic nerve injury. The "sniff test" is noninvasive and easy to perform. It involves fluoroscopic or ultrasonic evaluation of diaphragmatic motion during a rapid inspiratory maneuver with the patient in the supine position. This technique, however, is not useful if the patient requires positive-pressure mechanical ventilation. Phrenic nerve conduction studies provide a more direct method to assess phrenic nerve function and can be performed in mechanically ventilated patients [60]. Symptomatic phrenic nerve dysfunction may be managed with prolonged mechanical ventilation or the chronic use of noninvasive positive-pressure ventilation. Although dysfunction resulting from transection of the phrenic nerve is permanent, recovery of function is possible when stretch injury is the underlying mechanism.

Pleural complications

Pleural complications, especially pneumothorax, air leak, and pleural effusion, are common after lung transplantation. In a recent retrospective review of 100 consecutive lung transplant recipients, all patients had an early postoperative pleural effusion related to the allograft. Thirty-four patients developed additional acute pleural complications, including hemothorax (15), transient or persistent air leak (17), and empyema (3) [61].

Posttransplantation effusions may occur from increased alveolar capillary permeability, disruption of lymphatic drainage, and acute rejection [62]. Pleural effusions typically resolve within 2 to 3 weeks after the transplant procedure, although occasionally they may persist. An increasing effusion beyond the first few weeks after transplantation should prompt evaluation for infection, malignancy, or acute rejection [62–65].

The spontaneous resolution of most postoperative pleural effusions probably reflects improvement of ischemia-reperfusion–induced alveolar capillary injury and restoration of pulmonary lymphatics [66]. Sampling of pleural effusions in the immediate period after lung transplantation has shown that the effusion is initially bloody, exudative, and neutrophil-rich. Over the course of the next 7 days, the characteristics of the effusion evolve so that neutrophil, lactate dehydrogenase and protein concentrations decrease while macrophage and lymphocytes increase [67].

Pneumothoraces and air leaks are common early after transplantation but usually do not affect the recipient adversely. Approximately 10% of air leaks are persistent and require prolonged placement of a thoracostomy tube [61,68]. A recent study reported that this finding was associated with increased postoperative mortality [61]. If an air leak is persistent, increasing in size, or new, a bronchoscopy should be performed to evaluate for dehiscence of the bronchial anastomosis [62].

Hemothorax is a potentially life-threatening complication and should be suspected in patients who have bloody pleural output from indwelling chest tubes, opacification of the ipsilateral hemithorax, and decreasing hematocrit. This complication is more likely to occur in patients who required extensive lysis of pleural adhesions caused by previous pleurodesis or lung resection surgery during explantation of the native lung. Risk of pleural hemorrhage is increased further in recipients who require cardiopulmonary bypass, because of the requirement for intraoperative anticoagulation [61,62].

Lung cancer

Recipients of solid organ transplants have a three- to fourfold increased risk for developing posttransplantation malignancies such as skin cancer, posttransplantation lymphoproliferative disorder, sarcomas, renal cell carcinoma, and gynecologic cancers. Most of the data about the risk of cancer in transplant recipients, however, has come from large databases comprised predominantly of kidney transplant recipients. Because the major indications for lung transplantation are emphysema and idiopathic pulmonary fibrosis, diseases that are associated with an increased risk of lung cancer, single-lung recipients may be at particularly high risk for developing lung cancer.

A recent retrospective cohort study showed a bronchogenic carcinoma incidence of 1.2% in a cohort of lung transplant recipients who did not have cancer at the time of transplantation [69]. All tumors occurred in the native lung of former smokers who

received single-lung allografts (incidence of 2.4% in single-lung recipients). A large, retrospective, multicenter cohort study of 2168 consecutive lung transplant recipients (975 single-lung, 932 bilateral-lung, and 279 heart-lung transplants) from 1981 to 2001 reported a virtually identical incidence of bronchogenic carcinoma in single-lung recipients (2.5%) [70]. Again, all cases were seen in the native lung, and none were reported in patients who received bilateral or heart-lung transplants. Interestingly, the rates of lung cancer in these studies do not seem to be greater than those observed in high-risk patients (eg, smokers or patients who have COPD or idiopathic pulmonary fibrosis) in the general population [70–73]. Bronchogenic carcinoma arising in the allograft is rare, probably because of the careful donor selection process in which older age, significant history of tobacco use, and evidence of parenchymal lung disease identify organs that are unsuitable for transplantation [74].

Although the risk of developing lung cancer after lung transplantation relates largely to conventional risk factors, lung cancers that do arise seem to behave more aggressively under the influence of immunosuppression. In fact, tumor progression may be so rapid that it mimics an infectious process [69]. Whether it is the loss of antitumor immune surveillance in the immunosuppressed host or specific properties of administered immunosuppressive drugs that promote tumor growth is uncertain [75,76].

Drug toxicity

Sirolimus is a potent immunosuppressive agent that inhibits intracellular signals required for cell cycle progression, cell growth, and proliferation. It seems to impair wound healing through its inhibitory effects on fibroblast proliferation. Recently, two reports on the *de novo* administration of sirolimus after lung transplantation have showed an unusually high incidence of bronchial anastomotic dehiscence [77,78]. Pending further study, sirolimus should be used only after complete healing of the bronchial anastomosis [79].

Sirolimus-associated pulmonary toxicity has also been reported. Pathogenesis is unknown, and toxicity is not dependent on serum sirolimus levels [80,81]. Symptoms usually develop within 6 months of initiating sirolimus treatment and improve quickly with drug cessation. Patients typically present with dry cough, progressive dyspnea, fatigue, and weakness. Fever and hemoptysis may also be present [82]. Radiographic abnormalities include bilateral interstitial infiltrates, alveolar consolidation, and nodular opacities and may persist for several months after drug cessation [81]. Lymphocytic alveolitis and, less commonly, alveolar hemorrhage, are seen on analysis of bronchoalveolar lavage fluid. Histologic findings include bronchiolitis obliterans with organizing pneumonia, interstitial lymphocytic infiltrates, and alveolar hemorrhage [81–83].

Because sirolimus-associated pulmonary toxicity is potentially reversible, it is important to consider it in the differential diagnosis for dyspnea and radiographic infiltrates in the lung transplant recipient [84].

Exercise limitation

Although lung transplantation can lead to significant improvement in pulmonary function and exercise capacity, peak exercise performance remains suboptimal. Studies investigating exercise performance using cardiopulmonary exercise testing after single- and double-lung transplantation show a reduced anaerobic threshold and reduced maximum oxygen consumption despite the absence of significant cardiac or ventilatory limitations implicating peripheral skeletal muscle dysfunction as causes of exercise limitation [85–87]. A recent study using phosphorus magnetic resonance spectroscopy showed that transplant recipients asked to perform knee extension exercises to exhaustion had a lower resting pH in the quadriceps muscle and an earlier drop in pH than seen in healthy volunteers; this observation supports the notion that impaired peripheral muscle oxidative capacity is an important contributing factor [88]. These findings are consistent with the clinical observation that, after transplantation, many patients report leg fatigue, rather than dyspnea, as the predominant exercise-limiting symptom [86].

Patients who have advanced lung disease, especially COPD, are often profoundly deconditioned and have reduced skeletal muscle mass and weakness before transplantation [89]. Peripheral muscle biopsies from these patients reveal changes in skeletal muscle fiber-types. There is a marked reduction in fatigue-resistant, mitochondria-rich type I fibers and a shift toward type IIb fibers, which are better suited for anaerobic metabolism [90]. Posttransplantation interventions further contribute to reducing peripheral muscle oxidative phosphorylation. *In vivo* and *in vitro* studies have shown that the calcineurin inhibitor class of immunosuppressive drugs (cyclosporine, tacrolimus) can interfere directly with mitochondrial function [91–93]. Despite suboptimal peak exercise performance, most patients are able to resume an active lifestyle and report no limitations to exercise [11].

References

[1] Christie JD, Carby M, Bag R, et al. Report of the ISHLT Working Group: definition. J Heart Lung Transplant, in press.

[2] Levine SM, Angel LF. Primary graft failure: who is at risk? Chest 2003;124(4):1190–2.

[3] de Perrot M, Liu M, Waddell TK, et al. Ischemia-reperfusion-induced lung injury. Am J Respir Crit Care Med 2003;167(4):490–511.

[4] Christie JD, Ahya VN, Sager JS, et al. ISHLT PGD grade predicts differential mortality following lung transplantation [abstract # 90]. J Heart Lung Transplant 2005;24(2S):S71.

[5] Prekker ME, Nath DS, Johnson AC, et al. Validation of the proposed ISHLT grading system for primary graft dysfunction following lung transplantation [abstract #91]. J Heart Lung Transplant 2005;24(2S):S72.

[6] Christie JD, Kotloff RM, Pochettino A, et al. Clinical risk factors for primary graft failure following lung transplantation. Chest 2003;124(4):1232–41.

[7] Thabut G, Vinatier I, Stern JB, et al. Primary graft failure following lung transplantation: predictive factors of mortality. Chest 2002;121(6):1876–82.

[8] King RC, Binns OA, Rodriguez F, et al. Reperfusion injury significantly impacts clinical outcome after pulmonary transplantation. Ann Thorac Surg 2000;69(6):1681–5.

[9] Christie JD, Bavaria JE, Palevsky HI, et al. Primary graft failure following lung transplantation. Chest 1998;114(1):51–60.

[10] Thabut G, Mal H, Cerrina J, et al. Graft ischemic time and outcome of lung transplantation: a multicenter analysis. Am J Respir Crit Care Med 2005;171(7):786–91.

[11] Trulock EP, Edwards LB, Taylor DO, et al. The Registry of the International Society for Heart and Lung Transplantation: twenty-first official adult lung and heart-lung transplant report—2004. J Heart Lung Transplant 2004;23(7):804–15.

[12] Christie JD. Lung allograft ischemic time: crossing the threshold. Am J Respir Crit Care Med 2005;171(7):673–4.

[13] Pilcher DV, Scheinkestel CD, Snell GI, et al. High central venous pressure is associated with prolonged mechanical ventilation and increased mortality after lung transplantation. J Thorac Cardiovasc Surg 2005;129(4):912–8.

[14] Kotloff RM, Ahya VN, Crawford SW. Pulmonary complications of solid organ and hematopoietic stem cell transplantation. Am J Respir Crit Care Med 2004;170(1):22–48.

[15] Meade MO, Granton JT, Matte-Martyn A, et al. A

randomized trial of inhaled nitric oxide to prevent ischemia-reperfusion injury after lung transplantation. Am J Respir Crit Care Med 2003;167(11):1483–9.

[16] Nguyen DQ, Kulick DM, Bolman III RM, et al. Temporary ECMO support following lung and heart-lung transplantation. J Heart Lung Transplant 2000; 19(3):313–6.

[17] Oto T, Rosenfeldt F, Rowland M, et al. Extracorporeal membrane oxygenation after lung transplantation: evolving technique improves outcomes. Ann Thorac Surg 2004;78(4):1230–5.

[18] Novick RJ, Stitt LW, Al-Kattan K, et al. Pulmonary retransplantation: predictors of graft function and survival in 230 patients. Pulmonary Retransplant Registry. Ann Thorac Surg 1998;65(1):227–34.

[19] Christie JD, Sager JS, Kimmel SE, et al. Impact of primary graft failure on outcomes following lung transplantation. Chest 2005;127(1):161–5.

[20] Christie JD, Kotloff RM, Ahya VN, et al. The effect of primary graft dysfunction on survival after lung transplantation. Am J Respir Crit Care Med 2005;171(11): 1312–6.

[21] Toronto Lung Transplant Group. Unilateral lung transplantation for pulmonary fibrosis. N Engl J Med 1986; 314(18):1140–5.

[22] Stevens PM, Johnson PC, Bell RL, et al. Regional ventilation and perfusion after lung transplantation in patients with emphysema. N Engl J Med 1970;282(5):245–9.

[23] Veith FJ, Koerner SK, Siegelman SS, et al. Single lung transplantation in experimental and human emphysema. Ann Surg 1973;178(4):463–76.

[24] Mal H, Andreassian B, Pamela F, et al. Unilateral lung transplantation in end-stage pulmonary emphysema. Am Rev Respir Dis 1989;140(3):797–802.

[25] Marinelli WA, Hertz MI, Shumway SJ, et al. Single lung transplantation for severe emphysema. J Heart Lung Transplant 1992;11(3 Pt 1):577–82 [discussion: 582–3].

[26] Pochettino A, Kotloff RM, Rosengard BR, et al. Bilateral versus single lung transplantation for chronic obstructive pulmonary disease: intermediate-term results. Ann Thorac Surg 2000;70(6):1813–8 [discussion: 1818–9].

[27] Yonan NA, el-Gamel A, Egan J, et al. Single lung transplantation for emphysema: predictors for native lung hyperinflation. J Heart Lung Transplant 1998; 17(2):192–201.

[28] Weill D, Torres F, Hodges TN, et al. Acute native lung hyperinflation is not associated with poor outcomes after single lung transplant for emphysema. J Heart Lung Transplant 1999;18(11):1080–7.

[29] Mal H, Brugiere O, Sleiman C, et al. Morbidity and mortality related to the native lung in single lung transplantation for emphysema. J Heart Lung Transplant 2000;19(2):220–3.

[30] Mitchell JB, Shaw AD, Donald S, et al. Differential lung ventilation after single-lung transplantation for emphysema. J Cardiothorac Vasc Anesth 2002;16(4): 459–62.

[31] Gavazzeni V, Iapichino G, Mascheroni D, et al. Prolonged independent lung respiratory treatment after single lung transplantation in pulmonary emphysema. Chest 1993;103(1):96–100.

[32] Todd TR, Perron J, Winton TL, et al. Simultaneous single-lung transplantation and lung volume reduction. Ann Thorac Surg 1997;63(5):1468–70.

[33] Le Pimpec-Barthes F, Debrosse D, Cuenod CA, et al. Late contralateral lobectomy after single-lung transplantation for emphysema. Ann Thorac Surg 1996; 61(1):231–4.

[34] Kroshus TJ, Bolman III RM, Kshettry VR. Unilateral volume reduction after single-lung transplantation for emphysema. Ann Thorac Surg 1996;62(2):363–8.

[35] Fitton TP, Bethea BT, Borja MC, et al. Pulmonary resection following lung transplantation. Ann Thorac Surg 2003;76(5):1680–5 [discussion: 1685–6].

[36] Estenne M, Cassart M, Poncelet P, et al. Volume of graft and native lung after single-lung transplantation for emphysema. Am J Respir Crit Care Med 1999; 159(2):641–5.

[37] Venuta F, De Giacomo T, Rendina EA, et al. Thoracoscopic volume reduction of the native lung after single lung transplantation for emphysema. Am J Respir Crit Care Med 1998;157(1):292–3.

[38] Moy ML, Loring SH, Ingenito EP, et al. Causes of allograft dysfunction after single lung transplantation for emphysema: extrinsic restriction versus intrinsic obstruction. Brigham and Women's Hospital Lung Transplantation Group. J Heart Lung Transplant 1999; 18(10):986–93.

[39] Schulman LL, O'Hair DP, Cantu E, et al. Salvage by volume reduction of chronic allograft rejection in emphysema. J Heart Lung Transplant 1999;18(2): 107–12.

[40] Schmid RA, Boehler A, Speich R, et al. Bronchial anastomotic complications following lung transplantation: still a major cause of morbidity? Eur Respir J 1997;10(12):2872–5.

[41] Schroder C, Scholl F, Daon E, et al. A modified bronchial anastomosis technique for lung transplantation. Ann Thorac Surg 2003;75(6):1697–704.

[42] Chhajed PN, Malouf MA, Tamm M, et al. Interventional bronchoscopy for the management of airway complications following lung transplantation. Chest 2001;120(6):1894–9.

[43] Alvarez A, Algar J, Santos F, et al. Airway complications after lung transplantation: a review of 151 anastomoses. Eur J Cardiothorac Surg 2001;19(4): 381–7.

[44] Date H, Trulock EP, Arcidi JM, et al. Improved airway healing after lung transplantation. An analysis of 348 bronchial anastomoses. J Thorac Cardiovasc Surg 1995;110(5):1424–32 [discussion: 1432–3].

[45] Shennib H, Massard G. Airway complications in lung transplantation. Ann Thorac Surg 1994;57(2):506–11.

[46] Garfein ES, Ginsberg ME, Gorenstein L, et al. Superiority of end-to-end versus telescoped bronchial anastomosis in single lung transplantation for pulmo-

nary emphysema. J Thorac Cardiovasc Surg 2001; 121(1):149–54.

[47] Halkos ME, Godette KD, Lawrence EC, et al. High dose rate brachytherapy in the management of lung transplant airway stenosis. Ann Thorac Surg 2003; 76(2):381–4.

[48] Kennedy AS, Sonett JR, Orens JB, et al. High dose rate brachytherapy to prevent recurrent benign hyperplasia in lung transplant bronchi: theoretical and clinical considerations. J Heart Lung Transplant 2000;19(2):155–9.

[49] Leibowitz DW, Smith CR, Michler RE, et al. Incidence of pulmonary vein complications after lung transplantation: a prospective transesophageal echocardiographic study. J Am Coll Cardiol 1994;24(3):671–5.

[50] Schulman LL, Anandarangam T, Leibowitz DW, et al. Four-year prospective study of pulmonary venous thrombosis after lung transplantation. J Am Soc Echocardiogr 2001;14(8):806–12.

[51] Shah AS, Michler RE, Downey RJ, et al. Management strategies for pulmonary vein thrombosis following single lung transplantation. J Card Surg 1995;10(2): 169–78.

[52] Nagahiro I, Horton M, Wilson M, et al. Pulmonary vein thrombosis treated successfully by thrombectomy after bilateral sequential lung transplantation: report of a case. Surg Today 2003;33(4):282–4.

[53] Waurick PE, Kleber FX, Ewert R, et al. Pulmonary artery stenosis 5 years after single lung transplantation in primary pulmonary hypertension. J Heart Lung Transplant 1999;18(12):1243–5.

[54] Ferretti G, Boutelant M, Thony F, et al. Successful stenting of a pulmonary arterial stenosis after a single lung transplant. Thorax 1995;50(9):1011–2 [discussion: 1016–7].

[55] Soriano CM, Gaine SP, Conte JV, et al. Anastomotic pulmonary hypertension after lung transplantation for primary pulmonary hypertension: report of surgical correction. Chest 1999;116(2):564–6.

[56] Dorffner R, Eibenberger K, Youssefzadeh S, et al. Diaphragmatic dysfunction after heart or lung transplantation. J Heart Lung Transplant 1997;16(5):566–9.

[57] Sheridan Jr PH, Cheriyan A, Doud J, et al. Incidence of phrenic neuropathy after isolated lung transplantation. The Loyola University Lung Transplant Group. J Heart Lung Transplant 1995;14(4):684–91.

[58] Maziak DE, Maurer JR, Kesten S. Diaphragmatic paralysis: a complication of lung transplantation. Ann Thorac Surg 1996;61(1):170–3.

[59] Ferdinande P, Bruyninckx F, Van Raemdonck D, et al. Phrenic nerve dysfunction after heart-lung and lung transplantation. J Heart Lung Transplant 2004;23(1): 105–9.

[60] Dimopoulou I, Daganou M, Dafni U, et al. Phrenic nerve dysfunction after cardiac operations: electrophysiologic evaluation of risk factors. Chest 1998; 113(1):8–14.

[61] Ferrer J, Roldan J, Roman A, et al. Acute and chronic pleural complications in lung transplantation. J Heart Lung Transplant 2003;22(11):1217–25.

[62] Judson MA, Sahn SA. The pleural space and organ transplantation. Am J Respir Crit Care Med 1996; 153(3):1153–65.

[63] Bergin CJ, Castellino RA, Blank N, et al. Acute lung rejection after heart-lung transplantation: correlation of findings on chest radiographs with lung biopsy results. AJR Am J Roentgenol 1990;155(1):23–7.

[64] Judson MA, Handy JR, Sahn SA. Pleural effusion from acute lung rejection. Chest 1997;111(4):1128–30.

[65] Shitrit D, Izbicki G, Fink G, et al. Late postoperative pleural effusion following lung transplantation: characteristics and clinical implications. Eur J Cardiothorac Surg 2003;23(4):494–6.

[66] Ruggiero R, Fietsam Jr R, Thomas GA, et al. Detection of canine allograft lung rejection by pulmonary lymphoscintigraphy. J Thorac Cardiovasc Surg 1994; 108(2):253–8.

[67] Judson MA, Handy JR, Sahn SA. Pleural effusions following lung transplantation. Time course, characteristics, and clinical implications. Chest 1996;109(5): 1190–4.

[68] Herridge MS, de Hoyos AL, Chaparro C, et al. Pleural complications in lung transplant recipients. J Thorac Cardiovasc Surg 1995;110(1):22–6.

[69] Arcasoy SM, Hersh C, Christie JD, et al. Bronchogenic carcinoma complicating lung transplantation. J Heart Lung Transplant 2001;20(10):1044–53.

[70] Collins J, Kazerooni EA, Lacomis J, et al. Bronchogenic carcinoma after lung transplantation: frequency, clinical characteristics, and imaging findings. Radiology 2002;224(1):131–8.

[71] Henschke CI, McCauley DI, Yankelevitz DF, et al. Early Lung Cancer Action Project: overall design and findings from baseline screening. Lancet 1999; 354(9173):99–105.

[72] Ma Y, Seneviratne CK, Koss M. Idiopathic pulmonary fibrosis and malignancy. Curr Opin Pulm Med 2001; 7(5):278–82.

[73] Hubbard R, Venn A, Lewis S, et al. Lung cancer and cryptogenic fibrosing alveolitis. A population-based cohort study. Am J Respir Crit Care Med 2000;161(1): 5–8.

[74] Orens JB, Boehler A, de Perrot M, et al. A review of lung transplant donor acceptability criteria. J Heart Lung Transplant 2003;22(11):1183–200.

[75] Kotloff RM, Ahya VN. Medical complications of lung transplantation. Eur Respir J 2004;23(2):334–42.

[76] Hojo M, Morimoto T, Maluccio M, et al. Cyclosporine induces cancer progression by a cell-autonomous mechanism. Nature 1999;397(6719):530–4.

[77] Groetzner J, Kur F, Spelsberg F, et al. Airway anastomosis complications in de novo lung transplantation with sirolimus-based immunosuppression. J Heart Lung Transplant 2004;23(5):632–8.

[78] King-Biggs MB, Dunitz JM, Park SJ, et al. Airway anastomotic dehiscence associated with use of sirolimus immediately after lung transplantation. Transplantation 2003;75(9):1437–43.

[79] Bhorade SM, Ahya V, Kotloff RM, et al. Comparison

of sirolimus versus azathioprine in a tacrolimus based immunosuppressive regimen in lung transplantation. J Heart Lung Transplant 2004;23(2):S113.

[80] Singer SJ, Tiernan R, Sullivan EJ. Interstitial pneumonitis associated with sirolimus therapy in renal-transplant recipients. N Engl J Med 2000;343(24): 1815–6.

[81] Pham PT, Pham PC, Danovitch GM, et al. Sirolimus-associated pulmonary toxicity. Transplantation 2004; 77(8):1215–20.

[82] Morelon E, Stern M, Israel-Biet D, et al. Characteristics of sirolimus-associated interstitial pneumonitis in renal transplant patients. Transplantation 2001;72(5): 787–90.

[83] Vlahakis NE, Rickman OB, Morgenthaler T. Sirolimus-associated diffuse alveolar hemorrhage. Mayo Clin Proc 2004;79(4):541–5.

[84] McWilliams TJ, Levvey BJ, Russell PA, et al. Interstitial pneumonitis associated with sirolimus: a dilemma for lung transplantation. J Heart Lung Transplant 2003;22(2):210–3.

[85] Levy RD, Ernst P, Levine SM, et al. Exercise performance after lung transplantation. J Heart Lung Transplant 1993;12(1 Pt 1):27–33.

[86] Williams TJ, Patterson GA, McClean PA, et al. Maximal exercise testing in single and double lung transplant recipients. Am Rev Respir Dis 1992;145(1):101–5.

[87] Schwaiblmair M, Reichenspurner H, Muller C, et al.

Cardiopulmonary exercise testing before and after lung and heart-lung transplantation. Am J Respir Crit Care Med 1999;159(4 Pt 1):1277–83.

[88] Evans AB, Al-Himyary AJ, Hrovat MI, et al. Abnormal skeletal muscle oxidative capacity after lung transplantation by 31P-MRS. Am J Respir Crit Care Med 1997;155(2):615–21.

[89] Skeletal muscle dysfunction in chronic obstructive pulmonary disease. A statement of the American Thoracic Society and European Respiratory Society. Am J Respir Crit Care Med 1999;159(4 Pt 2):S1–40.

[90] Jacobsson P, Jorfeldt L, Brundin A. Skeletal muscle metabolites and fibre types in patients with advanced chronic obstructive pulmonary disease (COPD), with and without chronic respiratory failure. Eur Respir J 1990;3(2):192–6.

[91] McKenna MJ, Fraser SF, Li JL, et al. Impaired muscle Ca2 + and K + regulation contribute to poor exercise performance post-lung transplantation. J Appl Physiol 2003;95(4):1606–16.

[92] Wang XN, Williams TJ, McKenna MJ, et al. Skeletal muscle oxidative capacity, fiber type, and metabolites after lung transplantation. Am J Respir Crit Care Med 1999;160(1):57–63.

[93] Mercier JG, Hokanson JF, Brooks GA. Effects of cyclosporine A on skeletal muscle mitochondrial respiration and endurance time in rats. Am J Respir Crit Care Med 1995;151(5):1532–6.

Clin Chest Med 26 (2005) 623 – 629

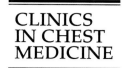

Noninfectious Pulmonary Complications of Liver, Heart, and Kidney Transplantation

Robert M. Kotloff, MD

Section of Advanced Lung Disease and Lung Transplantation, Pulmonary, Allergy, and Critical Care Division,
University of Pennsylvania Medical Center, 838 West Gates Building, 3400 Spruce Street, Philadelphia, PA 19104, USA

Because of their chronically immunosuppressed status, solid organ transplant recipients are continually at risk for infectious pulmonary complications. In addition, however, there are a number of noninfectious pulmonary complications that plague the transplant recipient. These complications arise because of numerous factors, including the underlying conditions that preceded transplantation, the transplant surgery itself, and toxicity of posttransplantation medications. This article focuses on noninfectious pulmonary complications in the three largest recipient populations: liver, kidney, and heart. Complications affecting the lung transplant population are discussed by Ahya and Kawut elsewhere in this volume.

Acute respiratory failure

Among the solid organ transplant populations under consideration in this article, the incidence of perioperative acute respiratory failure is highest in association with liver transplantation. A number of factors contribute to this risk, including the need for extensive upper abdominal surgery, marked intravascular volume shifts and volume overload, aggressive blood product support, and a relatively high frequency of postoperative pneumonia. Additionally, patients undergoing liver transplantation are often critically ill at the time of transplantation, and it is usual for patients to have been supported on mechanical ventilation for varying periods before trans-

plantation. Patients with fulminant hepatic failure are particularly predisposed to noncardiogenic pulmonary edema as a component of their liver failure. In a recent survey of 546 liver transplant recipients, Glanemann and colleagues [1] found that 11% of patients required mechanical ventilatory support beyond 24 hours. Risk factors for prolonged ventilator support included acute liver failure before transplantation, severe postoperative graft dysfunction, and retransplantation. All patients eventually were extubated, but 36% of those who had been ventilated longer than 24 hours and 12% of those ventilated for less than 24 hours required reintubation. The most common indications for reintubation were pneumonia, encephalopathy, and surgical bleeding [2]. The need for reintubation was associated with significantly poorer survival. In a small series of 44 liver transplant recipients, Pirat and colleagues [3] reported five episodes (11%) of acute postoperative respiratory failure, precipitated by pneumonia in three patients and by pulmonary edema resulting from volume overload in two.

Acute respiratory distress syndrome (ARDS) is a particularly lethal cause of postoperative respiratory failure after liver transplantation. The reported incidence ranges from 4% to 16%, with mortality as high as 80% to 100% [4,5]. Sepsis is the most common risk factor reported, but other potential risk factors include massive blood transfusions, transfusion-related acute lung injury, aspiration, and the use of muromonab-CD3 (OKT3) antilymphocyte therapy [6].

The risk of respiratory failure and acute lung injury is considerably lower after heart and kidney transplantation than after liver transplantation. In a

E-mail address: kotloff@mail.med.upenn.edu

0272-5231/05/$ – see front matter © 2005 Elsevier Inc. All rights reserved.
doi:10.1016/j.ccm.2005.06.011

chestmed.theclinics.com

series of 200 heart transplant procedures, prolonged respiratory failure requiring tracheostomy was reported in only seven cases (4.4%); five of the seven cases occurred within the first 6 months after transplantation. Perioperative respiratory failure was documented in 4% of 178 kidney transplant recipients from the University of Pittsburgh [7]. In a retrospective review of a national kidney transplant database encompassing more than 42,000 transplants, ARDS was documented in only 86 patients (0.2%), and only one of these cases occurred within the perioperative period [8]. Graft failure and the use of anti-lymphocyte globulin were associated with an increased risk of developing ARDS in multivariate analysis. Twenty-eight day mortality was 52% among the kidney transplant recipients who developed ARDS.

There has been a growing trend favoring use of noninvasive ventilation for a variety of patient populations with respiratory failure. The clinical efficacy of this modality in the solid organ transplant population was examined recently in a prospective, randomized trial [9]. Forty patients who had acute hypoxemic respiratory failure were enrolled; 20 patients were randomly assigned to receive noninvasive mechanical ventilation, and 20 were assigned to a standard-treatment group treated with supplemental oxygen using a Venturi mask. Major causes for respiratory failure included ARDS, mucus plugging/atelectasis, cardiogenic pulmonary edema, and pneumonia. Noninvasive ventilation was associated with a significant reduction in endotracheal intubation (20% versus 70%), severe sepsis and septic shock (20% versus 50%), and decreased ICU mortality (20% versus 50%), although there was no difference in overall in-hospital mortality. Based on this study and multiple studies documenting efficacy in other patient populations, the use of noninvasive ventilation is recommended as an initial ventilatory modality in appropriately selected organ transplant recipients who have hypoxemic respiratory failure.

Pleural effusions

Perioperative pleural effusions are present in 40% to 100% of liver transplant recipients [3,10]. Effusions are transudative and typically are right sided or bilateral but rarely are exclusively on the left. Disruption of diaphragmatic lymphatics during hepatectomy has been postulated to be the principal mechanism of fluid accumulation [10]. Other contributing mechanisms include volume overload, hypoalbuminemia, and atelectasis. Effusions may enlarge

during the first postoperative week but typically resolve by the third week. The need for drainage because of perceived respiratory compromise has been reported in up to 31% of patients [3,5,10]. Effusions that continue to enlarge beyond the first week, persist beyond 3 weeks, or involve only the left hemithorax should be sampled to rule out other causes [10]. Persistent or enlarging effusions should also prompt consideration of subdiaphragmatic processes including hematoma, biloma, or subphrenic abscess.

Small, bilateral or left-sided pleural effusions are a common perioperative phenomenon after cardiac surgery, and such effusions can transiently accompany heart transplantation. Beyond the perioperative period, noninfectious pleural effusions have been reported in 4% to 9% of heart transplant recipients [10,11]. A multitude of causes for these effusions have been identified, including malignancy, pericarditis, hemothorax, chylothorax, and idiopathic [10].

Pleural effusions encountered early after kidney transplantation are most likely caused by volume overload. A rare cause of early posttransplantation effusions in this patient population is urinothorax, arising from obstruction of the transplanted ureter [10,12,13]. The diagnosis of urinothorax rests on demonstration of a transudative effusion with a pH of less than 7.3 and a pleural fluid-to-serum creatinine ratio greater than 1.0 [10].

Diaphragmatic dysfunction

Right-sided diaphragmatic dysfunction is a common complication of liver transplantation. It is postulated to result from crush injury to the right phrenic nerve by the suprahepatic vena caval clamp placed during surgery [14]. To investigate the frequency and significance of this complication, McAlister and colleagues [14] used transcutaneous electrophysiologic testing of the phrenic nerves and diaphragmatic ultrasound in a prospective study of 48 liver transplant recipients. Evidence of delayed or absent right-sided phrenic nerve conduction was found in 79% of patients, whereas the left phrenic nerve conducted normally in all cases. In 38% of patients, associated right diaphragmatic paralysis was documented by ultrasound. Phrenic nerve injury was not associated with increased duration of mechanical ventilatory support or prolonged hospital stay. In a subset of patients followed with serial testing, abnormalities in phrenic nerve conduction and diaphragmatic excursion normalized by 9 months after surgery.

Limited data suggest that diaphragmatic dysfunction caused by phrenic nerve injury is also common after heart transplantation. Using ultrasound and fluoroscopy to assess diaphragmatic movement, Dorffner and colleagues [15] documented a 12% incidence of diaphragmatic dysfunction among 33 heart transplant recipients. Abnormalities predominantly involved the right hemidiaphragm. Diaphragmatic dysfunction was associated with an increased risk of pneumonia and a trend toward increased length of intubation compared with recipients with normal function.

Diaphragmatic hernia

Diaphragmatic hernias have been reported in heart transplant recipients who had left ventricular assist devices (LVAD) implanted before transplantation. These devices are placed either preperitoneally or intraperitoneally in the left upper quadrant. The inflow cannula penetrates the left hemidiaphragm and attaches to the left ventricle. The outflow cannula emerges from the ascending aorta and crosses anterior to the diaphragm near the midline. At the time of heart transplantation, the LVAD is explanted, and the left-sided diaphragmatic defect is routinely repaired. Repair of the anterior diaphragmatic defect is not necessarily standard practice, however; it has been argued this repair would add to the operative time and that midline scarring would close the rent naturally [16]. In the largest published series, Chatterjee and colleagues [16] reported diaphragmatic hernias in 8 of 67 heart transplant recipients with prior LVADs. The prevalence was 16% among the subset of patients in whom closure of the anterior midline diaphragmatic defect was not performed, and in all cases the hernia arose at the site of the unrepaired midline defect. In contrast, only 1 of 22 patients (4%) experienced this complication when the surgical procedure was modified to include routine closure of the anterior defect. That case, as well as others reported in the literature, involved herniation through a previously closed left-sided defect [16–18].

Patients with diaphragmatic hernias can be entirely asymptomatic, experience subacute gastrointestinal symptoms (abdominal pain, nausea, vomiting), or present emergently with colonic incarceration. Chest radiographs can be nonspecific, demonstrating only an ill-defined opacity at the base of the right or left lung (Fig. 1A). More suggestive findings include the presence of air within the opacity or actual visualization of colonic haustra. The diagnosis usually can be established definitively with CT of the chest and abdomen after administration of oral contrast agent (Fig. 1B). Surgical repair, using conventional laparotomy or performed laparoscopically, is indicated even in asymptomatic cases because of the risk of incarceration.

Metastatic pulmonary calcification

Deposition of calcium salts in the lung parenchyma and other organs is a well-described complication of chronic renal failure. In this setting, the deposition is thought to be caused by alterations in calcium and phosphate metabolism and associated secondary hyperparathyroidism. Since the initial descriptions, cases arising after kidney transplantation

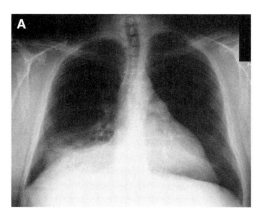
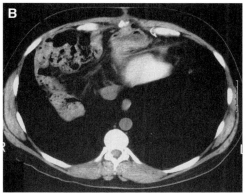

Fig. 1. Diaphragmatic hernia after heart transplantation. (*A*) Chest radiograph showing an opacity at the right base with ill-defined borders. (*B*) CT of the chest after oral administration of contrast agent demonstrates loops of bowel within the right hemithorax.

have been reported. In some of these cases, development of metastatic pulmonary calcification occurred in the setting of graft failure [19,20]. Less easily explained are reports of renal transplant recipients who developed this complication despite normal graft function and normal serum calcium and phosphate levels [21,22].

Metastatic pulmonary calcification also has been described in liver transplant recipients, with a reported incidence in two series of 5.2% and 47% [23,24]. Again, renal failure was a common but not invariable feature in these patients. Munoz and colleagues [24] found that all seven liver transplant recipients in their series had elevated serum parathyroid levels, including two patients who did not have renal insufficiency. Patients who developed metastatic calcification also had received significantly more blood products and elemental calcium than those without this complication, but no difference was detected in serum levels of calcium, phosphate, or vitamin D. The authors speculated that secondary hyperparathyroidism, caused by transient hypocalcemia induced by citrate-containing blood products and, in some cases, by renal insufficiency contributed to the soft tissue deposition of calcium.

Metastatic pulmonary calcification often is clinically silent but when extensive may cause restrictive physiology with impaired diffusion, hypoxemia, and, rarely, fulminant respiratory failure [19,25,26]. Chest radiographs typically reveal single or multiple nodular opacities or areas of alveolar consolidation (Fig. 2A) [27]. Because calcification often is not apparent on the plain-film radiographs, the radiographic picture is easily confused with more ominous processes such as infection, malignancy, or pulmonary edema. CT scan is helpful in establishing the diagnosis by demonstrating areas of high attenuation (>100 Hounsfield units), consistent with calcification, within the parenchymal opacities (Fig. 2B) [27]. There may be associated calcification of the bronchial walls, myocardium, or vessels of the chest wall [28]. Demonstration by bone scintigraphy of uptake of technetium-99m in the lung is another useful means of establishing a diagnosis. In rare instances of diagnostic uncertainty, transbronchial or surgical lung biopsy may be necessary. There is no established treatment for metastatic pulmonary calcification. Fortunately, the prognosis is generally quite favorable.

Pulmonary neoplasm

Posttransplantation lymphoproliferative disorder is the most common noncutaneous neoplasm encountered in the solid organ transplant populations, and it often presents with intrathoracic disease, particularly in heart transplant recipients. This topic is reviewed in detail by Loren and Tsai elsewhere in this issue. Among heart transplant recipients, bronchogenic carcinoma is the second most common noncutaneous neoplasm, with a prevalence of up to 4% reported in published series [29–31]. The relatively high prevalence in this transplant population seems to reflect a high rate of cigarette smoking, which predisposes patients to lung cancer and to ischemic cardiomyopathy, a common indication for heart transplantation. Indeed, a history of smoking was nearly universal

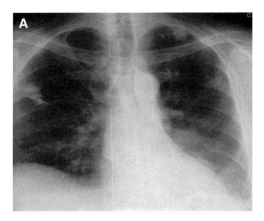
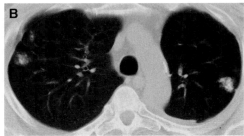

Fig. 2. Metastatic pulmonary calcification in an asymptomatic liver transplant recipient. (*A*) Chest radiograph demonstrates multifocal nodular opacities without obvious calcification. (*B*) CT scan reveals areas of high attenuation within the nodules, consistent with focal calcification. (*From* Kotloff RM, Ahya VN, Crawford SW. Pulmonary complications of solid organ and hematopoietic stem cell transplantation. Am J Respir Crit Care Med 2004;170:30; with permission.)

among the heart transplant recipients who had bronchogenic carcinoma reported in the literature [29,30]. Immunosuppression does not seem to pose an additional risk for development of lung cancer but may promote a more aggressive natural history once the disease is established [32].

Among liver transplant recipients with a pretransplantation history of hepatocellular carcinoma, the lung is the most common site of recurrence [33]. Recurrence usually occurs within 2 years of transplantation and appears radiographically as single or multiple lung nodules. An elevated alpha-fetoprotein level provides an important clue to the possibility of recurrent disease [33].

Drug toxicity

Sirolimus, also known as rapamycin, is a potent immunosuppressive agent recently introduced into clinical practice. Sirolimus seems to be far less nephrotoxic than the calcineurin inhibitors, and it is increasingly used either in combination with reduced doses of these agents or in their place. Since its release, numerous cases of interstitial pneumonitis developing in association with sirolimus administration have been reported [34–39]. The incidence of this complication remains unknown. Initial reports suggested that interstitial pneumonitis was largely a complication of excessive sirolimus blood concentrations, but more recent reports have documented cases in the setting of therapeutic drug levels [38,39]. Approximately 50% of cases develop within the first 6 months after initiation of sirolimus therapy [39]. Onset is usually insidious, but more acute and fulminant presentations have been described [40]. Common presenting symptoms include dyspnea and nonproductive cough; fever is present in 60% of cases [39]. Pulmonary function studies may reveal a restrictive pattern. Radiographic abnormalities include bilateral interstitial infiltrates, alveolar consolidation, ground-glass opacities, and nodules [34,37,39]. Bronchoalveolar lavage reveals evidence of a lymphocytic alveolitis and, less commonly, of alveolar hemorrhage. Histologic findings are diverse and include bronchiolitis obliterans with organizing pneumonia, interstitial lymphocytic infiltrates, alveolar hemorrhage, and non-necrotizing granulomas [34, 37,39]. Discontinuation of the drug leads to prompt clinical improvement, but radiographic abnormalities may take several months to resolve fully. In more severe cases, high doses of corticosteroids have been administered, but the true efficacy of these agents remains uncertain.

The murine monoclonal anti-CD3 antibody muromonab-CD3 (OKT3) was used commonly in the past for induction immunosuppression and treatment of refractory acute rejection. This agent is associated with a cytokine-release syndrome that is most pronounced with the first dose and that clinically presents with fever, rigors, nausea, hypotension, and dyspnea. A small number of patients have been reported to develop noncardiogenic pulmonary edema, which, rarely, can be fatal. Because of its toxicity and the availability of alternative agents, the use of muromonab-CD3 (OKT3) has diminished in recent years. The interleukin-2 receptor antagonists basilizimab and daclizumab are being used with increasing frequency as induction agents, in part because of generally favorable side-effect profiles. Three cases of noncardiogenic pulmonary edema in renal transplant recipients were recently reported in association with basilizimab infusion [41]. The mechanism underlying this reaction was not determined.

Pulmonary function abnormalities

Candidates awaiting heart transplantation typically demonstrate marked impairment in pulmonary function, attributed to chronic congestive heart failure with associated cardiomegaly, pleural effusions, interstitial edema, and engorgement of the bronchial vasculature. Restrictive and obstructive patterns occur with similar frequency; and a reduced diffusing capacity is seen commonly with both patterns. After heart transplantation, spirometric values improve dramatically, but, curiously, there typically is a worsening of the impairment in diffusing capacity that persists for years after transplantation [42–44]. Several studies have attempted to discern the relative contributions of abnormal membrane diffusion and pulmonary capillary blood volume, the two physiologic determinants of the diffusing capacity, to the observed decrement [42,45]. These studies suggest that the major factor is persistence of abnormal membrane diffusion, possibly reflecting irreversible changes in the alveolar capillary membrane induced by pretransplantation elevations in pulmonary vascular pressures. Additionally, transplantation results in a fall in pulmonary capillary blood volume as left-sided filling pressures normalize. Elevation in pulmonary capillary blood volume in patients who have congestive heart failure partially offsets the detrimental impact of abnormal membrane diffusion; conversely, normalization of pulmonary capillary blood volume after transplantation further unmasks the detrimental impact of impaired membrane diffusion. There are conflicting data on whether the observed impairment in diffusing capacity after heart transplantation contributes to exercise limitation [46,47].

Most long-term kidney transplant survivors also demonstrate impairment in diffusing capacity. There is no correlation between this physiologic abnormality and the presence or absence of interstitial lung disease on CT scans [48]. Beyond this negative observation, there are no studies that have elucidated a mechanism.

References

[1] Glanemann M, Langrehr J, Kaisers U, et al. Postoperative tracheal extubation after orthotopic liver transplantation. Acta Anaesthesiol Scand 2001;45(3): 333–9.

[2] Glanemann M, Kaisers U, Langrehr JM, et al. Incidence and indications for reintubation during postoperative care following orthotopic liver transplantation. J Clin Anesth 2001;13(5):377–82.

[3] Pirat A, Ozgur S, Torgay A, et al. Risk factors for postoperative respiratory complications in adult liver transplant recipients. Transplant Proc 2004;36(1):218–20.

[4] O'Brien JD, Ettinger NA. Pulmonary complications of liver transplantation. Clin Chest Med 1996;17(1): 99–114.

[5] Golfieri R, Giampalma E, Morselli Labate AM, et al. Pulmonary complications of liver transplantation: radiological appearance and statistical evaluation of risk factors in 300 cases. Eur Radiol 2000;10(7):1169–83.

[6] Yost CS, Matthay MA, Gropper MA. Etiology of acute pulmonary edema during liver transplantation: a series of cases with analysis of the edema fluid. Chest 2001; 119(1):219–23.

[7] Sadaghdar H, Chelluri L, Bowles SA, et al. Outcome of renal transplant recipients in the ICU. Chest 1995; 107(5):1402–5.

[8] Shorr AF, Abbott KC, Agadoa LY. Acute respiratory distress syndrome after kidney transplantation: epidemiology, risk factors, and outcomes. Crit Care Med 2003;31(5):1325–30.

[9] Antonelli M, Conti G, Bufi M, et al. Noninvasive ventilation for treatment of acute respiratory failure in patients undergoing solid organ transplantation: a randomized trial. JAMA 2000;283(2):235–41.

[10] Judson MA, Sahn SA. The pleural space and organ transplantation. Am J Respir Crit Care Med 1996; 153(3):1153–65.

[11] Lenner R, Padilla ML, Teirstein AS, et al. Pulmonary complications in cardiac transplant recipients. Chest 2001;120(2):508–13.

[12] Carcillo Jr J, Salcedo JR. Urinothorax as a manifestation of nondilated obstructive uropathy following renal transplantation. Am J Kidney Dis 1985;5(3): 211–3.

[13] Salcedo JR. Urinothorax: report of 4 cases and review of the literature. J Urol 1986;135(4):805–8.

[14] McAlister VC, Grant DR, Roy A, et al. Right phrenic nerve injury in orthotopic liver transplantation. Transplantation 1993;55(4):826–30.

[15] Dorffner R, Eibenberger K, Youssefzadeh S, et al. Diaphragmatic dysfunction after heart or lung transplantation. J Heart Lung Transplant 1997;16(5):566–9.

[16] Chatterjee S, Williams NN, Ohara ML, et al. Diaphragmatic hernias associated with ventricular assist devices and heart transplantation. Ann Thorac Surg 2004;77(6):2111–4.

[17] Farma J, Leeser D, Furukawa S, et al. Laparoscopic repair of diaphragmatic hernia after left ventricular assist device. J Laparoendosc Adv Surg Tech A 2003; 13(3):185–7.

[18] Mouly-Bandini A, Chalvignac V, Collart F, et al. Transdiaphragmatic hernia 1 year after heart transplantation following implantable LVAD. J Heart Lung Transplant 2002;21(10):1144–6.

[19] Kuhlman JE, Ren H, Hutchins GM, et al. Fulminant pulmonary calcification complicating renal transplantation: CT demonstration. Radiology 1989;173(2): 459–60.

[20] Ullmer E, Borer H, Sandoz P, et al. Diffuse pulmonary nodular infiltrates in a renal transplant recipient. Metastatic pulmonary calcification. Chest 2001;120(4): 1394–8.

[21] Murris-Espin M, Lacassagne L, Didier A, et al. Metastatic pulmonary calcification after renal transplantation. Eur Respir J 1997;10(8):1925–7.

[22] Breitz HB, Sirotta PS, Nelp WB, et al. Progressive pulmonary calcification complicating successful renal transplantation. Am Rev Respir Dis 1987;136(6): 1480–2.

[23] Libson E, Wechsler RJ, Steiner RM. Pulmonary calcinosis following orthotopic liver transplantation. J Thorac Imaging 1993;8(4):305–8.

[24] Munoz SJ, Nagelberg SB, Green PJ, et al. Ectopic soft tissue calcium deposition following liver transplantation. Hepatology 1988;8(3):476–83.

[25] Justrabo E, Genin R, Rifle G. Pulmonary metastatic calcification with respiratory insufficiency in patients on maintenance haemodialysis. Thorax 1979;34(3): 384–8.

[26] Giacobetti R, Feldman SA, Ivanovich P, et al. Sudden fatal pulmonary calcification following renal transplantation. Nephron 1977;19(5):295–300.

[27] Kotloff RM, Ahya VN, Crawford SW. Pulmonary complications of solid organ and hematopoietic stem cell transplantation. Am J Respir Crit Care Med 2004; 170:22–48.

[28] Lingam RK, Teh J, Sharma A, et al. Case report. Metastatic pulmonary calcification in renal failure: a new HRCT pattern. Br J Radiol 2002;75(889):74–7.

[29] Potaris K, Radovancevic B, Thomas CD, et al. Lung cancer after heart transplantation: a 17-year experience. Ann Thorac Surg 2005;79(3):980–3.

[30] de Perrot M, Wigle DA, Pierre AF, et al. Bronchogenic

carcinoma after solid organ transplantation. Ann Thorac Surg 2003;75(2):367–71.

[31] Dorent R, Mohammadi S, Tezenas S, et al. Lung cancer in heart transplant patients: a 16-year survey. Transplant Proc 2000;32(8):2752–4.

[32] Bagan P, Assouad J, Berna P, et al. Immediate and long-term survival after surgery for lung cancer in heart transplant recipients. Ann Thorac Surg 2005; 79(2):438–42.

[33] Paterson DL, Singh N, Gayowski T, et al. Pulmonary nodules in liver transplant recipients. Medicine (Baltimore) 1998;77(1):50–8.

[34] Morelon E, Stern M, Israel-Biet D, et al. Characteristics of sirolimus-associated interstitial pneumonitis in renal transplant patients. Transplantation 2001;72(5): 787–90.

[35] Singer SJ, Tiernan R, Sullivan EJ. Interstitial pneumonitis associated with sirolimus therapy in renal-transplant recipients. N Engl J Med 2000;343(24): 1815–6.

[36] Lennon A, Finan K, FitzGerald MX, et al. Interstitial pneumonitis associated with sirolimus (rapamycin) therapy after liver transplantation. Transplantation 2001;72(6):1166–7.

[37] McWilliams TJ, Levvey BJ, Russell PA, et al. Interstitial pneumonitis associated with sirolimus: a dilemma for lung transplantation. J Heart Lung Transplant 2003;22(2):210–3.

[38] Haydar AA, Denton M, West A, et al. Sirolimus-induced pneumonitis: three cases and a review of the literature. Am J Transplant 2004;4(1):137–9.

[39] Pham PT, Pham PC, Danovitch GM, et al. Sirolimus-associated pulmonary toxicity. Transplantation 2004; 77(8):1215–20.

[40] Manito N, Kaplinsky EJ, Bernat R, et al. Fatal interstitial pneumonitis associated with sirolimus therapy in a heart transplant recipient. J Heart Lung Transplant 2004;23(6):780–2.

[41] Bamgbola FO, Del Rio M, Kaskel FJ, et al. Noncardiogenic pulmonary edema during basiliximab induction in three adolescent renal transplant patients. Pediatr Transplant 2003;7(4):315–20.

[42] Mettauer B, Lampert E, Charloux A, et al. Lung membrane diffusing capacity, heart failure, and heart transplantation. Am J Cardiol 1999;83(1):62–7.

[43] Egan JJ, Lowe L, Yonan N, et al. Pulmonary diffusion impairment following heart transplantation: a prospective study. Eur Respir J 1996;9(4):663–8.

[44] Ewert R, Wensel R, Bettmann M, et al. Ventilatory and diffusion abnormalities in long-term survivors after orthotopic heart transplantation. Chest 1999;115(5): 1305–11.

[45] Al-Rawas OA, Carter R, Stevenson RD, et al. Mechanisms of pulmonary transfer factor decline following heart transplantation. Eur J Cardiothorac Surg 2000;17(4):355–61.

[46] Ewert R, Wensel R, Bruch L, et al. Relationship between impaired pulmonary diffusion and cardiopulmonary exercise capacity after heart transplantation. Chest 2000;117(4):968–75.

[47] Al-Rawas OA, Carter R, Stevenson RD, et al. Exercise intolerance following heart transplantation: the role of pulmonary diffusing capacity impairment. Chest 2000; 118(6):1661–70.

[48] Ewert R, Opitz C, Wensel R, et al. Abnormalities of pulmonary diffusion capacity in long-term survivors after kidney transplantation. Chest 2002;122(2):639–44.

Clin Chest Med 26 (2005) 631 – 645

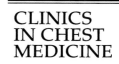

Post-Transplant Lymphoproliferative Disorder

Alison W. Loren, MD, MS[a,b], Donald E. Tsai, MD, PhD[a,*]

[a]Division of Hematology/Oncology, University of Pennsylvania School of Medicine, 16 Penn Tower, 3400 Spruce Street, Philadelphia, PA 19104, USA
[b]Center for Clinical Epidemiology and Biostatistics, University of Pennsylvania School of Medicine, Philadelphia, PA 19104, USA

Post-transplant lymphoproliferative disorder (PTLD) encompasses a heterogeneous group of abnormal lymphoid proliferations, generally of B cells, that occur in the setting of profound immunosuppression, such as primary immunodeficiency states, or after solid organ transplantation [1,2] or hematopoietic stem cell transplantation (HSCT) [3]. Nearly all PTLDs (80%–90%) are associated with Epstein-Barr virus (EBV) infection, manifested by the presence of EBV early RNA, EBV latent membrane protein, or EBV DNA in the neoplastic tissue. PTLD occurs in up to 15% of solid organ transplant recipients [4,5], with the highest rates occurring in recipients of lung and heart-lung transplants [4,6,7]. Incidence also varies depending on the type of transplant, the EBV status of donor and recipient, and the specific immunosuppressive regimen used. PTLD is reported in recipients of allogeneic and, rarely, autologous HSCT. Those at highest risk, with up to 24% of recipients affected, are patients who receive allogeneic T-cell–depleted, human leukocyte antigen (HLA)-mismatched grafts [8]. Pulmonary manifestations of PTLD are common and this disorder should be included in the differential diagnosis when lung nodules or masses, intrathoracic lymphadenopathy, or pleural effusions are encountered in solid organ or HSCT recipients.

This work was supported by grant no. CA76931 from the National Institutes of Health (to A.W. Loren) and by a Career Development Award from the American Society of Clinical Oncology (to D.E. Tsai).

* Corresponding author.
E-mail address: detsai@mail.med.upenn.edu (D.E. Tsai).

Pathophysiology

EBV first was implicated as a cause for malignancy in 1964, when viral particles were discovered in a patient who had Burkitt's lymphoma [9]. Since then, EBV has been implicated as a causative factor in nasopharyngeal carcinoma, Hodgkin's lymphoma, and PTLD. A member of the herpesvirus family, EBV infects and immortalizes B cells. EBV infection usually is asymptomatic in childhood. If the primary infection occurs during adolescence or adulthood, however, infectious mononucleosis occurs. Patients often demonstrate the classic triad of fever, posterior cervical lymphadenopathy, and pharyngitis. Activated T cells, apparent as atypical lymphocytes on the peripheral blood smear, are believed critical in modulating the proliferation of infected B cells during primary EBV infection. Ultimately, in immunocompetent people, the EBV genome forms an episome that remains latent in resting memory B cells. In certain immunocompromised patients, however, the critical T-cell control of B-cell growth is lacking, resulting in unchecked proliferation of EBV-infected B cells, and hyperplasia or frank malignancy follows [10].

Evidence is mounting that EBV-related B-cell proliferation is facilitated by an inadequate T-cell response. Higher levels of immunosuppression—in particular the use of specific anti–T-cell therapy, such as antithymocyte globulin or anti-CD3 monoclonal antibody—increase the risk of PTLD in solid organ and stem cell transplant recipients markedly. Renal allograft recipients who have PTLD and who achieve a complete remission after therapy show full

0272-5231/05/$ – see front matter © 2005 Elsevier Inc. All rights reserved.
doi:10.1016/j.ccm.2005.06.014

restoration of their CD8$^+$ T cells, some of which recognize EBV-specific proteins specifically [11]. In vitro studies demonstrate inhibition of EBV-induced lymphoproliferation by CD4$^+$ T cells [12]. Perhaps the most compelling evidence for the importance of T-cell regulation of EBV-driven B-cell proliferation is that one of the most successful therapies for PTLD is infusion of EBV-specific T cells (discussed later).

Classification

PTLD represents a spectrum of lymphoid hyper-proliferative states that includes benign conditions, such as infectious mononucleosis-like illnesses and lymphoid hyperplasia, and malignancies, such as B-cell (and, rarely, T-cell) lymphomas, which may take a fulminant course [5]. These disorders generally are associated with EBV infection (either primary infection or reactivation), but there are post-transplant lymphoid neoplasms that are not associated with EBV. Some studies suggest that EBV-negative tumors tend to occur at longer intervals post transplant and to portend a worse prognosis, with poor response to therapy [13,14].

Recommendations for a formal classification of PTLD were established by two international consensus groups and published in 1999 [15]. According to these guidelines, the term PTLD may encompass

Table 1
Pathologic classification of post-transplant lymphoproliferative disorder

Reference	Type of PTLD	Features
Frizzera et al	Hyperplasia	Polymorphic B-cell hyperplasia
(1981) [104]	Lymphoma	Polymorphic or monomorphic
		Nuclear atypia
		Necrosis
		Histologic invasiveness
Knowles et al	Plasmacytic hyperplasia	Polyclonal
(1995) [105]		Multiple EBV infection events
		No genetic mutations
	Polymorphic B-cell	Monoclonal
	hyperplasia/lymphoma	Single EBV infection event
		Variable oncogene/tumor suppressor gene mutations
	Immunoblastic lymphoma myeloma	Monoclonal disseminated disease
		Single EBV infection event
		One or more oncogene/tumor suppressor gene mutations
Harris et al	Early benign PTLD: plasmacytic or	Nodal disease with preservation of lymph node architecture
(1997) [16]	atypical lymphoid hyperplasia	<3 months post transplantation
	Infectious-mononucleosis-like syndrome	Polyclonal
	Polymorphic PTLD	Nodal disease with effacement of lymph node architecture or extranodal disease
		Full range of B-cell maturation
		Monoclonal
		Normal cytogenetics
		No oncogenic mutations
	Monomorphic PTLD (non-Hodgkin's B- or T-cell lymphoma)	Nodal disease with effacement of lymph node architecture or invasive extranodal disease
		Monomorphic sheets of transformed B-cells
		Monoclonal
		Some with abnormal cytogenetics or mutations in ras or p53
	T-cell-rich, large B-cell (Hodgkin's-like) lymphoma	Nodal disease
		Background of small T-cells with superimposed Reed-Sternberg–like cells
		Monoclonal
	Plasmacytoma-like lesions	Nodal disease with effacement of lymph node architecture by mature plasma cells with monoclonal immunoglobulin
		Monoclonal

From Loren AW, Porter DL, Stadtmauer ES, et al. Post-transplant lymphoproliferative disorder: a review. Bone Marrow Transplant 2003;31:145–55; with permission.

the full range of EBV-related lymphoproliferative states, including benign processes. When not otherwise specified, however, PTLD should refer to the neoplastic end of the PTLD spectrum. Neoplasia should be defined by two of the following three characteristics: (1) destruction of the underlying lymph node architecture, (2) monoclonality (regardless of morphology), and (3) evidence of EBV infection in the neoplastic cells. Several classification systems are described (Table 1), but that proposed by Harris and colleagues generally is accepted [16,17]. Typical monomorphic PTLD should be characterized further by World Health Organization or Revised European-American Lymphoma classification [17]. Fig. 1 depicts examples of monomorphic and polymorphic morphology and immunohistochemical staining for the presence of EBV. Most cells in polymorphic PTLD are reactive T cells, whereas the histology of monomorphic PTLD is composed predominantly of sheets of clonal B cells.

Two other rare forms of PTLD deserve mention. Occasionally, PTLD may take on a plasmacytic morphology. This form of PTLD resembles multiple myeloma and often presents with plasmacytomas. The malignant cells typically are CD20 negative. Alternatively, and somewhat surprisingly given the pathophysiology of EBV, there are reports of PTLDs of T-cell lineage, in which the malignant T cells are EBV positive [18–21]. T-cell PTLDs tend to present in an atypical and aggressive manner, often with fevers and other constitutional symptoms, such as weight loss and night sweats, organ infiltration, and cytopenias, but sometimes without lymphadenopathy. This entity, which can be difficult to identify, must be entertained specifically when considering the differential diagnosis of ill transplant patients. Management of these two atypical forms of PTLD is challenging, because they do not respond to anti-CD20 antibody therapy (rituximab), which is becoming a mainstay of therapy in many patients.

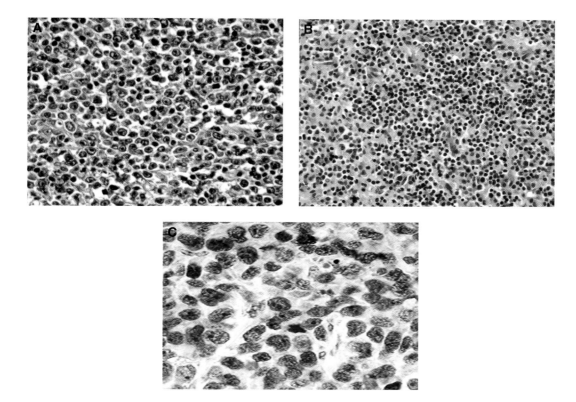

Fig. 1. Morphology and immunophenotype of PTLD (unless indicated otherwise, the images represent ×400 magnification). (A) Hematoxylin-eosin stain at ×40 magnification of monomorphic PTLD, an infiltrate of mostly intermediate cells with high mitotic rate and interspersed coagulative necrosis. (B) Polymorphic PTLD. (C) Expression of the EBV-encoded, nuclear RNA (EBER-1).

Diagnosis and staging

As is the case with all suspected lymphomas, it is critically important to obtain sufficient tissue for diagnosis, usually by excisional biopsy of the involved tissue or lymph node. Current recommendations for identifying a PTLD lesion are described in Table 2.

Noninvasive diagnosis of PTLD is not yet possible, although two blood tests may have some use. Polymerase chain reaction (PCR) testing of the peripheral blood for the presence of EBV-derived DNA is one promising method, but published studies of solid organ transplantation yield conflicting results; no data are available for the HSCT population. A recent study of 35 adult solid organ transplant patients referred for possible PTLD evaluates the usefulness of peripheral blood EBV PCR for diagnosing PTLD [22]. A viral load of greater than 1000 copies/2×10^6 peripheral blood lymphocytes was considered a positive test. The final diagnosis of PTLD was made by tissue biopsy. Of the 35 patients, seven had a positive EBV PCR, and all of these were diagnosed with PTLD by biopsy. An additional 11 patients had a negative EBV PCR and had biopsy-proven PTLD [22]. The sensitivity was 39%, with specificity and positive predictive value of 100%. Studies of pediatric transplantation, however, show higher sensitivity and lower specificity for detecting EBV disease [23]. There are some critical unresolved issues regarding the use of serum EBV PCR, including the absence of universal standards for detecting EBV DNA, lack of consensus on which portion of the genome should be targeted by PCR primers, disagreement on what consists of a positive versus a negative test, and inability to compare results across different laboratories. There may be significant differences between adult and pediatric immune systems—an adult may be able to mount a sufficient immune response to clear circulating EBV, even in the setting of immunosuppression, whereas a child may be unable to do so. This may explain the apparent usefulness of EBV PCR in the pediatric, but not the adult, population. In patients who have a positive EBV PCR, following these levels closely correlates with disease response, a finding supported by some [24,25], but not all [26], studies. Thus, although EBV PCR is a useful adjunctive diagnostic tool, it cannot replace excisional biopsy; however, in patients who have high levels of circulating EBV DNA, it may be used to monitor response to therapy. Another marker that has garnered attention is serum protein electrophoresis (SPEP) to detect and monitor PTLD [27–29]. EBV loads are higher in patients who have monoclonal gammopathy after organ transplantation [28]. In a study of more than 900 liver transplant recipients, 114 patients had a gammopathy, 10% of whom developed PTLD; successful therapy correlated with disappearance of the monoclonal protein in half of the patients. Monoclonal gammopathy does not predict histology (ie, PTLD patients who have gammopathies do not have plasmacytic tumors). SPEP is a more widely available test that is less subject to individual laboratory variation and may have some use in early detection of a higher-risk population. In patients who have monoclonal proteins associated with PTLD, disease course may be monitored with SPEP [27].

Although staging of PTLD is not defined formally, the authors recommend following World Health Organization guidelines for lymphoma staging by obtaining contrast-enhanced CT of the chest, abdomen, and pelvis; serum lactate dehydrogenase (LDH) for prognostic purposes [6]; and EBV PCR on peripheral blood, as this may be useful for follow-up [22] (discussed previously). Unlike for non-PTLD lymphomas, however, the authors believe that bone marrow biopsy is not required for staging.

Table 2
Diagnostic studies for post-transplant lymphoproliferative disorder

Specimen	Study	Goal
Excisional biopsy of mass/node	Routine morphologic examination	Assess for polymorphic versus monomorphic histology Evaluate lymph node architecture
	Immunophenotyping: flow cytometry or immunohistochemistry	Assess for polyclonality vs. monoclonality Determine lineage (B- versus T-cell) Stain for EBV-specific proteins
	Molecular studies: fluorescent in-situ hybridization for EBV early RNA or PCR for the EBV genome	Assess for the presence of EBV in the lesion
Serum	Viral capsid antigen or EBV nuclear antigen IgM and IgG PCR for EBV DNA (viral load)	Assess for active (primary or reactivated) EBV infection Possible role for surveillance and pre-emptive therapy

Post-transplant lymphoproliferative disorder in solid organ transplant recipients

The risk of developing PTLD after solid organ transplantation is variable and is most dependent on the level of immunosuppression, particularly with specific antilymphocyte therapy. All solid organ transplant recipients are at increased risk for many malignancies, especially those of lymphoid origin [30]. Table 3 lists the observed risk factors for the development of PTLD in solid organ transplant patients. Although many younger patients have not yet been exposed to EBV, it is not clear if the increased risk of PTLD in pediatric transplant recipients is related to the fact that they are more likely EBV negative [5,31]. One recent study estimates the relative risk of non-Hodgkin's lymphoma (NHL) in solid organ transplant recipients compared with an age-matched population [7]. The lowest-risk group comprised those patients receiving cadaveric kidney transplants, with a relative risk of 12.6 and a 10-year cumulative incidence of 1.6%. Recipients of other transplanted organs, in increasing order of PTLD risk, are pancreas, liver, heart, and lung, with combined heart-lung transplant recipients at the highest risk (relative risk 239.5) (Fig. 2) [7]. These findings closely mirror those of other investigators and are believed related to the higher degree of immunosuppression in heart and lung transplant

Table 3
Risk factors for developing post-transplant lymphoproliferative disorder

Solid organ transplantation	Hematopoietic stem cell transplantation
Lung or heart-lung transplant	T-cell depletion
EBV-seronegative recipient (especially with EBV-seropositive donor)	HLA mismatching: related or unrelated (synergistic with T-cell depletion)
Primary or reactivated EBV infection after transplant	Specific anti–T-cell therapy (conditioning regimen or GVHD prophylaxis or treatment)
High-dose immunosuppression including anti–T-cell therapy and calcineurin inhibitors	Primary immunodeficiency as indication for transplant
Cytomegalovirus disease	

From Loren AW, Porter DL, Stadtmauer ES, et al. Post-transplant lymphoproliferative disorder: a review. Bone Marrow Transplant 2003;31:145–55; with permission.

recipients, owing to the high mortality resulting from graft rejection in the early post-transplant period [32]. The incidence of PTLD after lung transplantation is reportedly as low as 3% [33,34], although most series report rates of approximately 6% [33,35,36].

Although PTLD occurs most frequently within the first year after solid organ transplantation, with a median onset of 6 months [5,6], cases are reported as early as 1 week and as late as 9 years post transplant [6]. Clinical features vary widely, requiring a high index of suspicion to make the diagnosis of PTLD. Patients who have benign B-cell proliferations may have infectious mononucleosis-like symptoms, with fever, lymphadenopathy, pharyngitis, and tonsillar enlargement. The illness can be severe, and laryngeal edema may occur. Patients who have malignant PTLD frequently also have fever, weight loss, fatigue, and lymphadenopathy and mass effects from the tumor itself, often in the central nervous system [37], gastrointestinal tract, and head and neck. PTLD frequently involves the transplanted organ itself [7], and allograft dysfunction is a common presentation. Distinguishing PTLD from organ rejection on clinical grounds can be difficult, highlighting the crucial importance of biopsy in ascertaining the diagnosis. PTLD should be considered strongly when empiric increases in immunosuppression result in worsening organ dysfunction [5]. Patients who have disseminated disease may develop diffuse organ infiltration with lymphoma or multiorgan system failure with a septic or a systemic inflammatory reaction syndrome presentation.

Intrathoracic involvement may be seen in any solid organ transplant recipient but is encountered most commonly after heart, lung, and heart-lung transplantation. PTLD presents most commonly as single or multiple pulmonary nodules or masses that may have smooth or irregular margins. Nodules may be surrounded by a rim of ground glass density (halo sign), mimicking the features of invasive aspergillosis. Other intrathoracic findings seen in a minority of patients include hilar and mediastinal adenopathy and pleural effusions. Cavitation is distinctly unusual and its presence should prompt consideration of alternative causes.

Overall mortality of PTLD in the solid organ transplant population is difficult to establish, given the heterogeneity of presentations, underlying conditions, and therapies. Mortality rates of approximately 40% to 70% are reported [38], although with recent improvements in the understanding of the pathogenesis of this disease and the development of new therapies, survival seems to be improving. Lymphoproliferative disorders occurring in the post-

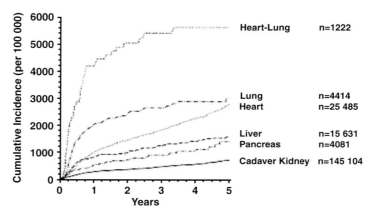

Fig. 2. Five-year incidence of NHL in organ transplant recipients. Relative risk: heart-lung 239.5, lung 58.6, heart 27.6, liver 29.9, pancreas 34.9, and cadaver kidney 12.6. (*From* Opelz G, Döhler B. Lymphomas after solid organ transplantation: a collaborative transplant study report. Am J Transplant 2003;4:222–30; with permission.)

transplant setting that are not associated with EBV may comprise a distinct subgroup of PTLD: they tend to occur later after transplant (median of 50 months post transplant), to have a more malignant-appearing histology, and to behave more aggressively, with reported median survival of 1 month [13,14], although these findings are not uniform [7].

Prognosis seems to be related to the site of disease and possibly the timing of onset. Patients who have nodal disease or disease affecting the allograft itself, which is common, have a more favorable prognosis compared with those patients who have extranodal, nonallograft or disseminated disease [7]. Controversy exists as to whether or not "late" PTLDs (occurring more than 1 year post transplant) are truly different from "early" lesions (less than 1 year post transplant). Some investigators suggest that early PTLDs more frequently are EBV positive and have a better prognosis [13,14], although this is not borne out by the single case series in which these groups are compared explicitly [36].

With improved understanding of the pathogenesis and optimal therapies for PTLD (discussed later), clinical questions regarding retransplantation in patients who have a history of PTLD have arisen. These issues are relevant primarily in the renal transplant population, as patients can be "bridged" with hemodialysis if removal of the allograft is required for therapy (which is done frequently). One small study suggests that retransplantation may be safe, provided that there is an appropriately long interval (ie, 1–2 years) between resolution of PTLD and retransplantation [39,40]. Performance of a second lung transplantation in a patient who has a history of PTLD never has been described.

Post-transplant lymphoproliferative disorder in hematopoietic stem cell transplant recipients

HSCT is performed primarily to cure malignancies and less commonly to treat severe autoimmune, immune deficiency, or metabolic diseases. (For a detailed discussion of HSCT, see the article by Cutler and Antin elsewhere in this issue.) Briefly, HSCT involves the administration of myeloablative doses of chemotherapy or radiation, followed by infusion of stem cells which return to the marrow and reconstitute hematopoiesis in 10 to 21 days, depending on the conditioning regimen and source of cells. Stem cells may derive from patients themselves (autologous HSCT) or they may derive from donors (allogeneic), either family members or an unrelated volunteers. Allogeneic transplant donors are matched to recipients at HLA class I and class II loci. Sometimes stem cell grafts are manipulated to select the most primitive hematopoietic stem cells (CD34+ selection) or to deplete the graft of T cells, which are powerful mediators of graft-versus-host disease (GVHD), a severe complication of allogeneic HSCT that occurs in 40% to 70% of transplant recipients. A recent advance in HSCT is the use of nonmyeloablative conditioning regimens, in which recipients receive treatment that is intended to be profoundly immunosuppressive but does not ablate the bone marrow. Regimens may include chemotherapy, radiation, or antibody therapy, followed by infusion of donor stem cells. The primary goal of this therapy is to harness the graft-versus-tumor effect, a potent form of immunotherapy, which occurs when the donor's T cells (and possibly B cells) attack the recipient's malignancy.

PTLD is reported after all types of HSCT and is related strongly to the use of immunosuppressive agents, which may occur before transplant as part of the conditioning regimen or post transplant for GVHD prophylaxis or treatment [41]. PTLD in HSCT differs in several important ways, however, from PTLD in the solid organ transplant population. First, unlike solid organ recipients, in whom the malignant PTLD cells are of recipient origin, PTLDs in allogeneic HSCT patients generally are of donor origin [8,42,43]. Second, although EBV is the causative agent in HSCT-related PTLD, there is no relationship between EBV exposure status (of either the donor or the recipient) and development of PTLD in HSCTs. Finally, patients who receive allogeneic HSCT eventually develop a fully reconstituted, donor-derived immune system. This allows for the unique opportunity to treat these patients who have donor-derived cellular immunotherapy.

Although most commonly described in the myeloablative allogeneic HSCT population, EBV-related lymphoid tumors are described in recipients of autologous [44–47] and nonmyeloablative transplants [48–50]. PTLD is a rare complication of autologous HSCT and likely is related to profound chemotherapy-induced immunosuppression. Alternatively, the explicit goal of nonmyeloablative transplantation is profound host immunosuppression. Hence, the conditioning regimens frequently include low to moderate doses of total body irradiation, antilymphocyte antibodies, such as antithymocyte globulin, or profoundly immunosuppressive chemotherapy, such as fludarabine and cyclophosphamide. The incidence of PTLD after these types of transplants is expected to be high. The relatively recent development of this strategy, and the use of alemtuzumab, an anti-CD52 antibody that depletes T and B lymphocytes [51,52], may account for the few cases of PTLD reported after nonmyeloablative transplantation.

The incidence of PTLD in standard (myeloablative) allogeneic HSCT recipients varies greatly depending on the donor type and degree of HLA matching, conditioning regimen, GVHD prophylaxis, and underlying disease. Overall, PTLD occurs in approximately 1% to 2% of all allogeneic HSCT recipients [3,8,42], but rates as high as 24% are described in recipients of T-cell–depleted, HLA-mismatched, or unrelated grafts [8]. The onset of PTLD in HSCT patients is on average much earlier than that for solid organ recipients, with a median onset of 70 to 90 days. In addition, mortality of PTLD in these patients is far greater, exceeding 90% in all reported series. In one study, the risk factors that affected survival adversely were stem cell rather than solid organ transplant, HSCT for hematologic malignancy rather than immunodeficiency, and four or more sites of disease [53]. It is not uncommon for these patients to be diagnosed with PTLD at autopsy. Risk factors for the development of PTLD in this setting are enumerated in Table 3 [8,42,54–56].

Clinical features of PTLD in allogeneic HSCT recipients are similar to those of solid organ transplant recipients, and include fever, lymphadenopathy, pharyngitis, hepatosplenomegaly, and neurologic symptoms. There seems to be a greater incidence of the fulminant, disseminated form of PTLD, perhaps accounting for the increased mortality seen in this population. Pulmonary involvement occurs in approximately 20% of cases, usually as a component of disseminated disease. Infection, usually involving aspergillus or cytomegalovirus, complicates many cases.

Given the intriguing finding that PTLD in the allogeneic HSCT population is nearly always of donor origin, several hypotheses are proposed regarding the role of EBV in these malignancies. Profound immunosuppression is the major risk factor for developing PTLD in all settings, and the role of T cells in regulating the B-cell proliferation induced by EBV seems to be the most critical part of the immune response. Most cases of PTLD in allogeneic HSCT involve seropositive donors and recipients. The lymphoproliferation is donor derived because the host lymphoid system has been eradicated successfully by the conditioning regimen. In cases where the donor is seronegative, however, the PTLD still may be of donor origin, suggesting that donor cells may become infected with EBV after the transplant [8,42,57]. This may occur via environmental exposure (either through the usual routes of exposure to infected saliva or blood transfusions) or, if recipients are EBV seropositive, through exposure of donor-derived lymphocytes to latent EBV in recipient B cells or nasopharyngeal epithelial cells [42].

Recommendations for diagnosing PTLD in the setting of HSCT are nearly identical to those for solid organ transplant recipients. Because HSCT patients who have PTLD tend to have a more fulminant course, with more rapid development of disease and disseminated organ involvement, however, the urgency of making the diagnosis is greater in this population. The authors recommend that a high index of suspicion be maintained, with PTLD considered in the differential diagnosis of any (allogeneic) HSCT recipients who have fever, organ dysfunction, lymphadenopathy, or hepatosplenomegaly. The authors emphasize that adequate biopsy specimens are essential, given the multitude of studies that are required to make the diagnosis, and that the material should be evaluated by pathologists who are experienced in diagnosing PTLD. In addition to the studies described previously, the authors recommend assessing the tissue for donor versus host origin.

Surveillance

There recently has been interest in surveillance, prophylaxis, and early treatment of PTLD. Experience with monitoring for PTLD is limited, and there are no prospective randomized clinical trials of early interventions. Several compelling reports, however, suggest that surveillance for the presence of primary or reactivated EBV infection may prove useful, and there are small series suggesting that preemptive therapy may prevent PTLD effectively.

Several groups have examined solid organ transplant and HSCT recipients for evidence of active EBV infection. EBV activity can be assessed in various ways, including evaluation of EBV viral load in the peripheral blood (as measured by PCR amplification), measurement of the number of EBV-infected peripheral blood mononuclear cells, and ex vivo spontaneous growth of EBV-transformed B cells [24,25, 58–61]. Serology for antibodies to EBV viral capsid antigen or nuclear antigen is less sensitive than these methods but is specific for EBV disease. By all of these measures, it is demonstrated that EBV activity is greater in transplant recipients who have PTLD than in transplant recipients who do not have PTLD, healthy EBV-seropositive adults, and healthy adults who have infectious mononucleosis [62]. Furthermore, these EBV-related markers tend to rise in the weeks before development of clinical PTLD and to peak at the time of diagnosis of PTLD [24,59, 61,63], implying that they may be used as predictors of the development of PTLD. Although the studies are small, negative predictive values were high (94%–100%); sensitivity was more variable [25,61,64].

Prophylaxis, pre-emptive therapy, and treatment

Antiviral therapy

Initial attempts to prevent PTLD in the solid organ transplant population focused primarily on using thymidine kinase inhibitors, such as ganciclovir or acyclovir, to eradicate or control EBV in a prophylactic setting for high-risk patients [25,64–67]. These drugs inhibit the replication of the EBV-related herpes viruses, herpes simplex, and cytomegalovirus. In vivo, however, these drugs are ineffective against EBV, because EBV-associated lymphomas do not express thymidine kinase, the target of these drugs. In addition, EBV survives as an episome outside of the lymphocyte's genome, and these drugs do not eradicate EBV from latently infected B cells [68,69]. Clinical reports of prophylactic antiviral drugs are unconvincing, involving small numbers of patients in observational studies. Each investigator defines "high-risk" differently, complicating the interpretation of these studies. Anecdotal reports of acyclovir or ganciclovir for treatment of PTLD are not substantiated [38]. In general, antiviral therapies consistently are combined with other interventions, making an estimate of the efficacy of antiviral therapy difficult. Many other therapies (discussed later) were combined with high-dose antiviral therapy, usually acyclovir. Thus, it also is difficult to assess the true usefulness of antivirals as adjuncts to other treatments. An approach using arginine butyrate to induce latent EBV thymidine kinase expression, followed by treatment with ganciclovir [70], produced a response in five of six patients in an early trial. The recently reported results of a larger trial included 15 heavily pretreated and highly refractory PTLD patients, ten of whom sustained a partial or complete response to therapy [71]; further studies are ongoing.

Reduction of immunosuppression

The mainstay of therapy for PTLD in solid organ transplant recipients is reduction of immunosuppression. The effectiveness of this intervention was described initially by Starzl and colleagues in 1984 [72] and recently has been substantiated [6]. Predictors of lack of response to reduction of immunosuppression include a serum LDH greater than 2.5 times the upper limit of normal, organ dysfunction, and multiple visceral sites of disease. Patients who lacked all of these risk factors had an 89% response rate, whereas the presence of two or more risk factors portended a poor prognosis, with no patients responding [6]. Although early reports suggested that patients who had PTLD who were diagnosed more than 1 year after transplantation were unlikely to respond to reduction in immunosuppression, later series show that is not the case [6]. EBV status also does not predict response to reduction of immunosuppression [6]; in fact, EBV-negative PTLDs are shown to respond to reduction in immunosuppression [13,14]. The authors emphasize that this maneuver should be attempted in patients who have EBV-negative tumors and in those who have classic EBV-related PTLD, regardless of time from organ transplantation.

Reduction in immunosuppression should be individualized for each patient based on factors, such as their allograft type, immunosuppressive regimen, and severity of disease. As a general guideline, azathioprine or mycophenolate mofetil should be discontinued and the doses of calcineurin inhibitor (cyclosporine and tacrolimus) and prednisone reduced. Patients who have liver or renal allografts may tolerate greater reduction or even cessation of immunosuppression. Their organ function can be followed by serial liver function studies or creatinine; thus, early rejection can be identified, allowing appropriate immunosuppression to be reinstituted in time to salvage the allograft while allowing a period of time under maximum reduction in immunosuppression. Renal transplant patients have the additional advantage of hemodialysis should catastrophic rejection occur. Retransplantation of a renal allograft after eradication of PTLD has been performed successfully and may provide the ultimate backup for aggressive reduction in immunosuppression [40]. Unfortunately, lung and cardiac allografts do not tolerate such aggressive reduction in immunosuppression because of complications, such as cardiac arrythmias and bronchiolitis obliterans, respectively. Measured reduction in immunosuppressive medications on an individual basis should be attempted. Allograft rejection occurs as an infrequent complication in responders and nonresponders to reduction in immunosuppression. With close monitoring for allograft dysfunction, acute rejection is an uncommon and easily treated event [6]. Clinical response may be delayed after reduction in immunosuppression. Studies show that clinical response should occur within 4 weeks of reduced immunosuppression [6], although patients often note symptomatic improvement within 1 to 2 weeks.

Reduction in immunosuppression is an appropriate first-line strategy for patients who have a high likelihood of response (ie, those who lack the risk factors predictive of poor response [described previously]), are free of active allograft rejection, and are sufficiently stable to permit a 2 to 4 week period of observation for clinical response. In patients who have risk factors predicting a low likelihood of response, aggressive disease, or inability to tolerate reduction in immunosuppression, immediate treatment with rituximab or cytotoxic chemotherapy is an option.

Local therapy

When possible, complete surgical excision of localized disease is highly effective, including, in the case of renal transplantation, graft nephrectomy. Localized disease treated with definitive local therapy (surgery or radiation), combined with reduction of immunosuppression, has an excellent prognosis, with PTLD-related mortality rates reported between 0% and 26% [6,38,73,74]. Renal transplant patients in whom the allograft is the only affected site do particularly well with this therapy, as graft nephrectomy also permits complete cessation of immunosuppression.

Cytokine therapy

Given the importance of a competent immune system in controlling EBV-related lymphoproliferation, several case series and case reports describe experience with various immune modulators. Responses to interferon-α alone or in combination with intravenous immunoglobulin have been reported [8,54,73,75]. Patients frequently experience graft rejection, reflecting nonspecific T-cell stimulation resulting from this therapy. Inhibition of interleukin-6, a cytokine that promotes the growth and proliferation of B cells, has resulted in moderate success [8,38, 73,75,76].

Cytotoxic chemotherapy

Chemotherapy also is used to treat PTLD, often after failure to respond to surgical excision or reduction of immunosuppression. Regimens are similar to those used for NHL, such as CHOP and ProMACE-CytaBOM. Although generally effective and rapid in controlling PTLD, they result in extremely high infection and mortality rates [74,77, 78], although one group recently reported a complete remission rate of 63% and median disease-free survival of 10.5 years using CHOP chemotherapy after cessation of immunosuppression in kidney transplant recipients [79]. Invariably, transplant patients have at least one vital organ that is not functioning well and are immunosuppressed at baseline, complicating the use of chemotherapy. In addition, they frequently are colonized with nosocomial pathogens; thus, infections often result from highly resistant organisms, such as methicillin-resistant *Staphylococcus aureus* or multidrug-resistant *Pseudomonas* species. The mortality rate for PTLD patients receiving chemotherapy is approximately 20% to 30%, in stark contrast to the good outcomes in healthy patients who have newly diagnosed NHL who receive identical chemotherapy regimens. In these healthy patients, chemotherapy-related neutropenic infections, organ toxicity, and hospitalizations are rare. Organ transplant patients undergoing chemotherapy should be monitored closely for infectious complications and may benefit from prophylactic antibiotic and filgrastim support.

Anti–B-cell antibodies

A logical therapeutic option to control B-cell proliferation is anti–B-cell antibody therapy. Expression of B-cell antigens is variable in PTLD, most likely because of dysregulation by EBV infection. Nevertheless, results are promising, with response rates of 50% to 80% [53,80–83]. Predictors of poor response to anti–B-cell therapy include multivisceral disease, late-onset PTLD (more than 1 year post transplant), and central nervous system involvement. Successes with the initial use of murine monoclonal antibodies led to use of several specific anti–B-cell therapies, with promising results. An early study of 58 solid organ and stem cell transplant recipients treated with anti-CD21 and anti-CD24 described a 63% complete response rate and 46% overall survival with a median follow-up of 61 months [53]. More recently, rituximab (human-mouse chimeric monoclonal anti-CD20 antibody) has been used [83], with favorable toxicity and response profiles. Again, PTLD behaves differently from de novo NHL in its response to rituximab. Rituximab seems to cure many patients who have PTLD, although it is a useful adjunct, but not curative, in nontransplant patients who have NHL. The reasons for this contrast are unclear but may relate to its mechanism of action. Rituximab binds to CD20 and results in clearance of these cells, either by simple apoptosis or via antibody-dependent complement-mediated lysis. One hypothesis is that rituximab may "activate" the immune system in patients who have PTLD, which prevents recurrence of disease. A report of five patients who had PTLD treated with rituximab demonstrated a decrease in EBV viral load in all patients but progression of the PTLD tumor in three patients [26], questioning the accuracy of following EBV DNA levels in patients receiving rituximab. In addition to "naked" monoclonal antibodies, such as rituximab, anti–B-cell antibodies linked to radionuclides, such as tositumomab (anti-CD20 linked to iodine-131) and ibritumomab tiuxetan (anti-CD20 linked to yttrium-90), seem hopeful and warrant additional studies.

Cellular immunotherapy

The use of cellular therapy to prevent and treat PTLD was developed first in the allogeneic HSCT population, in which PTLDs generally are of donor origin and donor lymphocytes can be collected and infused, with or without prior manipulations to generate EBV-specificity, into the recipient. This strategy has been extrapolated to solid organ transplant recipients, with modifications.

Recipients of T-cell depleted or HLA-mismatched HSCT have decreased T- and B-cell counts markedly for at least 6 months and possibly several years after transplant [84–87]. As the frequency of EBV-specific $CD8^+$ T cells rises after HSCT, a decrease in EBV viral load [88] and regression of PTLD [85,89,90] are observed. In addition, the efficacy of unselected donor leukocytes in reconstituting recipients' immune systems are well described [86]. These two observations incited investigators to attempt prophylaxis and treatment of PTLD who had donor leukocyte infusions. Initial treatment with unselected donor mononuclear cells resulted in high rates of GVHD and significant toxicity, but EBV-specific cytotoxic T lymphocytes (CTL) are more efficacious and far safer [60,91–94].

The use of EBV-specific CTL to treat PTLD after solid organ transplantation is feasible and effective but requires some key modifications. First, most cases of PTLD in solid organ allograft patients are of recipient, not donor, origin [95]. Because donors and recipients are not HLA identical, and T-cell killing is HLA-restricted, the infused cells should be HLA identical to the recipient [96]. An informative case report describes an 11-year-old boy who had central nervous system PTLD after a cadaveric (HLA-mismatched) lung transplant and who was treated with his HLA-identical brother's peripheral blood mononuclear cells and achieved complete remission, although his course was complicated by several bouts of acute rejection of the transplanted lungs [97]. In a seven-patient series, Nalesnik and co-workers collected peripheral blood mononuclear cells from solid organ transplant patients who had PTLD, cultured them with recombinant human IL-2, and reinfused them. The four patients who had EBV-positive tumors all sustained involution of their tumors; two patients suffered organ rejection as a complication of this therapy [98]. In a proof-of-principle experiment, T cells were harvested from three patients before solid organ transplantation. EBV-specific cell lines were cultured and reinfused into the patients after transplant as PTLD prophylaxis. Their circulating EBV DNA levels were suppressed below pretransplant levels, and EBV-specific CTL were measurable in the patients' blood for 3 months after transplant [99]. It subsequently was demonstrated that EBV-specific CTL could be generated from allograft recipients after transplant, despite ongoing immunosuppression [100], which has been replicated by other groups [101]. The only large clinical experience with reinfusion of these CTL is in patients who had high levels of circulating EBV DNA but not clinical PTLD [102]. Sixty solid organ transplant recipients who had high circulating levels of EBV DNA provided peripheral blood samples, but EBV-specific CTL lines were able to be generated in only 23 patients. Seven patients were reinfused for persistently high circulating EBV DNA levels, and in five, EBV DNA levels fell greater than 2 logs or to below the limits of detection. Unfortunately, the expertise, expense, and time required to generate these cell lines may limit the general applicability of this therapy. In addition, this strategy is not applicable to EBV-seronegative solid organ transplant recipients. A small trial of partially HLA-matched allogeneic highly EBV-specific CTL taken from a pre-existing tissue bank and used with continued immunosuppression demonstrated complete response in four of eight transplant patients who had EBV-positive PTLD: liver/small bowel (3), liver only (2), kidney (2), and stem cells (1) [103]. None experienced GVHD or graft rejection. Thus, use of either autologous or partly HLA-matched allogeneic CTL may have a promising future in effective treatment or prevention of PTLD in solid organ transplant patients.

Summary

PTLD is an increasingly recognized complication of solid organ transplantation and HSCT. Prompt diagnosis is key and requires high levels of clinical vigilance. Surveillance for PTLD by monthly PCR for circulating EBV DNA may be appropriate, particularly in such high-risk settings as EBV-seromismatched (donor-positive, recipient-negative) solid organ transplants and T-cell–depleted, HLA-mismatched stem cell transplants. When possible, surgical excision of the node, mass, or affected organ should be undertaken and combined with reduced immunosuppression and possibly radiotherapy. Rituximab is a recent and highly promising therapy for all patients who have PTLD, whereas cytotoxic chemotherapy should be reserved for cases refractory to these interventions because of its relatively high risk of infectious complications and mor-

tality. Cellular immunotherapy with EBV-specific T cells is highly effective and feasible in solid organ and stem cell transplant patients. Noninvasive diagnostic testing or monitoring for PTLD using EBV PCR or other serologic studies is an active area of investigation. Prophylaxis against PTLD with pre-emptive infusion of EBV-specific CTL either in all high-risk recipients or in patients who have increasing EBV viral loads also may be successful. In general, therapies for PTLD are resulting in improved outcomes. This diagnosis, once devastating, is moving toward becoming a complication of transplant that can be managed and often cured.

References

[1] Starzl TE. Discussion of: Murray JE, Wilson RE, Tilney NL, et al. Five years' experience in renal transplantation with immunosuppressive drugs: survival, function, complications and the role of lymphocyte depletion by thoracic duct fistula. Ann Surg 1968;168:416–35.

[2] Penn I, Hammond W, Brettschneider L, et al. Malignant lymphomas in transplantation patients. Transplant Proc 1969;1:106–12.

[3] Bhatia S, Ramsay NK, Steinbuch M, et al. Malignant neoplasms following bone marrow transplantation. Blood 1996;87:3633–9.

[4] Armitage JM, Kormos RL, Stuart RS, et al. Posttransplant lymphoproliferative disease in thoracic organ transplant patients: ten years of cyclosporine-based immunosuppression. J Heart Lung Transplant 1991; 10:877–86 [discussion: 886–7].

[5] Nalesnik MA. Posttransplantation lymphoproliferative disorders (PTLD): current perspectives. Semin Thorac Cardiovasc Surg 1996;8:139–48.

[6] Tsai DE, Hardy CL, Tomaszewski JE, et al. Reduction in immunosuppression as initial therapy for posttransplant lymphoproliferative disorder: analysis of prognostic variables and long- term follow-up of 42 adult patients. Transplantation 2001;71:1076–88.

[7] Opelz G, Dohler B. Lymphomas after solid organ transplantation: a collaborative transplant study report. Am J Transplant 2003;4:222–30.

[8] Shapiro RS, McClain K, Frizzera G, et al. Epstein-Barr virus associated B cell lymphoproliferative disorders following bone marrow transplantation. Blood 1988;71:1234–43.

[9] Epstein MA, Achong BG, Barr YM. Virus particles in cultured lymphoblasts from Burkitt's lymphoma. Lancet 1964;1:702–3.

[10] Cohen JI. Epstein-Barr virus infection. N Engl J Med 2000;343:481–92.

[11] Porcu P, Eisenbeis CF, Pelletier RP, et al. Successful treatment of posttransplantation lymphoproliferative disorder (PTLD) following renal allografting is

associated with sustained CD8(+) T-cell restoration. Blood 2002;100:2341–8.

[12] Omiya R, Buteau C, Kobayashi H, Paya CV, Celis E. Inhibition of EBV-induced lymphoproliferation by CD4(+) T cells specific for an MHC class II promiscuous epitope. J Immunol 2002;169:2172–9.

[13] Leblond V, Davi F, Charlotte F, et al. Posttransplant lymphoproliferative disorders not associated with Epstein-Barr virus: a distinct entity? J Clin Oncol 1998;16:2052–9.

[14] Nelson BP, Nalesnik MA, Bahler DW, et al. Epstein-Barr virus-negative post-transplant lymphoproliferative disorders: a distinct entity? Am J Surg Pathol 2000;24:375–85.

[15] Paya CV, Fung JJ, Nalesnik MA, et al. Epstein-Barr virus-induced posttransplant lymphoproliferative disorders. ASTS/ASTP EBV-PTLD Task Force and The Mayo Clinic Organized International Consensus Development Meeting. Transplantation 1999;68:1517–25.

[16] Harris NL, Ferry JA, Swerdlow SH. Posttransplant lymphoproliferative disorders: summary of Society for Hematopathology Workshop. Semin Diagn Pathol 1997;14:8–14.

[17] Harris NL, Jaffe ES, Diebold J, et al. World Health Organization classification of neoplastic diseases of the hematopoietic and lymphoid tissues: report of the Clinical Advisory Committee meeting-Airlie House, Virginia, November 1997. J Clin Oncol 1999;17:3835–49.

[18] George TI, Jeng M, Berquist W, et al. Epstein-Barr virus-associated peripheral T-cell lymphoma and hemophagocytic syndrome arising after liver transplantation: case report and review of the literature. Pediatr Blood Cancer 2005;44:270–6.

[19] Lee HK, Kim HJ, Lee EH, et al. Epstein-Barr virus-associated peripheral T-Cell lymphoma involving spleen in a renal transplant patient. J Korean Med Sci 2003;18:272–6.

[20] Rajakariar R, Bhattacharyya M, Norton A, et al. Post transplant T-cell lymphoma: a case series of four patients from a single unit and review of the literature. Am J Transplant 2004;4:1534–8.

[21] Tsai DE, Aqui NA, Vogl DT, et al. Successful treatment of T-cell posttransplant lymphoproliferative disorder with retinoid analog, bexarotene. Am J Transplant 2005;5:2070–3.

[22] Tsai DE, Nearey M, Hardy CL, et al. Use of EBV PCR for the diagnosis and monitoring of posttransplant lymphoproliferative disorder in adult solid organ transplant patients. Am J Transplant 2002;2:946–54.

[23] Green M, Webber SA. EBV viral load monitoring: unanswered questions. Am J Transplant 2002;2:894–5.

[24] Kenagy DN, Schlesinger Y, Weck K, et al. Epstein-Barr virus DNA in peripheral blood leukocytes of patients with posttransplant lymphoproliferative disease. Transplantation 1995;60:547–54.

[25] McDiarmid SV, Jordan S, Kim GS, et al. Prevention and preemptive therapy of postransplant lymphoproliferative disease in pediatric liver recipients. Transplantation 1998;66:1604–11.

[26] Yang J, Tao Q, Flinn IW, et al. Characterization of Epstein-Barr virus-infected B cells in patients with posttransplantation lymphoproliferative disease: disappearance after rituximab therapy does not predict clinical response. Blood 2000;96:4055–63.

[27] Aqui NA, Tomaszewski JE, Goodman D, et al. Use of serum protein electrophoresis to monitor patients with post-transplant lymphoproliferative disorder. Am J Transplant 2003;3:1308–11.

[28] Babel N, Schwarzmann F, Pruss A, et al. Monoclonal gammopathy of undetermined significance (MGUS) is associated with an increased frequency of Epstein-Barr Virus (EBV) latently infected B lymphocytes in long-term renal transplant patients. Transplant Proc 2004;36:2679–82.

[29] Lemoine A, Pham P, Azoulay D, et al. Detection of gammopathy by serum protein electrophoresis for predicting and managing therapy of lymphoproliferative disorder in 911 recipients of liver transplants. Blood 2001;98:1332–8.

[30] Feng S, Buell JF, Chari RS, et al. Tumors and transplantation: the 2003 Third Annual ASTS State-of-the-Art Winter Symposium. Am J Transplant 2003;3:1481–7.

[31] Nalesnik MA, Makowka L, Starzl TE. The diagnosis and treatment of posttransplant lymphoproliferative disorders. Curr Probl Surg 1988;25:367–472.

[32] Opelz G, Henderson R. Incidence of non-Hodgkin lymphoma in kidney and heart transplant recipients. Lancet 1993;342:1514–6.

[33] Ramalingam P, Rybicki L, Smith MD, et al. Post-transplant lymphoproliferative disorders in lung transplant patients: the Cleveland Clinic experience. Mod Pathol 2002;15:647–56.

[34] Reams BD, McAdams HP, Howell DN, et al. Post-transplant lymphoproliferative disorder: incidence, presentation, and response to treatment in lung transplant recipients. Chest 2003;124:1242–9.

[35] Gao SZ, Chaparro SV, Perlroth M, et al. Post-transplantation lymphoproliferative disease in heart and heart-lung transplant recipients: 30-year experience at Stanford University. J Heart Lung Transplant 2003;22:505–14.

[36] Paranjothi S, Yusen RD, Kraus MD, et al. Lymphoproliferative disease after lung transplantation: comparison of presentation and outcome of early and late cases. J Heart Lung Transplant 2001;20:1054–63.

[37] Castellano-Sanchez AA, Li S, Qian J, et al. Primary central nervous system posttransplant lymphoproliferative disorders. Am J Clin Pathol 2004;121:246–53.

[38] Benkerrou M, Durandy A, Fischer A. Therapy for transplant-related lymphoproliferative diseases. Hematol Oncol Clin North Am 1993;7:467–75.

[39] Hanto DW. Retransplantation after post-transplant

lymphoproliferative diseases (PTLD): when is it safe? Am J Transplant 2004;4:1733–4.

[40] Karras A, Thervet E, Meur YL, et al. Successful renal retransplantation after post-transplant lymphoproliferative disease. Am J Transplant 2004;4:1904–9.

[41] Juvonen E, Aalto SM, Tarkkanen J, et al. High incidence of PTLD after non-T-cell-depleted allogeneic haematopoietic stem cell transplantation as a consequence of intensive immunosuppressive treatment. Bone Marrow Transplant 2003;32:97–102.

[42] Zutter MM, Martin PJ, Sale GE, et al. Epstein-Barr virus lymphoproliferation after bone marrow transplantation. Blood 1988;72:520–9.

[43] Lones MA, Lopez-Terrada D, Shintaku IP, et al. Posttransplant lymphoproliferative disorder in pediatric bone marrow transplant recipients: disseminated disease of donor origin demonstrated by fluorescence in situ hybridization. Arch Pathol Lab Med 1998;122:708–14.

[44] Shepherd JD, Gascoyne RD, Barnett MJ, et al. Polyclonal Epstein-Barr virus-associated lymphoproliferative disorder following autografting for chronic myeloid leukemia. Bone Marrow Transplant 1995;15:639–41.

[45] Hauke RJ, Greiner TC, Smir BN, et al. Epstein-Barr virus-associated lymphoproliferative disorder after autologous bone marrow transplantation: report of two cases. Bone Marrow Transplant 1998;21:1271–4.

[46] Lones MA, Kirov I, Said JW, et al. Post-transplant lymphoproliferative disorder after autologous peripheral stem cell transplantation in a pediatric patient. Bone Marrow Transplant 2000;26:1021–4.

[47] Nash RA, Dansey R, Storek J, et al. Epstein-Barr virus-associated posttransplantation lymphoproliferative disorder after high-dose immunosuppressive therapy and autologous CD34-selected hematopoietic stem cell transplantation for severe autoimmune diseases. Biol Blood Marrow Transplant 2003;9:583–91.

[48] Ho AY, Adams S, Shaikh H, et al. Fatal donor-derived Epstein-Barr virus-associated post-transplant lymphoproliferative disorder following reduced intensity volunteer-unrelated bone marrow transplant for myelodysplastic syndrome. Bone Marrow Transplant 2002;29:867–9.

[49] Lange A, Klimczak A, Dlubek D, et al. B-cell lymphoproliferative syndrome and peripheral blood CD20 + cells expansion after hematopoietic stem cell transplantation: association with fludarabine and anti-thymocyte globulin containing conditioning regimen. Transplant Proc 2003;35:3093–5.

[50] Snyder MJ, Stenzel TT, Buckley PJ, et al. Posttransplant lymphoproliferative disorder following non-myeloablative allogeneic stem cell transplantation. Am J Surg Pathol 2004;28:794–800.

[51] Hale G, Waldmann H. Risks of developing Epstein-Barr virus-related lymphoproliferative disorders after T-cell-depleted marrow transplants. CAMPATH Users. Blood 1998;91:3079–83.

[52] Heslop HE. Preventing Epstein-Barr virus lymphoproliferative disease after bone marrow transplantation. J Immunother 2001;24:283–4.

[53] Benkerrou M, Jais JP, Leblond V, et al. Anti-B-cell monoclonal antibody treatment of severe posttransplant B- lymphoproliferative disorder: prognostic factors and long-term outcome. Blood 1998;92:3137–47.

[54] Gross TG, Steinbuch M, DeFor T, et al. B cell lymphoproliferative disorders following hematopoietic stem cell transplantation: risk factors, treatment and outcome. Bone Marrow Transplant 1999;23:251–8.

[55] Micallef IN, Chhanabhai M, Gascoyne RD, et al. Lymphoproliferative disorders following allogeneic bone marrow transplantation: the Vancouver experience. Bone Marrow Transplant 1998;22:981–7.

[56] Curtis RE, Travis LB, Rowlings PA, et al. Risk of lymphoproliferative disorders after bone marrow transplantation: a multi-institutional study. Blood 1999;94:2208–16.

[57] Parry-Jones N, Haque T, Ismail M, et al. Epstein-Barr virus (EBV) associated B-cell lymphoproliferative disease following HLA identical sibling marrow transplantation for aplastic anaemia in a patient with an EBV seronegative donor. Transplantation 1999;67:1373–5.

[58] Riddler SA, Breinig MC, McKnight JL. Increased levels of circulating Epstein-Barr virus (EBV)-infected lymphocytes and decreased EBV nuclear antigen antibody responses are associated with the development of posttransplant lymphoproliferative disease in solid-organ transplant recipients. Blood 1994;84:972–84.

[59] Savoie A, Perpete C, Carpentier L, et al. Direct correlation between the load of Epstein-Barr virus-infected lymphocytes in the peripheral blood of pediatric transplant patients and risk of lymphoproliferative disease. Blood 1994;83:2715–22.

[60] Rooney CM, Smith CA, Ng CY, et al. Use of gene-modified virus-specific T lymphocytes to control Epstein- Barr-virus-related lymphoproliferation. Lancet 1995;345:9–13.

[61] Lucas KG, Burton RL, Zimmerman SE, et al. Semiquantitative Epstein-Barr virus (EBV) polymerase chain reaction for the determination of patients at risk for EBV-induced lymphoproliferative disease after stem cell transplantation. Blood 1998;91:3654–61.

[62] Baldanti F, Grossi P, Furione M, et al. High levels of Epstein-Barr virus DNA in blood of solid-organ transplant recipients and their value in predicting posttransplant lymphoproliferative disorders. J Clin Microbiol 2000;38:613–9.

[63] Rooney CM, Loftin SK, Holladay MS, et al. Early identification of Epstein-Barr virus-associated post- transplantation lymphoproliferative disease. Br J Haematol 1995;89:98–103.

[64] Green M, Bueno J, Rowe D, et al. Predictive negative value of persistent low Epstein-Barr virus viral

load after intestinal transplantation in children. Transplantation 2000;70:593–6.

[65] Birkeland SA, Andersen HK, Hamilton-Dutoit SJ. Preventing acute rejection, Epstein-Barr virus infection, and posttransplant lymphoproliferative disorders after kidney transplantation: use of aciclovir and mycophenolate mofetil in a steroid-free immunosuppressive protocol. Transplantation 1999;67:1209–14.

[66] Darenkov IA, Marcarelli MA, Basadonna GP, et al. Reduced incidence of Epstein-Barr virus-associated posttransplant lymphoproliferative disorder using preemptive antiviral therapy. Transplantation 1997;64:848–52.

[67] Davis CL, Harrison KL, McVicar JP, et al. Antiviral prophylaxis and the Epstein Barr virus-related posttransplant lymphoproliferative disorder. Clin Transplant 1995;9:53–9.

[68] Colby BM, Shaw JE, Elion GB, et al. Effect of acyclovir [9-(2-hydroxyethoxymethyl)guanine] on Epstein-Barr virus DNA replication. J Virol 1980;34:560–8.

[69] Crumpacker CS. Ganciclovir. N Engl J Med 1996;335:721–9.

[70] Faller DV, Mentzer SJ, Perrine SP. Induction of the Epstein-Barr virus thymidine kinase gene with concomitant nucleoside antivirals as a therapeutic strategy for Epstein- Barr virus-associated malignancies. Curr Opin Oncol 2001;13:360–7.

[71] Perrine SP, Hermine O, Mentzer SJ, et al. A phase I/II study of arginine butyrate and ganciclovir in patients with Epstein-Barr virus-associated lymphoid malignancies. Blood 2004;104:176a.

[72] Starzl TE, Nalesnik MA, Porter KA, et al. Reversibility of lymphomas and lymphoproliferative lesions developing under cyclosporin-steroid therapy. Lancet 1984;1:583–7.

[73] Davis CL, Wood BL, Sabath DE, et al. Interferon-alpha treatment of posttransplant lymphoproliferative disorder in recipients of solid organ transplants. Transplantation 1998;66:1770–9.

[74] Dotti G, Fiocchi R, Motta T, et al. Lymphomas occurring late after solid-organ transplantation: influence of treatment on the clinical outcome. Transplantation 2002;74:1095–102.

[75] Faro A, Kurland G, Michaels MG, et al. Interferon-alpha affects the immune response in post-transplant lymphoproliferative disorder. Am J Respir Crit Care Med 1996;153(4 Pt 1):1442–7.

[76] Haddad E, Paczesny S, Leblond V, et al. Treatment of B-lymphoproliferative disorder with a monoclonal anti- interleukin-6 antibody in 12 patients: a multicenter phase 1–2 clinical trial. Blood 2001;97:1590–7.

[77] Swinnen LJ, Mullen GM, Carr TJ, et al. Aggressive treatment for postcardiac transplant lymphoproliferation. Blood 1995;86:3333–40.

[78] Mamzer-Bruneel MF, Lome C, Morelon E, et al. Durable remission after aggressive chemotherapy for very late post-kidney transplant lymphoprolifera-

tion: a report of 16 cases observed in a single center. J Clin Oncol 2000;18:3622–32.

[79] Gill D, Juffs HG, Herzig KA, et al. Durable and high rates of remission following chemotherapy in posttransplantation lymphoproliferative disorders after renal transplantation. Transplant Proc 2003;35:256–7.

[80] Faye A, Van Den Abeele T, Peuchmaur M, et al. Anti-CD20 monoclonal antibody for post-transplant lymphoproliferative disorders. Lancet 1998;352:1285.

[81] Fischer A, Blanche S, Le Bidois J, et al. Anti-B-cell monoclonal antibodies in the treatment of severe B-cell lymphoproliferative syndrome following bone marrow and organ transplantation. N Engl J Med 1991;324:1451–6.

[82] Kuehnle I, Huls MH, Liu Z, et al. CD20 monoclonal antibody (rituximab) for therapy of Epstein-Barr virus lymphoma after hemopoietic stem-cell transplantation. Blood 2000;95:1502–5.

[83] Milpied N, Vasseur B, Parquet N, et al. Humanized anti-CD20 monoclonal antibody (Rituximab) in post transplant B-lymphoproliferative disorder: a retrospective analysis on 32 patients. Ann Oncol 2000;11(Suppl 1):113–6.

[84] Crawford DH, Mulholland N, Iliescu V, et al. Epstein-Barr virus infection and immunity in bone marrow transplant recipients. Transplantation 1986;42:50–4.

[85] Kook H, Goldman F, Padley D, et al. Reconstruction of the immune system after unrelated or partially matched T-cell-depleted bone marrow transplantation in children: immunophenotypic analysis and factors affecting the speed of recovery. Blood 1996;88:1089–97.

[86] Small TN, Papadopoulos EB, Boulad F, et al. Comparison of immune reconstitution after unrelated and related T-cell- depleted bone marrow transplantation: effect of patient age and donor leukocyte infusions. Blood 1999;93:467–80.

[87] Marshall NA, Howe JG, Formica R, et al. Rapid reconstitution of Epstein-Barr virus-specific T lymphocytes following allogeneic stem cell transplantation. Blood 2000;96:2814–21.

[88] Kuzushima K, Kimura H, Hoshino Y, et al. Longitudinal dynamics of Epstein-Barr virus-specific cytotoxic T lymphocytes during posttransplant lymphoproliferative disorder. J Infect Dis 2000;182:937–40.

[89] Lucas KG, Small TN, Heller G, Dupont B, O'Reilly RJ. The development of cellular immunity to Epstein-Barr virus after allogeneic bone marrow transplantation. Blood 1996;87:2594–603.

[90] Khatri VP, Baiocchi RA, Peng R, et al. Endogenous CD8 + T cell expansion during regression of monoclonal EBV- associated posttransplant lymphoproliferative disorder. J Immunol 1999;163:500–6.

[91] Porter DL, Orloff GJ, Antin JH. Donor mononuclear cell infusions as therapy for B-cell lymphoproliferative disorder following allogeneic bone marrow transplant. Transplant Sci 1994;4:12–4 [discussion 14–6].

[92] Papadopoulos EB, Ladanyi M, Emanuel D, et al. Infusions of donor leukocytes to treat Epstein-Barr virus-associated lymphoproliferative disorders after allogeneic bone marrow transplantation. N Engl J Med 1994;330:1185–91.

[93] Rooney CM, Smith CA, Ng CY, et al. Infusion of cytotoxic T cells for the prevention and treatment of Epstein-Barr virus-induced lymphoma in allogeneic transplant recipients. Blood 1998;92:1549–55.

[94] Gustafsson A, Levitsky V, Zou JZ, et al. Epstein-Barr virus (EBV) load in bone marrow transplant recipients at risk to develop posttransplant lymphoproliferative disease: prophylactic infusion of EBV-specific cytotoxic T cells. Blood 2000;95: 807–14.

[95] Gulley ML, Swinnen LJ, Plaisance Jr KT, et al. Tumor origin and CD20 expression in posttransplant lymphoproliferative disorder occurring in solid organ transplant recipients: implications for immune-based therapy. Transplantation 2003;76:959–64.

[96] Bollard CM, Savoldo B, Rooney CM, et al. Adoptive T-cell therapy for EBV-associated post-transplant lymphoproliferative disease. Acta Haematol 2003; 110:139–48.

[97] Emanuel DJ, Lucas KG, Mallory Jr GB, et al. Treatment of posttransplant lymphoproliferative disease in the central nervous system of a lung transplant recipient using allogeneic leukocytes. Transplantation 1997;63:1691–4.

[98] Nalesnik MA, Rao AS, Zeevi A, et al. Autologous lymphokine-activated killer cell therapy of lymphoproliferative disorders arising in organ transplant recipients. Transplant Proc 1997;29:1905–6.

[99] Haque T, Amlot PL, Helling N, et al. Reconstitution of EBV-specific T cell immunity in solid organ transplant recipients. J Immunol 1998;160: 6204–9.

[100] Khanna R, Bell S, Sherritt M, et al. Activation and adoptive transfer of Epstein-Barr virus-specific cytotoxic T cells in solid organ transplant patients with posttransplant lymphoproliferative disease. Proc Natl Acad Sci USA 1999;96:10391–6.

[101] Savoldo B, Goss J, Liu Z, et al. Generation of autologous Epstein-Barr virus-specific cytotoxic T cells for adoptive immunotherapy in solid organ transplant recipients. Transplantation 2001;72:1078–86.

[102] Comoli P, Labirio M, Basso S, et al. Infusion of autologous Epstein-Barr virus (EBV)-specific cytotoxic T cells for prevention of EBV-related lymphoproliferative disorder in solid organ transplant recipients with evidence of active virus replication. Blood 2002;99:2592–8.

[103] Haque T, Wilkie GM, Taylor C, et al. Treatment of Epstein-Barr-virus-positive post-transplantation lymphoproliferative disease with partly HLA-matched allogeneic cytotoxic T cells. Lancet 2002;360:436–42.

[104] Frizzera G, Hanto DW, Gajl-Peczalska KJ, et al. Polymorphic diffuse B-cell hyperplasias and lymphomas in renal transplant recipients. Cancer Res 1981; 41(11 Pt 1):4262–79.

[105] Knowles DM, Cesarman E, Chadburn A, et al. Correlative morphologic and molecular genetic analysis demonstrates three distinct categories of post-transplantation lymphoproliferative disorders. Blood 1995;85:552–65.

ELSEVIER
SAUNDERS

Clin Chest Med 26 (2005) 647–659

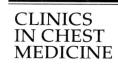

CLINICS
IN CHEST
MEDICINE

Bacterial and Mycobacterial Pneumonia in Transplant Recipients

Leanne B. Gasink, MD*, Emily A. Blumberg, MD

*Division of Infectious Diseases, Department of Medicine, University of Pennsylvania, 3 Silverstein, Suite E,
3400 Spruce Street, Philadelphia, PA 19104, USA*

Pulmonary infections are the most common infectious complication in lung and heart transplant recipients, the second most common infectious complication in liver transplant patients, and the most common cause of infectious death after hematopoietic stem cell transplant (HSCT) [1–5]. Bacteria and mycobacteria are important pulmonary pathogens in transplant recipients and are the focus of this article. Although considerable overlap exists, there are significant differences in the epidemiology and clinical presentation of these organisms in solid organ transplant (SOT) and HSCT recipients. The first section of this article focuses on infections in SOT recipients (predominantly heart, liver, lung, and kidney transplant recipients), and the latter addresses these infections in HSCT recipients.

Pyogenic gram-negative and gram-positive bacteria, both nosocomially and community acquired, reportedly account for more than one third of pneumonia episodes in renal, liver, heart, and lung transplant recipients and occur with an incidence of 15% in HSCT recipients [2,6–9]. Because the cause of infectious pneumonias frequently is not identified (and identification often depends on the extent to which specific diagnoses are pursued), it is difficult to determine the frequency with which specific pathogens cause infection. In some cases, pathogens remain unknown despite aggressive diagnostic attempts. For example, one prospective study that performed bronchoalveolar lavage on all liver transplant recipients with pulmonary infiltrates reported that no microbiologic cause was identified in 30% of pneumonias that met clinical and other confirmatory criteria for infection [7]. Hospital-acquired pneumonias (HAP) can be especially difficult to diagnose definitively, and methods to determine causative organisms are controversial and often unreliable [10]. Community-acquired pneumonias (CAP) are common in transplant recipients, but loss to follow-up may prevent diagnosis and identification in transplant centers, resulting in an underestimation of the actual incidence. Like HAP, observational studies have found that a cause of CAP is defined in only 6% of outpatients and 25% of inpatients [11]. Therefore, although existing data suggest that bacterial HAP and CAP are significant and important infections in transplant recipients, the extent to which they cause morbidity and mortality is unknown.

Although rare, mycobacterial infections occur with increased frequency and severity in transplant recipients, and the clinical manifestations are varied. Despite overlapping risk factors, transplant recipients manifest infection less often and quite differently than do persons with AIDS [12]. Management of mycobacterial infection is complex, controversial, and evolving, currently with little transplant recipient–specific data to guide therapy. Infection with *Mycobacterium tuberculosis* is particularly important for transplant recipients in countries where tuberculosis (TB) is endemic, and active infection in these patients has serious implications for public health and safety.

* Corresponding author.
E-mail address: leanne.gasink@uphs.upenn.edu
(L.B. Gasink).

0272-5231/05/$ – see front matter © 2005 Elsevier Inc. All rights reserved.
doi:10.1016/j.ccm.2005.06.003

Solid organ transplant recipients

Timelines for infectious complications after SOT are useful tools to identify periods of greatest risk for infection, but specific host, pathogen, and environmental factors may provide additional clues to diagnosis [13]. Potential sources of bacterial or mycobacterial pulmonary infection include reactivation of latent disease, new infection, or acquisition from a donor with pneumonia or bacteremia. The risk of pulmonary infections varies depending on the type of organ transplanted. Renal transplant recipients are at the lowest risk, reflecting the less invasive surgical process and generally lower levels of immunosuppression [2]. The risk of pulmonary infection in lung transplant recipients is far greater than for other SOT recipients [2,14]. In addition to immunosuppression, factors unique to lung transplant recipients that predispose them to pulmonary infection include exposure of the allograft to the external environment, poor lymphatic drainage, impaired mucociliary clearance, blunted cough caused by postoperative pain and lung denervation, narrowing of the bronchial anastomosis, and the potential for direct transfer from the donated lung [14]. Recurrent or chronic rejection in SOT recipients results in increased exposure to immunosuppressive therapy, further increasing the risk of infection. [13].

Hospital- and community-acquired pneumonias in solid organ transplant recipients

Post-SOT bacterial pneumonias have been classified as those that occur in the early postoperative period and those that occur much later. This bimodal distribution roughly correlates with HAP and CAP, respectively, but infection can occur at any time. *Legionella* infection may be acquired from hospital or community sources.

Hospital-acquired pneumonia

HAP most commonly is a perioperative complication with incidence rates estimated at 10% for liver and heart transplant recipients and 15% for lung transplant recipients [2]. The incidence has declined in recent years, probably because of the widespread implementation of prophylactic antibiotics [15]. Risk factors for HAP have not been specifically determined for SOT recipients but presumably are similar to those noted for other postoperative and hospitalized patients. Prolonged mechanical ventilation and impaired clearance of pulmonary secretions related to surgery and pain are major risk factors [2,10].

Although occult pneumonia in donated lungs seemingly increases the risk of postoperative pneumonia in lung transplant recipients, the presence of bacterial organisms on Gram stain of donor bronchial washings is not in itself predictive of posttransplant pneumonia [2,13]. Despite the presence of virulent and often highly resistant bacteria in the airways of patients who had cystic fibrosis before lung transplantation, no overall increase in the risk of postoperative pneumonia has been identified. The one exception involves patients who have cystic fibrosis and are infected with organisms from the *Burkholderia Cepacia* complex (especially genomovar 3, also known as *Burkholderia cenocepacia*). Transplantation in this particular subgroup of patients is associated with a high rate of posttransplantation pneumonia and a markedly inferior posttransplantation survival rate [16,17]. Consequently, infection with this organism precludes transplantation at most centers.

As in all HAP, commonly isolated organisms include gram-negative pathogens, such as *Pseudomonas aeruginosa*, *Escherichia coli*, *Klebsiella pneumoniae,* and *Enterobacter, Acinetobacter*, and *Legionella* species, but gram-positive infections are increasingly common [5–8,10]. Of particular concern is the emergence of multidrug-resistant bacteria. General risk factors for resistant bacteria in HAP include antimicrobial therapy in the preceding 90 days, hospitalization for more than 5 days, high prevalence of hospital-specific resistance, and immunosuppressive disease or therapy [10].

Recommendations for prevention of HAP include infection-control measures (ie, standard precautions, isolation of resistant pathogens, routine surveillance of ICUs), minimization of aspiration, avoidance of unnecessary and prolonged intubation, and aggressive pulmonary toilet [10,18]. Empiric, broad-spectrum antibiotic therapy should be started immediately in all suspected cases, and the choice of agents should depend on institutional resistance patterns. Because most bacterial pulmonary infections are treatable, an early, aggressive pursuit of an etiologic diagnosis is strongly advocated so that directed and definitive therapy can be administered [13].

Community-acquired pneumonia

CAP can occur at any time after transplantation, although it tends to be noted after 6 months [13]. *Streptococcus pneumoniae* (the most common cause of CAP in the general population), *Haemophilus influenza*, and *Legionella* species are the most common pathogens identified, and infection is usually well tolerated and easily treatable [2,5,7,13,19]. Risk factors for acquisition of *S pneumoniae*, such as immunosuppression, liver disease, chronic lung disease, chronic cardiovascular disease, and renal disease, are commonly present in SOT and may increase the risk of severe disease and death [20]. *P aeruginosa* is an uncommon cause of CAP but is a particular concern in lung transplant recipients who have cystic fibrosis or chronic rejection.

Pneumococcal polysaccharide vaccination is recommended for all SOT candidates before transplantation [21]. Although revaccination is recommended every 5 years, antibody titers in response to vaccination are often lower in transplant recipients, and antibody levels are more likely to decline rapidly [20,22,23]. Therefore, revaccination may be considered at 2- to 3-year intervals [21]. Pneumococcal conjugate vaccine may be more immunogenic in SOT recipients, but there are inadequate data to recommend its routine use at this time [21,24]. Given the propensity for secondary bacterial pneumonias in the setting of influenza infection, yearly influenza vaccination may also help prevent the development of bacterial pneumonias. Finally, *H influenza* type B conjugate vaccine (HIB) should be administered to all children before SOT transplant. Asplenic or other immunosuppressed patients may exhibit reduced antibody responses to HIB, and revaccination based on measured HIB titers has been suggested [21].

Pursuit of an etiologic diagnosis in SOT recipients with CAP through Gram stain and culture of respiratory secretions is encouraged, but in most cases, as in immunocompetent individuals, no organism can be identified. Therefore, the American Thoracic Society (ATS) and the Infectious Disease Society of America have provided guidelines for the empiric treatment of CAP [25,26]. For SOT, a beta-lactam plus a macrolide or a quinolone generally is recommended. An antipseudomonal beta-lactam should be considered in persons at high risk such as lung transplant recipients who have cystic fibrosis or bronchiolitis obliterans syndrome. Of major concern is the emergence of drug-resistant *S pneumoniae*. Although 40% of isolates are resistant by in vitro criteria, controversy exists regarding the clinical significance of pneumococcal isolates with reduced sensitivity to beta-lactams [26]. When pneumonia is being treated, all but the most resistant *S pneumoniae* isolates (amoxicillin minimum inhibitory concentration ≥4) may respond favorably to beta-lactams [26]. Quinolone resistance is currently rare but may be increasing [26].

Pneumonia in lung transplant recipients who have bronchiolitis obliterans syndrome

Bacterial pneumonias are a common late complication in lung transplant recipients who develop chronic rejection, functionally defined as bronchiolitis obliterans syndrome [2,14]. Pulmonary function progressively deteriorates, and the lower respiratory tract becomes colonized with organisms that are often resistant to multiple antibiotics. Patients present with recurrent lower respiratory tract infections and evidence of bronchiectasis on chest imaging [14,27]. *P aeruginosa* is most frequently identified as the causative agent, but other gram-negative organisms, including *Acinetobacter* species, are frequently found [2–4]. Eradication of these pathogens can be extremely difficult [3].

Legionella *pneumonia*

Legionella species are important causes of both HAP and CAP in SOT recipients. Major transplant centers report that 35% to 80% of identified *Legionella* infections occur in SOT recipients [28,29]. In some centers, *Legionella* is the most frequent cause of pneumonia in SOT recipients, accounting for 25% to 50% of cases [30]. Estimating the incidence of *Legionella* in transplant recipients, as in nontransplant populations, is limited by the absence of a pathognomonic clinical presentation, the lack of reliable and rapid diagnostic testing for all species, and the need for specialized culture methods that may not be available in all hospitals. As a result, *Legionella* may be significantly underdiagnosed [30]. In fact, numerous studies document that the incidence of *Legionella* is proportional to the intensity of application of diagnostic testing [31]. *L pneumophila* subtype 1 accounts for 80% of isolates in the general population, but SOT recipients may be predisposed to non–*L pneumophila* infection, and a variety of species have been reported [32].

Deficiencies in cellular immune function are thought to increase the risk of *Legionella* infections, which have been reported in all organ transplant groups [28,32–40]. *Legionella* is acquired through the inhalation or aspiration of contaminated water, which often occurs nosocomially [32,41]. Although infections can occur at any time, cases usually are identified in the early posttransplantation interval and during periods of augmented immunosuppression, reflecting increased susceptibility secondary to intensified immunosuppression, exposure to potentially contaminated in-hospital water sources, and, perhaps, a more aggressive approach to diagnosis [32]. Corticosteroid dose in renal transplant recipients was found to be an independent risk factor for the development of legionellosis [42]. Surgery has also been implicated as a risk factor, and in the peritransplantation period *Legionella* may be transmitted to

SOT recipients through mechanical ventilators and nasogastric tubes [43,44]. Several nosocomial outbreaks have been documented in SOT units [38,45].

Legionella pneumonia presents with a broad spectrum of illness but can be quite severe in both immunosuppressed and normal hosts. Fever and pulmonary symptoms are most prominent with gastrointestinal symptoms often preceding respiratory findings. Surprisingly, SOT recipients do not seem to have increased morbidity or mortality compared with non-transplant patients [32]. Treatment failures in SOT recipients have been documented, however, and there have been multiple reports of progression to cavitation [35]. In a retrospective assessment of 40 cases that included 14 SOT recipients, nosocomial infection, intubation, and the development of lung abscess, cavitation, or pleural effusion were statistically significant predictors of mortality, but SOT was not [28].

Legionella should be considered in all SOT patients presenting with CAP, especially in those who fail to respond to beta-lactam therapy. Diagnosis of *Legionella* infection can be confirmed by culture of respiratory specimens, examination of urine for the presence of *Legionella pneumophila* serotype 1 antigen, or direct fluorescent antibody testing of respiratory specimens [32]. Culture is the most sensitive and specific method of diagnostic testing, followed by the urinary antigen test. For maximal sensitivity of culture, several types of selective media must be used [44]. Because culture is not performed routinely in all centers, care must be taken to ensure that proper diagnostic tests are ordered and performed. Detection of urinary antigen has an estimated sensitivity of 70% and a specificity of 100% [32]. It is extremely useful for rapid diagnosis but identifies only *L pneumophila* serotype 1 antigen. Thus, the urinary antigen assay may be less useful in SOT recipients, who more often are infected with other species of *Legionella*, than in normal hosts. All patients suspected of *Legionella* infection should undergo testing with both culture and urinary antigen identification to maximize sensitivity [32]. Serologic diagnosis, which requires acute and convalescent serum, is not helpful clinically but can be useful for epidemiologic investigations.

Because *Legionella* frequently is acquired through contaminated hospital water systems, the Centers for Disease Control (CDC) and the Health care Infection Control Advisory Committee have suggested that facilities with transplant programs periodically perform cultures for *Legionella* in water samples as part of a comprehensive strategy to prevent disease in high-risk patients. No guidelines regarding the frequency or number of testing sites are provided, however

[18]. The CDC does recommend that an epidemiologic and environmental investigation be initiated (1) when a single inpatient on a transplant unit develops a case of laboratory-confirmed, definite (ie, after ≥10 days of continuous inpatient stay) or possible (ie, within 2 to 9 days of inpatient stay) health-care–associated *Legionella* infection, or (2) when two or more patients develop laboratory-confirmed legionnaires' disease within 6 months of each other and after having visited an outpatient transplant unit during the 10-day period before illness onset. Using serology, one transplant center diagnosed *L micdadei* in nine SOT recipients over a 6-month period after an epidemiologic investigation was prompted by the identification of nosocomial infection in two renal transplant recipients [45]. A hospital hot-water source was identified. This and other reports underscore the importance of maintaining a high index of suspicion and continued monitoring for *Legionella*, especially in centers caring for immunocompromised patients. It is possible that hospitals may experience nosocomial cases over an extended period of time without being aware that a problem exists [32]. Appropriate responses to the identification of *Legionella* species in a transplant unit are described in the CDC guidelines and should be performed in conjunction with the facility's infection control team and, if necessary, state and local health departments [18]. An extensive investigation in the event of an isolated nosocomial case of *Legionella* occurring outside the transplant unit is not recommended by the CDC, but this recommendation remains controversial given the possibility of simultaneous, unrecognized infections and the potential for prevention of nosocomial outbreaks [30].

Delayed therapy of *Legionella* has been associated with increased mortality. Thus, prompt empiric therapy should be initiated in all patients suspected of infection [46]. The preferred treatment of *Legionella* is azithromycin or a fluoroquinolone. Although erythromycin is active against *Legionella* species, it should be avoided in SOT patients because of drug interactions with calcineurin inhibitors. Despite in vitro data demonstrating activity of imipenem and rifampin against *Legionella*, these antimicrobial agents are not clinically effective for *Legionella* infections and should not be used [31,32]. Although initially 21 days was recommended for immunosuppressed hosts, 10 to 14 days of therapy now is considered the standard duration of treatment [47]. Although treatment failures have been reported, development of antibiotic resistance has not been documented as an underlying cause [35,47]. Some experts recommend prolonged therapy only when the patient has not responded clinically within 5 days of therapy [31].

Nocardia *infections in solid organ transplant recipients*

Nocardia species are ubiquitous environmental saprophytes belonging to the genus *Actinomycetes*. Immunosuppression is the major risk factor, and infections are seen most often in SOT recipients, patients who have lymphoreticular malignancy or advanced HIV infection, and persons receiving chronic steroid therapy [48]. In the SOT population, the reported frequency of infection varies widely but falls between 0.7% and 3% in most reports [48,49]. Concomitant infection with Cytomegalovirus, profound hypogammaglobulinemia, and aggressive immunosuppression, such as the use of antilymphocyte immunoglobulin preparations, have been proposed as risk factors for nocardial infection in SOT recipients [13,48,50].

Transmission occurs primarily through inhalation, resulting in pulmonary infection and subsequent dissemination to other tissues, especially the brain. Penetrating injury can result in primary cutaneous infection [51]. In SOT recipients, infections occur most often between 1 and 6 months after transplantation and are associated with prolonged periods of immunosuppression [52]. Pulmonary nocardiosis may result in granulomatous or pyogenic processes and is caused by *Nocardia asteroides* complex in 90% of infections [48,53]. Chest radiography most often shows nodular lesions that often progress to cavitation, but diffuse infiltrates and consolidation can also occur [48,54]. Definitive diagnosis requires identification of typical gram-positive, aerobic, modified acid-fast–positive, branching and beading bacteria on tissue culture. Diagnosis or suspicion of pulmonary nocardiosis always should prompt evaluation of the brain to exclude abscess and a careful search for other sites of dissemination.

The use of trimethoprim-sulfamethoxazole (TMP-SMX) as prophylaxis against *Pneumocystis jiroveci* pneumonia may reduce the incidence of nocardial infection. Breakthrough infection may still occur, however, possibly more often in patients taking TMP-SMX every other day than in those on a daily regimen [48,49]. Although susceptibility testing is recommended, TMP-SMX is also the preferred treatment for established nocardial infections. Recommended dosing is 15 mg/kg/day divided into two to four doses daily and may be given orally or intravenously [48]. Other therapeutic options include sulfonamides alone, which are equally effective in high

doses, and a variety of other agents (imipenem, meropenem, amikacin, minocycline, third-generation cephalosporins, linezolid, ciprofloxacin, and amoxicillin-clavulanate), but these agents have been less well studied, and certain *Nocardia* species may be more likely to demonstrate resistance [48]. Some authors have recommended the use of amikacin with second-line agents, based on in vitro data that suggest synergy [55]. Duration of treatment varies depending on the level of immunosuppression, site of infection, and rapidity of clinical response. In general, pulmonary and soft tissue infections should be treated for 6 to 12 months, and central nervous system infection should be treated for 9 to 12 months [56,57]. Brain abscesses may require surgical drainage, and immunosuppression should be reduced, if possible [48]. After completion of therapy, follow-up imaging should be performed, and prolonged or lifelong secondary prophylaxis is often provided [48,58].

Mycobacterial infections in solid organ transplant recipients

Tuberculosis

Although the incidence of TB after SOT is low in developed countries, SOT recipients have a 50- to 100-fold higher risk of infection compared with the general population [2,59]. In endemic countries, rates of infection are much higher. In India, 12% to 20% of SOT recipients develop TB [60]. TB-related mortality rates are high. In a recent report, mortality after TB diagnosis in renal transplant recipients in the United States was 23% at 1 year, with an adjusted hazard ratio of 4.13 compared with recipients without TB [61]. Other authors have reported infection-related mortality rates ranging from 10% to 30% [60,62,63]. Despite differences in incidence among countries, TB clearly causes significant morbidity and mortality in SOT recipients worldwide and also poses public health risks.

Most cases occur in the first year after transplantation and are probably the result of reactivation of latent infection [2,59,64], although 20% to 25% of cases occur in patients who have positive tuberculin skin tests before transplantation. Although high false-negative rates are expected in patients who have end-stage organ dysfunction, less than 50% of published cases underwent skin testing before transplantation, an important step in the pretransplantation evaluation [64]. TB can also be acquired through infected donor organs and postoperatively [65]. Specific risk factors for TB after SOT have not been well established. A prospective evaluation of 1414 renal transplant recipients in India that identified 27 (13.3%) cases of active TB implicated receipt of cyclosporine (versus prenisolone plus azathioprine), diabetes mellitus, and chronic liver disease as potential risk factors [60]. Prior residence in an endemic country should alert practitioners to the high risk of prior exposure and latent TB infection [64].

A comprehensive literature review that identified 511 cases of TB in SOT recipients reported that 51% of patients had pulmonary TB, 16% had extrapulmonary TB, and 33% had disseminated TB [64]. In normal hosts, rates of disseminated disease are about 15% [59]. Receipt of OKT3 was a significant risk factor for dissemination. Among patients who had disseminated disease, more than 50% had pulmonary involvement. Fever was the most common symptom, occurring in 90% of patients who had disseminated disease and 66% of those with pulmonary disease. Only 4% had cavitary lung disease, but radiographic abnormalities were found in virtually all cases. Because clinical and radiographic findings of TB may be atypical in SOT recipients, a high index of suspicion should be maintained so that diagnosis and treatment are not delayed. Factors potentially associated with high mortality are rejection and treatment of rejection, shorter duration of TB treatment, and other opportunistic infections [63].

Given the potential for significant morbidity and mortality, a thorough, pretransplantation assessment of candidates and, if possible, donors, is mandatory. A detailed and careful history regarding potential TB exposures, prior TB infection, and prior treatment for latent or active TB should be performed. Chest radiographs should be examined for evidence of prior infection. All patients should undergo tuberculin skin testing, including candidates with a history of bacille Calmette-Guérin vaccination [59]. Although the likelihood of diagnosing latent infection by skin testing would seem to be higher before transplantation and initiation of antirejection drugs, many latently infected transplant candidates fail to mount a response to skin testing because of underlying chronic disease, malnutrition, and the use of corticosteroids to treat many of the conditions that lead to transplantation [2]. An area of induration of 5 mm or larger should be considered positive in all patients. Treatment for latent TB should be considered for any patient with a positive skin test who was not previously treated and for those with history of prior active TB who did not receive a complete course of appropriate therapy, regardless of skin testing results [59]. These categories include patients who have evidence of prior infection on chest radiography or significant TB exposures (ie, close family contact or

receipt of an organ from a donor with a positive skin test), even if skin testing is negative.

The approach to treatment of both latent and active TB is complicated by a number of factors present in the SOT patient. High mortality rates in SOT have been attributed to the disease itself and also to direct consequences of TB therapy [2]. In particular, rejection and graft loss have been reported frequently in patients treated with rifamycins [66]. Rifamycins dramatically increase hepatic metabolism of calcineurin inhibitors and consequently lower the blood levels of these agents. In one report, more than 25% of treated renal, heart, and liver transplant recipients experienced graft failure while receiving rifamycin therapy [63]. Interactions between calcineurin inhibitors and isoniazid have also been reported, but this interaction generally is not clinically significant and should not preclude the use of isoniazid [59]. Drug-induced hepatotoxicity remains an important concern in patients taking isoniazid and may lead to discontinuation of therapy [67]. As discussed later, drug-induced hepatotoxicity is a particular issue in liver transplant recipients, in whom development of abnormal liver function studies while taking isoniazid leads to discontinuation of the drug in 41% to 83% of patients [2].

The American Society of Transplantation (AST) has published recommendations regarding the treatment of TB infection, although many issues remain unresolved [59]. In general, rifampin as treatment for latent TB infection or in combination with other drugs for active TB therapy should not be used in SOT recipients. Avoidance of rifamycins will extend the duration of therapy beyond the standard 6-month course. All transplant recipients taking isoniazid should be monitored routinely for hepatotoxicity, but asymptomatic elevations in transaminases that are still less than five times the normal range should prompt enhanced monitoring rather than discontinuation of therapy.

Treatment of latent infection should be considered for all transplant recipients with a positive tuberculin skin test and is more urgent when donors or recipients are recent converters [59]. Initiation in transplant candidates is more controversial. AST guidelines recommend initiation of latent TB therapy in renal transplant candidates who face long wait times and already have an increased risk of active TB, lung transplant candidates in whom active TB may be difficult to identify in the setting of other pulmonary processes, and other candidates already receiving immunosuppressive therapy [59]. Otherwise, the recommendations suggest that it may be preferable to begin therapy after SOT, when the patients may be more medically stable and the risk of active TB increases because of immunosuppression. In light of the prolonged waiting times to transplantation for all but the most severely ill candidates, other authors advocate pretransplantation initiation of treatment for latent TB for all candidates for whom therapy is not contraindicated. In this way, the 9-month course of therapy often can be completed before initiation of other potentially hepatotoxic drugs (eg, calcineurin inhibitors, azathioprine, azole antifungal agents) that complicate the administration and monitoring of isoniazid [2].

The use of isoniazid for the treatment of latent TB infection in liver transplant candidates and recipients raises additional considerations. When isoniazid is administered after transplantation, elevation in hepatic transaminases should not be attributed automatically to drug toxicity but should always prompt an aggressive pursuit of a definitive diagnosis [2,59]. To minimize uncertainty, isoniazid therapy should not be started, ideally, until liver enzymes have stabilized [59,63]. There is an understandable reluctance to use isoniazid before liver transplantation, because of the universal presence of severe liver disease among candidates. In one published series of 18 liver transplant candidates, however, isoniazid was well tolerated by all patients, suggesting that it can be safely administered even in the setting of severe liver disease [68]. Obviously liver transplant candidates receiving isoniazid should be monitored closely, and decisions to treat should be weighed carefully against the risk for hepatotoxicity.

Nontuberculous mycobacteria

Nontuberculous mycobacteria (NTM) are ubiquitous organisms that have recently emerged as disease-causing pathogens in immunosuppressed persons. NTM infections have been well documented in SOT recipients and are increasing in frequency and severity [12,69]. Risk factors for infection are not well studied, but exposure to contaminated water or soil is the presumed method of acquisition for many species.

Species most commonly isolated from SOT recipients include *Mycobacterium avium* complex, *M kansasii, M marinum, M haemophilum, M fortuitum, M chelonae,* and *M abscessus* [12]. In lung transplant patients, NTM infection may be particularly common, occurring more often than TB in the largest published series [70]. In this series, 23 (8.8%) of 261 patients were diagnosed with 17 and six pulmonary and extrapulmonary mycobacterial infections, respectively. Pulmonary infections included *M avium* complex (n = 13), TB (n = 2), *M abscessus*

(n = 2), and one each of *M intracellulare, kansasii,* and *asiaticum* [70]. *M avium* complex and other NTM are common in persons with underlying lung diseases, and these organisms colonize or infect the lungs of many candidates awaiting lung transplantation [12]. For example, NTM has been cultured from the lungs of 13% of cystic fibrosis patients older than 10 years old [71]. It is uncertain whether the significant rate of pretransplantation carriage of these organisms enhances the risk of posttransplantation infection.

In other SOT recipients, the incidence of NTM infection seems to be much lower [72,73]. Furthermore, the ratio of pulmonary-to-extrapulmonary infection is also lower. In renal and heart transplant recipients, cutaneous disease is the most commonly reported manifestation of disease [69]. A recent review summarizes the distribution of all NTM pathogens and sites of infection that have been reported in SOT recipients [69].

The outcome of infection with NTM is highly variable and, in general, treatment requires prolonged combination antimicrobial therapy specific to the identified species [12,69,70,72,73]. Therapy is complicated by variable resistance patterns, drug interactions with immunosuppressive medications, lack of data specific to the SOT population, and sometimes unpredictable responses to treatment [12]. Furthermore, because NTM can colonize the lung without invasive disease, the decision to initiate therapy may be complicated [12,70]. Postoperative therapy may not be necessary in a lung transplant recipient whose colonized lung was explanted during transplantation, but the risks for subsequent symptomatic infection and the need for therapy should be assessed on a case-by-case basis [12,70].

Guidelines for the diagnosis of invasive NTM disease have been published by the ATS and rely on clinical, radiographic, and bacteriologic criteria [74]. Commonly recommended treatment regimens for NTM use the rifamycins and clarithromycin, both of which have dramatic effects on the metabolism of calcineurin inhibitors. Thus, care must be taken when choosing therapy, and patients must be monitored closely. Other commonly recommended drug classes, such as the aminoglycosides, have significant associated toxicities as well. Severe infections may require three or more drugs, and recommended durations vary, often contingent on the clinical response to therapy [12,69]. Initiation of treatment with more than one drug is advised to avoid development of resistance during therapy [12]. Susceptibility testing is available only at specialty laboratories, and guidelines for the testing of specific NTM species and particular antimicrobial agents have been published by the National Committee of Clinical Laboratory Standards [75]. General information and recommended drugs for NTM in SOT recipients can be found in the AST Infectious Diseases guidelines [12].

Hematopoietic stem cell transplant recipients

A myriad of infectious and noninfectious pulmonary complications occur in 40% to 60% of HSCT recipients after transplantation [76]. Timelines describing the sequence of specific pulmonary complications in HSCT recipients may be even more useful than infectious disease timelines in SOT recipients, because pulmonary processes are more likely to occur within well-defined periods, and permanent suppression of immune function by antirejection medication is often absent [2,76]. As in SOT recipients, however, specific patient, pathogen, and environmental factors may influence the duration of these intervals [2,77]. Deficiencies in cellular and humoral immunity in HSCT recipients place these patients at high risk for bacterial and mycobacterial infections. Factors affecting susceptibility to infection in HSCT recipients include pretransplantation immune status, type of conditioning regimen, degree and duration of neutropenia, and development of graft-versus-host disease (GVHD) [76,77]. Allogeneic transplantation is associated with a higher risk of infection than autologous transplantation, and matched, unrelated-donor transplants carry the greatest risk [2,76,77]. Differences between these groups are related to the degree of minor differences in histocompatibility between donor and recipient. Greater mismatch results in slower immune reconstitution and a greater risk of GVHD [77]. GVHD is accompanied by impaired opsonization and impaired reticuloendothelial function. In addition, immunosuppressive agents that are administered to treat or prevent GVHD in high-risk patients result in defects in cellular immunity [77]. Alternative strategies to obtain stem cells for allogeneic transplantation, such as umbilical cord and placenta tissues and T-cell depletion from the donor stem cell product, are also associated with delays in humoral and cellular immune recovery [77].

Hospital- and community-acquired pneumonias in hematopoietic stem cell transplant recipients

Pre-engraftment (neutropenic phase)

Although hospital-acquired bacterial infections are common during the first 30 days after transplantation, the exact incidence of bacterial pneumonia is unknown [76]. Neutropenic fevers are most likely caused by bacterial pathogens, but only rarely is an organism identified [78]. Pneumonias may not be recognized, because a blunted inflammatory response often results in minimal clinical and radiographic signs [79]. Difficulties inherent in the identification of specific causes of pneumonia and differences in the definition of HAP further complicate diagnosis [10,80]. Determination of a microbiologic cause may be particularly difficult during this period because of the empiric use of broad-spectrum antibiotics to treat neutropenic fevers [76]. Reported incidences of bacterial pneumonia vary widely, from less than 5% to more than 30%, and are predominately caused by gram-negative bacteria, such as *P aeruginosa* and *K pneumoniae*, but gram-positive organisms and anaerobes are often seen as well, and outbreaks of *Legionella* infections have been reported [76,80–83]. Risk factors for pneumonia during this period include neutropenia, disruption of mucosal integrity, and an increased risk of aspiration caused by oropharyngeal mucositis and the use of narcotic analgesia [76]. Treatment with broad-spectrum antipseudomonal antibiotics should be initiated immediately in all patients suspected of bacterial pneumonia and in febrile neutropenic patients [78]. The emergence of drug-resistant bacteria is concerning, and the choice of empiric antibiotic depends on institutional resistance patterns [78]. Chest radiographs should be obtained as part of the initial evaluation of patients suspected of having pneumonia. A negative chest radiograph, however, should prompt performance of CT, because infiltrates may be demonstrated in up to 50% of febrile neutropenic patients who have a normal chest radiograph [84].

Early postengraftment (day 30–100)

Except in recipients who have GVHD, bacterial infections are less frequent 30 to 100 days after HSCT, during which time engraftment has occurred and neutropenia has resolved in most patients [76]. Allogeneic transplant recipients are at higher risk than autologous recipients for infection during this period because of slower engraftment and a higher incidence of GVHD. Localized pneumonias seen on chest radiograph most commonly are caused by bacteria, whereas the most commonly identified cause of interstitial pneumonitis is Cytomegalovirus [76]. No cause is identified in 50% of cases [76]. Therapy should be based on site of acquisition (HAP or CAP), degree of immunosuppression, severity of illness, and local resistance patterns in conjunction with established guidelines [10,25,26].

Late postengraftment (beyond 100 days)

The risk of bacterial pneumonia beyond 3 months after transplantation is generally low except in recipients of T-cell–depleted allogeneic transplants and recipients with chronic GVHD [77]. Chronic GVHD occurs in 20% to 45% of HSCT recipients after 6 months, resulting in defects in opsonization and reticuloendothelial function and mandating ongoing administration of immunosuppressive agents. These factors, in turn, confer an increased risk of pulmonary infections [76]. A recent study of 1359 HSCT recipients followed prospectively after discharge from the Fred Hutchinson Cancer Research Center offers insight into the epidemiology of and risk factors for late pneumonias [85]. Three hundred forty-one recipients (25%) experienced at least one episode of pneumonia after discharge. Causative agents were established in only 42% of cases. Bacteria were the second most common cause of pneumonia (following viral infection), accounting for 9% of all cases and 22% of cases in which a cause was identified. Commonly identified organisms in patients who have late bacterial pneumonia include encapsulated organisms such as *H influenza* and *S pneumoniae*, but gram-negative pathogens were reported in one fourth of the patients in the Fred Hutchinson Cancer Research Center series [2,76,77,80,85]. Late bacterial pneumonias were almost exclusively seen in allogeneic recipients, the majority of whom had chronic GVHD. Survival rates after an episode of late bacterial pneumonia were quite favorable [85].

Intensive monitoring for infection and a low threshold for initiating therapy are the general rules for patients who have chronic GVHD. Broad-spectrum antibiotics should be administered when pneumonia is suspected and narrowed if an etiologic agent is identified. Guidelines for severe pneumonia suggest beta-lactams (antipseudomonal if at risk) and a quinolone to cover encapsulated organisms [10,25,26].

For prevention, the CDC advocates antibiotic prophylaxis against encapsulated organisms in allogeneic transplant recipients during treatment for chronic GVHD [78]. TMP-SMX administered for *Pneumocystis* infection may also provide protection against pneumococcal infection [78]. The 23-valent pneumococcal vaccine has limited immunogenicity among HSCT recipients, but it may be beneficial to some patients and should be administered 12 and 24 months after HSCT [78]. The seven-valent conjugate vaccine may be more advantageous, but there are no current data to support its use. HIB vaccination should be given 12, 14, and 24 months after HSCT [78].

Legionella pneumonia

HSCT recipients seem to be at lower risk for *Legionella* pneumonia than SOT recipients, perhaps because they are not mechanically ventilated during transplantation [30]. However, *L pneumophila* and non–*L pneumophila* infections have been documented, infection can result in substantial morbidity and mortality, and outbreaks on transplant units have occurred [81,82]. There is little information regarding *Legionella* in HSCT recipients, but the risk of infection is expected to persist after engraftment, because cell-mediated defects predominate, particularly among patients have GVHD [79].

As in the case of SOT, clinical symptoms are not reliable predictors of *Legionella* infection, and a low threshold for a complete diagnostic work-up (culture and urine antigen testing) and initiation of azithromycin or quinolone therapy should be maintained. CDC recommendations regarding the surveillance and response to identified cases are identical to guidelines in place for SOT [78].

Nocardia infections in hematopoietic stem cell transplant recipients

Nocardia infections have been reported almost exclusively in allogeneic bone marrow transplant recipients. In a retrospective review of 301 allogeneic bone marrow transplants, five cases (1.7%) were identified, all in patients who had severe chronic GVHD and were receiving intense immunosuppressive therapy [55]. In the largest study to date, comprised of 6759 HSCT recipients, 22 cases of proven or probable *Nocardia* infection were diagnosed a mean of 210 days after HSCT [86]. *N asteroides* was the causative species in all but one patient. Pulmonary involvement occurred in 56%, and eight patients had coinfection with other opportunistic pathogens (Cytomegalovirus and *Aspergillus*). No independent risk factors for infection were identified.

As in SOT and other populations, prolonged administration of TMP-SMX is the recommended treatment for established nocardial infections, but second-line agents are also available if myelosuppression is of concern or an allergy to sulfa exists. Although formal preventative strategies to minimize the risk of *Nocardia* infection are not currently employed, the use of low-dose TMP-SMX for *P jiroveci* prophylaxis may have the added benefit of reducing the risk of *Nocardia* infection and is strongly preferred over other *Pneumocystis* regimens in patients who have chronic GVHD.

Mycobacterial infections in hematopoietic stem cell transplant recipients

Tuberculosis

Although impaired T-cell responses would be expected to result in a high incidence of TB, this infection is uncommon in HSCT recipients. Nonetheless, rates of infection in HSCT recipients are 10 to 40 times higher than expected compared with the general population [87]. Retrospective determination of infection may underestimate the incidence of TB in HSCT, but reported rates are often less than 1%, even in multicenter surveys [87–89]. Surprisingly, some highly endemic areas, such as India, also have reported a very low prevalence (1.28%) [90]. Higher rates have been reported in Hong Kong, where investigators prospectively identified TB in 5.5% of HSCT recipients, and in Taiwan, where HSCT rates were 13.1-fold higher than in the normal population [91,92].

Allogeneic HSCT, total body irradiation, chronic GVHD, and corticosteroid therapy have been implicated as potential risk factors for TB [87,91–93]. Onset of disease can be highly variable, with two studies reporting medians of 150 and 324 days and ranges from 11 to 3337 days [87,91]. A recent review of all English-language reported cases in HSCT recipients reported that 80% of TB cases were pulmonary, whereas only 2% of cases were disseminated [93]. Although 25% of patients who had TB died, mortality was largely attributed to other causes, and response to therapy was reportedly generally satisfactory.

Although the clinical and radiographic presentation of TB in the HSCT population usually mimics that in the nontransplant population, atypical presentations have been described. In one case report, an early and rapidly progressive case of TB was mistaken for diffuse alveolar hemorrhage after autologous HSCT and was ultimately fatal 2 weeks after corticosteroid therapy was initiated [94].

As with SOT, the diagnosis of latent TB infection in HSCT recipients can be difficult because of the compromised validity of skin testing in the setting of immunosuppression. A positive result of skin testing is defined as induration of 5 mm or more, but any patient with a significant exposure to persons with active TB should be considered for latent TB treatment, regardless of skin testing results [78]. Specific guidelines for the treatment of latent TB infection in HSCT recipients are provided by the CDC [78]. First-line therapy is isoniazid for 9 months.

Rifampin generally is not recommended after HSCT because of the potential interactions with commonly administered medications including corticosteroids, fluconazole, analgesics, and calcineurin inhibitors [78]. As such, treatment regimens for active TB infection often must be modified, and patients receiving regimens excluding rifamycins are not candidates for 6-month courses of therapy. General guidelines for treatment are available, and recommendations regarding the approach to treatment in SOT may be helpful [59,95].

Nontuberculous mycobacteria

The incidence of NTM infection is generally less than 1% in HSCT centers [69,88]. However, Memorial Sloan-Kettering Cancer Center identified 16 (2.8%) definite cases of NTM and 34 (6%) possible or probable cases of NTM among 561 allogeneic HSCT recipients over a 9-year period [96]. Factors implicated in the five- to 20-fold increased incidence of NTM at Sloan-Kettering include nosocomial exposure and the use of T-cell–depleted grafts, but ascertainment bias may have also contributed. A recent review identified 93 reported cases of NTM infection in HSCT recipients [69]. Compared with SOT recipients, infections in HSCT recipients were more likely to be caused by rapid growers (45% of identified isolates) or *M haemophilum* (24%) and most often caused central venous catheter-related blood stream infection (37%) rather than pulmonary disease (30%), cutaneous disease (18%), or disseminated disease (12%). Median time to diagnosis was 140 days.

In addition to diagnostic criteria established for immunosuppressed patients by the ATS, the CDC has developed formal criteria specifically for the diagnosis of NTM pulmonary, catheter-related, and "other" infections in HSCT recipients [96]. The type and duration of therapy must be carefully chosen, based on the site of infection, identified species, susceptibility profiles, severity of infection, degree of immunosuppression, and potential drug interactions. Prolonged combination therapy is generally the rule, but some blood stream infections can be treated successfully with much shorter courses [97]. Clinicians should refer to the ATS treatment guidelines for general treatment recommendations [74]. Additional sources of guidance include recommendations from the AST [12], as well as a review by Doucette and Fishman [69] that provides detailed recommendations specific to NTM infection in SOT and HSCT recipients.

References

[1] Kusne S, Dummer JS, Singh N, et al. Infections after liver transplantation. An analysis of 101 consecutive cases. Medicine (Baltimore) 1988;67(2):132–43.

[2] Kotloff RM, Ahya VN, Crawford SW. Pulmonary complications of solid organ and hematopoietic stem cell transplantation. Am J Respir Crit Care Med 2004; 170(1):22–48.

[3] Kramer MR, Marshall SE, Starnes VA, et al. Infectious complications in heart-lung transplantation. Analysis of 200 episodes. Arch Intern Med 1993;153(17): 2010–6.

[4] Maurer JR, Tullis DE, Grossman RF, et al. Infectious complications following isolated lung transplantation. Chest 1992;101(4):1056–9.

[5] Cisneros JM, Munoz P, Torre-Cisneros J, et al. Pneumonia after heart transplantation: a multi-institutional study. Spanish Transplantation Infection Study Group. Clin Infect Dis 1998;27(2):324–31.

[6] Chang GC, Wu CL, Pan SH, et al. The diagnosis of pneumonia in renal transplant recipients using invasive and noninvasive procedures. Chest 2004; 125(2):541–7.

[7] Torres A, Ewig S, Insausti J, et al. Etiology and microbial patterns of pulmonary infiltrates in patients with orthotopic liver transplantation. Chest 2000; 117(2):494–502.

[8] Montoya JG, Giraldo LF, Efron B, et al. Infectious complications among 620 consecutive heart transplant patients at Stanford University Medical Center. Clin Infect Dis 2001;33(5):629–40.

[9] Speich R, van der Bij W. Epidemiology and management of infections after lung transplantation. Clin Infect Dis 2001;33(Suppl 1):S58–65.

[10] American Thoracic Society; Infectious Diseases Society of America. Guidelines for the management of adults with hospital-acquired ventilator-associated, and healthcare-associated pneumonia. Am J Respir Crit Care Med 2005;171(4):388–416.

[11] Fine MJ, Stone RA, Singer DE, et al. Processes and outcomes of care for patients with community-acquired pneumonia: results from the Pneumonia Patient Outcomes Research Team (PORT) cohort study. Arch Intern Med 1999;159(9):970–80.

[12] Nontuberculous mycobacteria. Am J Transplant 2004; 4(Suppl 10):42–6.

[13] Fishman JA, Rubin RH. Infection in organ-transplant recipients. N Engl J Med 1998;338(24):1741–51.

[14] Arcasoy SM, Kotloff RM. Lung transplantation. N Engl J Med 1999;340(14):1081–91.

[15] Paradis IL, Williams P. Infection after lung transplantation. Semin Respir Infect 1993;8(3):207–15.

[16] Aris RM, Routh JC, LiPuma JJ, et al. Lung transplantation for cystic fibrosis patients with Burkholderia cepacia complex. Survival linked to genomovar type. Am J Respir Crit Care Med 2001;164(11): 2102–6.

[17] Chaparro C, Maurer J, Gutierrez C, et al. Infection with Burkholderia cepacia in cystic fibrosis. Outcome following lung transplantation. Am J Respir Crit Care Med 2001;163:43–8.

[18] Tablan OC, Anderson LJ, Besser R, et al. Guidelines for preventing health-care–associated pneumonia, 2003: recommendations of CDC and the Healthcare Infection Control Practices Advisory Committee. MMWR Recomm Rep 2004;53(RR-3):1–36.

[19] Singh N, Gayowski T, Wagener M, et al. Pulmonary infections in liver transplant recipients receiving tacrolimus. Changing pattern of microbial etiologies. Transplantation 1996;61(3):396–401.

[20] Prevention of pneumococcal disease: recommendations of the Advisory Committee on Immunization Practices (ACIP). MMWR Recomm Rep 1997;46(RR-8): 1–24.

[21] Avery RK, Ljungman P. Prophylactic measures in the solid-organ recipient before transplantation. Clin Infect Dis 2001;33(Suppl 1):S15–21.

[22] Linnemann Jr CC, First MR, Schiffman G. Response to pneumococcal vaccine in renal transplant and hemodialysis patients. Arch Intern Med 1981;141(12): 1637–40.

[23] Blumberg EA, Brozena SC, Stutman P, et al. Immunogenicity of pneumococcal vaccine in heart transplant recipients. Clin Infect Dis 2001;32(2):307–10.

[24] Kumar D, Rotstein C, Miyata G, et al. Randomized, double-blind, controlled trial of pneumococcal vaccination in renal transplant recipients. J Infect Dis 2003;187(10):1639–45.

[25] Mandell LA, Bartlett JG, Dowell SF, et al. Update of practice guidelines for the management of community-acquired pneumonia in immunocompetent adults. Clin Infect Dis 2003;37(11):1405–33.

[26] Niederman MS, Mandell LA, Anzueto A, et al. Guidelines for the management of adults with community-acquired pneumonia. Diagnosis, assessment of severity, antimicrobial therapy, and prevention. Am J Respir Crit Care Med 2001;163(7):1730–54.

[27] Multiply antibiotic-resistant gram-negative bacteria. Am J Transplant 2004;4(Suppl 10):21–4.

[28] Tkatch LS, Kusne S, Irish WD, et al. Epidemiology of Legionella pneumonia and factors associated with Legionella-related mortality at a tertiary care center. Clin Infect Dis 1998;27(6):1479–86.

[29] Chow JW, Yu VL. Legionella: a major opportunistic pathogen in transplant recipients. Semin Respir Infect 1998;13(2):132–9.

[30] Muder RR, Stout JE, Yu VL. Nosocomial Legionella micdadei infection in transplant patients: fortune favors the prepared mind. Am J Med 2000;108(4):346–8.

[31] Yu VL, Ramirez J, Roig J, Sabria M. Legionnaires disease and the updated IDSA guidelines for community-acquired pneumonia. Clin Infect Dis 2004;39(11):1734–7 [author reply 1737–8].

[32] Legionella. Am J Transplant 2004;4(Suppl 10):25–7.

[33] Bangsborg JM, Uldum S, Jensen JS, et al. Nosocomial legionellosis in three heart-lung transplant patients: case reports and environmental observations. Eur J Clin Microbiol Infect Dis 1995;14(2):99–104.

[34] Ernst A, Gordon FD, Hayek J, et al. Lung abscess complicating Legionella micdadei pneumonia in an adult liver transplant recipient: case report and review. Transplantation 1998;65(1):130–4.

[35] Fraser TG, Zembower TR, Lynch P, et al. Cavitary Legionella pneumonia in a liver transplant recipient. Transpl Infect Dis 2004;6(2):77–80.

[36] Horbach I, Fehrenbach FJ. Legionellosis in heart transplant recipients. Infection 1990;18(6):361–3.

[37] Nichols L, Strollo DC, Kusne S. Legionellosis in a lung transplant recipient obscured by cytomegalovirus infection and Clostridium difficile colitis. Transpl Infect Dis 2002;4(1):41–5.

[38] Prodinger WM, Bonatti H, Allerberger F, et al. Legionella pneumonia in transplant recipients: a cluster of cases of eight years' duration. J Hosp Infect 1994; 26(3):191–202.

[39] Singh N, Muder RR, Yu VL, et al. Legionella infection in liver transplant recipients: implications for management. Transplantation 1993;56(6):1549–51.

[40] Winston DJ, Seu P, Busuttil RW. Legionella pneumonia in liver transplant recipients. Transplantation 1998;66(3):410.

[41] Rangel-Frausto MS, Rhomberg P, Hollis RJ, et al. Persistence of Legionella pneumophila in a hospital's water system: a 13-year survey. Infect Control Hosp Epidemiol 1999;20(12):793–7.

[42] Le Saux NM, Sekla L, McLeod J, et al. Epidemic of nosocomial Legionnaires' disease in renal transplant recipients: a case-control and environmental study. CMAJ 1989;140(9):1047–53.

[43] Venezia RA, Agresta MD, Hanley EM, et al. Nosocomial legionellosis associated with aspiration of nasogastric feedings diluted in tap water. Infect Control Hosp Epidemiol 1994;15(8):529–33.

[44] Stout JE, Yu VL. Legionellosis. N Engl J Med 1997;337(10):682–7.

[45] Knirsch CA, Jakob K, Schoonmaker D, et al. An outbreak of Legionella micdadei pneumonia in transplant patients: evaluation, molecular epidemiology, and control. Am J Med 2000;108(4):290–5.

[46] Heath CH, Grove DI, Looke DF. Delay in appropriate therapy of Legionella pneumonia associated with increased mortality. Eur J Clin Microbiol Infect Dis 1996;15(4):286–90.

[47] Singh N, Stout JE, Yu VL. Prevention of Legionnaires' disease in transplant recipients: recommendations for a standardized approach. Transpl Infect Dis 2004;6(2): 58–62.

[48] Nocardia infections. Am J Transplant 2004; 4(Suppl 10):47–50.

[49] Husain S, McCurry K, Dauber J, et al. Nocardia infection in lung transplant recipients. J Heart Lung Transplant 2002;21(3):354–9.

[50] Patel R, Paya CV. Infections in solid-organ transplant recipients. Clin Microbiol Rev 1997;10(1):86–124.

[51] Merigou D, Beylot-Barry M, Ly S, et al. Primary cutaneous Nocardia asteroides infection after heart transplantation. Dermatology 1998;196(2):246–7.

[52] Singh N, Husain S. Infections of the central nervous system in transplant recipients. Transpl Infect Dis 2000;2(3):101–11.

[53] Arduino RC, Johnson PC, Miranda AG. Nocardiosis

[54] Conces Jr DJ. Bacterial pneumonia in immunocompromised patients. J Thorac Imaging 1998;13(4): 261–70.

[55] Daly AS, McGeer A, Lipton JH. Systemic nocardiosis following allogeneic bone marrow transplantation. Transpl Infect Dis 2003;5(1):16–20.

[56] Chapman SW, Wilson JP. Nocardiosis in transplant recipients. Semin Respir Infect 1990;5(1):74–9.

[57] Wallace Jr RJ, Septimus EJ, Williams Jr TW, et al. Use of trimethoprim-sulfamethoxazole for treatment of infections due to Nocardia. Rev Infect Dis 1982; 4(2):315–25.

[58] Sabeel A, Alrabiah F, Alfurayh O, et al. Nocardial brain abscess in a renal transplant recipient successfully treated with triple antimicrobials. Clin Nephrol 1998;50(2):128–30.

[59] Mycobacterium tuberculosis. Am J Transplant 2004; 4(Suppl 10):37–41.

[60] John GT, Shankar V, Abraham AM, et al. Risk factors for post-transplant tuberculosis. Kidney Int 2001; 60(3):1148–53.

[61] Klote MM, Agodoa LY, Abbott K. Mycobacterium tuberculosis infection incidence in hospitalized renal transplant patients in the United States, 1998–2000. Am J Transplant 2004;4(9):1523–8.

[62] Lattes R, Radisic M, Rial M, et al. Tuberculosis in renal transplant recipients. Transpl Infect Dis 1999; 1(2):98–104.

[63] Aguado JM, Herrero JA, Gavalda J, et al. Clinical presentation and outcome of tuberculosis in kidney, liver, and heart transplant recipients in Spain. Spanish Transplantation Infection Study Group, GESITRA. Transplantation 1997;63(9):1278–86.

[64] Singh N, Paterson DL. Mycobacterium tuberculosis infection in solid-organ transplant recipients: impact and implications for management. Clin Infect Dis 1998;27(5):1266–77.

[65] Winthrop KL, Kubak BM, Pegues DA, et al. Transmission of mycobacterium tuberculosis via lung transplantation. Am J Transplant 2004;4(9):1529–33.

[66] Modry DL, Stinson EB, Oyer PE, et al. Acute rejection and massive cyclosporine requirements in heart transplant recipients treated with rifampin. Transplantation 1985;39(3):313–4.

[67] Meyers BR, Papanicolaou GA, Sheiner P, et al. Tuberculosis in orthotopic liver transplant patients: increased toxicity of recommended agents; cure of disseminated infection with nonconventional regimens. Transplantation 2000;69(1):64–9.

[68] Singh N, Wagener MM, Gayowski T. Safety and efficacy of isoniazid chemoprophylaxis administered during liver transplant candidacy for the prevention of posttransplant tuberculosis. Transplantation 2002; 74(6):892–5.

[69] Doucette K, Fishman JA. Nontuberculous mycobacterial infection in hematopoietic stem cell and solid or-

gan transplant recipients. Clin Infect Dis 2004;38(10): 1428–39.

[70] Malouf MA, Glanville AR. The spectrum of myco-bacterial infection after lung transplantation. Am J Respir Crit Care Med 1999;160(5 Pt 1):1611–6.

[71] Olivier KN, Weber DJ, Wallace Jr RJ, et al. Non-tuberculous mycobacteria. I: multicenter prevalence study in cystic fibrosis. Am J Respir Crit Care Med 2003;167(6):828–34.

[72] Novick RJ, Moreno-Cabral CE, Stinson EB, et al. Nontuberculous mycobacterial infections in heart transplant recipients: a seventeen-year experience. J Heart Transplant 1990;9(4):357–63.

[73] Queipo JA, Broseta E, Santos M, et al. Mycobacte-rial infection in a series of 1261 renal transplant re-cipients. Clin Microbiol Infect 2003;9(6):518–25.

[74] Wallace Jr RJ, Griffith D, Olivier KN, et al. Diagnosis and treatment of disease caused by nontuberculous mycobacteria. Medical Section of the American Lung Association. Am J Respir Crit Care Med 1997;156: S1–25.

[75] National Committee of Clinical Laboratory Standards. Susceptibility testing of mycobacteria, Nocardiae, and other aerobic actinomycetes: approved guideline. Wayne (PA): National Committee of Clinical Labora-tory Standards; 2003.

[76] Soubani AO, Miller KB, Hassoun PM. Pulmonary complications of bone marrow transplantation. Chest 1996;109(4):1066–77.

[77] Wingard JR. Opportunistic infections after blood and marrow transplantation. Transpl Infect Dis 1999;1(1): 3–20.

[78] Guidelines for preventing opportunistic infections among hematopoietic stem cell transplant recipients. MMWR Recomm Rep 2000;49(RR-10):1–128.

[79] Rolston KV. The spectrum of pulmonary infections in cancer patients. Curr Opin Oncol 2001;13(4):218–23.

[80] Lossos IS, Breuer R, Or R, et al. Bacterial pneumonia in recipients of bone marrow transplantation. A five-year prospective study. Transplantation 1995;60(7): 672–8.

[81] Oren I, Zuckerman T, Avivi I, et al. Nosocomial outbreak of Legionella pneumophila serogroup 3 pneu-monia in a new bone marrow transplant unit: evalua-tion, treatment and control. Bone Marrow Transplant 2002;30(3):175–9.

[82] Harrington RD, Woolfrey AE, Bowden R, et al. Le-gionellosis in a bone marrow transplant center. Bone Marrow Transplant 1996;18(2):361–8.

[83] Leung AN, Gosselin MV, Napper CH, et al. Pulmo-nary infections after bone marrow transplantation: clin-ical and radiographic findings. Radiology 1999;210(3): 699–710.

[84] Heussel CP, Kauczor HU, Heussel G, et al. Early

detection of pneumonia in febrile neutropenic patients: use of thin-section CT. AJR Am J Roentgenol 1997; 169(5):1347–53.

[85] Chen CS, Boeckh M, Seidel K, et al. Incidence, risk factors, and mortality from pneumonia developing late after hematopoietic stem cell transplantation. Bone Marrow Transplant 2003;32(5):515–22.

[86] van Burik JA, Hackman RC, Nadeem SQ, et al. No-cardiosis after bone marrow transplantation: a retro-spective study. Clin Infect Dis 1997;24(6):1154–60.

[87] de la Camara R, Martino R, Granados E, et al. Tuberculosis after hematopoietic stem cell transplanta-tion: incidence, clinical characteristics and outcome. Spanish Group on Infectious Complications in He-matopoietic Transplantation. Bone Marrow Transplant 2000;26(3):291–8.

[88] Roy V, Weisdorf D. Mycobacterial infections follow-ing bone marrow transplantation: a 20 year retrospec-tive review. Bone Marrow Transplant 1997;19(5): 467–70.

[89] Cordonnier C, Martino R, Trabasso P, et al. Myco-bacterial infection: a difficult and late diagnosis in stem cell transplant recipients. Clin Infect Dis 2004; 38(9):1229–36.

[90] George B, Mathews V, Srivastava V, Srivastava A, et al. Tuberculosis among allogeneic bone marrow transplant recipients in India. Bone Marrow Transplant 2001;27(9):973–5.

[91] Ip MS, Yuen KY, Woo PC, et al. Risk factors for pul-monary tuberculosis in bone marrow transplant recipi-ents. Am J Respir Crit Care Med 1998;158(4):1173–7.

[92] Ku SC, Tang JL, Hsueh PR, et al. Pulmonary tuber-culosis in allogeneic hematopoietic stem cell transplan-tation. Bone Marrow Transplant 2001;27(12):1293–7.

[93] Yuen KY, Woo PC. Tuberculosis in blood and mar-row transplant recipients. Hematol Oncol 2002;20(2): 51–62.

[94] Keung YK, Nugent K, Jumper C, et al. Mycobacte-rium tuberculosis infection masquerading as diffuse alveolar hemorrhage after autologous stem cell trans-plant. Bone Marrow Transplant 1999;23(7):737–8.

[95] Caminero JA, de March P. Statements of ATS, CDC, and IDSA on treatment of tuberculosis. Am J Respir Crit Care Med 2004;169(2):316–7 [author reply: 317].

[96] Weinstock DM, Feinstein MB, Sepkowitz KA, et al. High rates of infection and colonization by non-tuberculous mycobacteria after allogeneic hematopoietic stem cell transplantation. Bone Marrow Transplant 2003;31(11):1015–21.

[97] Gaviria JM, Garcia PJ, Garrido SM, et al. Non-tuberculous mycobacterial infections in hematopoietic stem cell transplant recipients: characteristics of respiratory and catheter-related infections. Biol Blood Marrow Transplant 2000;6(4):361–9.

Clin Chest Med 26 (2005) 661 – 674

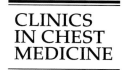

Aspergillus Pulmonary Infections in Transplant Recipients

Dorothy A. White, MD[a,b,*]

[a]*Department of Medicine, Memorial Sloan Kettering Cancer Center, 1275 York Avenue, New York, NY 10021, USA*
[b]*Department of Medicine, Weill Medical College of Cornell University, 1300 York Avenue, New York, NY 10021, USA*

Aspergillus infections are increasing in frequency in those undergoing solid organ and hematopoietic stem cell transplantation (HSCT) [1,2]. This increase is in sharp distinction to many other infections in transplant recipients whose impact has been decreased because of prophylaxis or early surveillance. The incidence of *Aspergillus* infection in HSCT recipients is approximately 10% to 15% [3–7]. In solid organ transplantation the infection occurs in 1% to 8% of recipients [8–13]. It is estimated that 9% to 17% of all deaths in transplant recipients in the first year are attributable to invasive aspergillosis [9]. The ongoing impact of *Aspergillus* infection on morbidity and mortality after transplantation makes this subject an area of intense clinical and research interest. The epidemiologic features of the infection as well as its management and diagnosis have been evolving.

Organism

Aspergillus species are saprophytic filamentous fungi ubiquitous in many environments. Conidia, the infectious form, are 2 to 3 microns in size. They are aerosolized into the environment and are inhaled. Because of their small size, they can deposit in the alveoli. Once in the lung, they may germinate into hyphal forms, which can invade the lung and pulmonary vasculature and disseminate hematogenously. The fungus appears in tissue specimens as hyphae, which are characteristically acute-angle branching and septated, measuring 2 to 4 microns in size (Fig. 1).

A fumigatus has been the most common disease-causing species and has been implicated in most invasive pneumonia cases reported in the literature. Other species seen are *A flavus*, *A terreus*, *A niger*, and *A nidulans*. Compared with *A fumigatus,* other species are more likely to be colonizers or associated with sinus disease only. Recently, however, an increasing frequency of invasive disease caused by non-*fumigatus Aspergillus* species has been noted. In HSCT recipients, positive bronchoalveolar lavage (BAL) or biopsy cultures yielded a non-*fumigatus Aspergillus* species in 33.4% of specimens between 1996 and 1998, compared with 18.3% from 1993 to 1995 [6]. In another report, *A terreus* accounted for 20% of the *Aspergillus* species recovered [14].

Host defense

Innate immune response against *Aspergillus* species consists of alveolar macrophages and peripheral neutrophils. Resident pulmonary macrophages ingest conidia, kill germinating cells, and secrete cytokines and chemokines to coordinate secondary defense. Neutrophils attack and damage germinating conidia and hyphae by oxidative mechanisms [15–17]. Patients with neutropenia or defects in phagocytic function have long been recognized to be susceptible to aspergillosis. High cumulative doses of corticosteroids, which impair macrophage function, are associated with an increased risk of invasive aspergillosis [18].

---

* Department of Medicine, Memorial Sloan Kettering Cancer Center, 1275 York Avenue, New York, NY 10021.
E-mail address: whited@mskcc.org

0272-5231/05/$ – see front matter © 2005 Elsevier Inc. All rights reserved.
doi:10.1016/j.ccm.2005.06.007

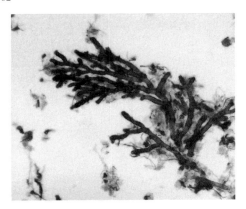

Fig. 1. Silver stain shows the septated hyphae of *Aspergillus fumigatus* with characteristic angle branching.

There is also evidence that T-helper (Th) cell cytokines play a role in adaptive defense against *Aspergillus* [18–23]. Th1 cytokines, such as tumor necrosis factor alpha, gamma interferon, interleukin-12, and interleukin-15, augment superoxide production and enhance the antifungal activity of polymorphonuclear and mononuclear phagocytes against *Aspergillus* species. Immunocompetent mice exposed to a sublethal inoculum of *Aspergillus* conidia developed resistance to subsequent local and systemic infection. The protective Th1 response that the mice demonstrated was characterized by antigen-specific CD4$^+$ T cells that produced gamma interferon and interleukin-2 [19]. Adoptive transfer of *Aspergillus*-specific CD4$^+$ splenic T cells from these animals conferred protection to naive animals [23]. Th2 responses have been associated with progression of *Aspergillus* infection, and their neutralization has been associated with amelioration of infection [24]. Signal transduction mediated by Toll-like receptors (TLR) also plays a role [25]. *Aspergillus* conidia stimulate TLR2 and TLR4 to release a protective Th1 response. Germination of hyphae, however, leads to loss of TLR4-mediated signals and to TLR2 stimulation, resulting in a predominantly Th2 response. This switch from a proinflammatory to an anti-inflammatory immune response during fungal germination may represent a mechanism for *Aspergillus* to evade recognition [25].

Many *Aspergillus* infections in transplant patients occur outside well-defined neutropenic periods or in the absence of high doses of corticosteroids and may be related to defects in T-cell function. These observations on host defense also suggest potential for immunomodulation strategies, such as enhancing Th1 responses or neutralizing suppressive cytokines as adjuvants to treatment of *Aspergillus* infections.

Epidemiology

Hematopoietic stem cell transplantation

Aspergillosis occurs in approximately 10% to 15% of patients undergoing HSCT [1–7]. The impact is marked, with a mortality rate ranging up to 80% [1,3–7]. A major trend in *Aspergillus* infection after HSCT is that the infection now occurs predominantly late after engraftment in non-neutropenic patients, in whom graft-versus-host disease (GVHD) requires the use of immunosuppressive agents [7,26]. Traditionally, invasive pulmonary aspergillosis occurred during periods of neutropenia. Use of peripheral rather than bone marrow stem cells has led to faster repopulation and less early infection. The incidence of chronic GVHD, however, may be higher with this type of transplant, leading to an increased risk of late aspergillosis [6,27]. The mean time to onset of *Aspergillus* infection after myeloablative allogeneic transplant is 78 days, with a bimodal incidence characterized by peaks associated with neutropenia and GVHD [1]. Nonmyeloablative grafts have a decreased incidence of myelopoietic toxicity, but these regimens are otherwise immunosuppressive, and rates of *Aspergillus* infection are comparable or somewhat higher than with conventional myeloablative grafts [8]. The mean time to onset of *Aspergillus* infection is 107 days after nonmyeloablative transplantations, with the major risk factor being the presence and severity of GVHD [1]. The overall risk of *Aspergillus* infection is much lower (~5%) in autologous stem cell transplants and is associated with neutropenia [3].

With T-cell–depleted or CD34-selected grafts, there may be a trend toward higher rates of invasive aspergillosis because of delayed lymphocyte reconstitution [28,29]. Cord blood recipients, alternatively, may have a high incidence of aspergillosis early after transplantation because of a delay in reconstitution of neutrophil function [6]. Overall, the HLA match of the graft, stem cell source, and the presence and severity of GVHD and cytomegalovirus (CMV) disease all affect the risk and timing of *Aspergillus* infection [6,7]. Additionally, the types of agents used to treat GVHD can contribute to the risk of fungal infection. Alemtuzumab, an anti-DC52 monoclonal antibody that depletes peripheral blood T and B cells, has been associated with increased risk of *Aspergillus* infection [1]. Infliximab, an anti-tumor necrosis factor alpha antibody, is also associated with an increased risk of A*spergillus* infection [30].

Solid organ transplantation

The incidence of *Aspergillus* infection is approximately 5% to 8% in liver, lung, and heart transplant recipients, with a lower percentage in kidney, pancreas, and small bowel transplant recipients [1,8–13]. Infection is most common in the first 6 months after transplantation and almost always involves the lung. In solid organ transplant recipients, there is a significant risk of dissemination, and central nervous system disease is the most common site. A change in the type of agents used to suppress rejection may affect the clinical presentation and the risk of dissemination of *Aspergillus* infection. Tacrolimus and sirolimus, although potent immunosuppressive agents, also enhance the activities of antifungal drugs and may affect tissue tropism of the fungus [31]. In an animal model of invasive aspergillosis, mice receiving cyclosporin had widely disseminated disease, including in the brain, whereas those receiving tacrolimus and sirolimus showed disseminated infection but nearly complete absence of hyphae in the brain [32].

In lung transplant recipients, *Aspergillus* can be detected in airway cultures in up to 30% of cases, but invasive aspergillosis occurs in only 3% to 15% of cases, with an average about 6% [2,9,11]. Approximately 58% of the infections are tracheobronchitis or bronchial anastomotic infections, 32% are invasive pulmonary aspergillosis, and 22% are disseminated [33]. Most tracheobronchitis or anastomotic infection occurs within 3 months of transplantation, with pulmonary or systemic infections occurring later. Infection usually occurs in the transplanted lung and only rarely occurs in the native lung. The risk of invasive pulmonary aspergillosis is greater in single-lung transplantations than in double-lung transplantations, especially when the single-lung transplantation is done for chronic obstructive pulmonary disease [33]. Bilateral and right-lung transplants have a higher incidence of bronchial anastomotic infection [34]. Other risk factors identified for development of *Aspergillus* infections are CMV infection and posttransplantation colonization with *Aspergillus* [34–37]. Colonization before transplantation does not predispose the patient to invasive disease [36,37]. Mortality for invasive aspergillosis is approximately 50% to 55%, with the highest rates reported in association with disseminated infections [11,33]. Death from localized anastomotic or airways infection is rare, but fatal erosion into the adjacent pulmonary artery has been reported.

Heart transplant recipients have approximately the same risk of *Aspergillus* infection as lung transplant recipients [38–40]. Approximately 75% of cases occur within the initial 3 months [10,37–40]. Recovery of the organism from the respiratory tract is highly predictive of infection [10]. Risk factors for development of *Aspergillus* infection include reoperation, hemodialysis after transplantation, and CMV disease [38–41]. Mortality ranges from 50% to 80% [38–40].

Aspergillus infections develop in up to 8% of liver transplants recipients [8,9,13]. Recovery of the organism from the respiratory tract is uncommon but has a high positive predictive value for invasive disease [9]. Risk factors for development of infection are retransplantation, renal failure, and fulminant hepatic failure as the indication for transplantation [9,13,42]. Traditionally *Aspergillus* infection developed very early after transplantation, with a median onset of less than 3 weeks [33,42]. Dissemination, most commonly to the central nervous system, was reported in up to 60% of infections [9,42,43]. *Aspergillus* infection is the most common cause of brain abscess in persons undergoing liver transplantation [44]. Recent studies have suggested that *Aspergillus* infection after liver transplantation now may occur at a later period and that the risk of dissemination is lower. One study comparing the periods 1998 to 2002 and 1990 to 1995 found that 55% of the infections occurred after day 90 in the latter years, compared with 23% in the early period. Dissemination decreased from 62% to 30% [45]. Possible explanations are improved surgical techniques and medical management and changes in the immunosuppressive agents. CMV disease may also be occurring later because of use of prophylaxis, leading to delayed *Aspergillus* infections. A recent study found a mortality rate of 60% [46].

Renal transplant recipients have the lowest incidence of *Aspergillus* infection among solid organ transplant recipients, with the infection occurring in about 1% of cases [9,47,48]. The mortality rate is high, however, in the range of 75% to 80% [9,48]. High-dose corticosteroids, graft failure, and use of potent immunosuppressive agents have identified as risk factors [9,49,50].

Clinical presentation

Aspergillus infection can present with allergic manifestations, saprophytic involvement, or invasive disease. In the transplant population, almost all

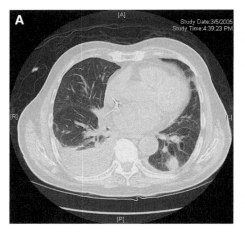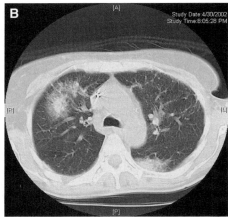

Fig. 2. Radiographic findings of *Aspergillus* infection. (*A*) Chest CT on the left shows solitary nodule in the left lower lobe. (*B*) The scan on the right shows bilateral, patchy, wedge-shaped infiltrates.

disease is caused by invasive aspergillosis, which includes invasive pulmonary aspergillosis (IPA), tracheobronchitis, sinusitis, and disseminated disease. The clinical presentation of IPA is variable and can initially be subtle, making early detection difficult. Fever, cough, and dyspnea are the most common symptoms but are not specific [51,52]. Both hemoptysis and pleuritic chest pain should suggest the possibility of *Aspergillus* infection given the angio-invasive nature of the infection, but these symptoms occur in only some patients. IPA may also present with central nervous system disease resulting from dissemination. In one series of HSCT recipients, the presentation was with respiratory symptoms in 50% of cases, fever alone in 32%, and signs of dissemination in the remainder [52]. Absence of fever should not exclude consideration of infection [52].

Radiographic features characteristically are single or multiple nodules, wedge-shaped pleural-based densities, or cavities (Fig. 2). Diffuse infiltrates also are described. Findings on CT scans include the halo sign, an area of low attenuation surrounding a nodular lung lesion; and the crescent sign, an air crescent near the periphery of lung nodules caused by contraction of infarcted tissues (Figs. 3 and 4) [53]. The halo sign occurs early and may not be present in non-neutropenic patients or later in the course of infection. The air crescent occurs late in the course of the infection, often after resolution of neutropenia. Chest CT scans have been found to be much more sensitive than chest radiographs in detecting the presence of *Aspergillus* infection and should be used early when infection is suspected [54]. CT abnormalities have been best documented in neutropenic HSCT

recipients, and atypical findings may occur in other settings.

In addition to IPA, *Aspergillus* infection can be localized to the airways. Obstructing bronchial aspergillosis is characterized by large mucoid *Aspergillus*-containing casts that can obstruct the airways. Progression to a more inflammatory and invasive bronchitis leads to formation of plaques and ulceration [11,55–57]. The appearance varies from mucosal plugs with minimal inflammation to mild ulceration and to extensive inflammation with pseudomembranes of necrotic cells and fungal hyphae covering the airway (Fig. 5). Tracheobronchitis can cause atelectasis if extensive. Tracheobronchial infection has been seen occasionally in HSCT, leukemia, and patients who have HIV infection, but

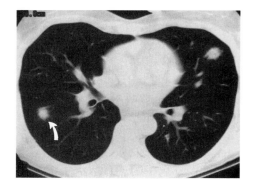

Fig. 3. Halo sign. An area of low attenuation (*arrow*) surrounding a nodular lesion, which occurs early and transiently in *Aspergillus* infection, predominantly in neutropenic patients.

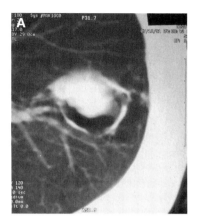
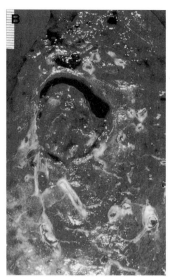

Fig. 4. Air crescent (*A*) radiographically and (*B*) pathologically. (*A*) A rim of air occurs near the periphery of a lung nodule. This presentation is highly suggestive of *Aspergillus* infection, although it occurs late in the course. (*B*) Pathology of a lesion with an air crescent shows contraction of infarcted lung tissue containing inflammatory cells and fungi. This presentation is associated with a risk of life-threatening hemoptysis.

there is a special predisposition to this form of infection in lung transplant recipients, who develop this ulcerative and pseudomembranous bronchitis at the anastomotic site [11,34,57]. Devitalized cartilage and foreign suture material create an environment that makes local *Aspergillus* infection more likely.

Clinical manifestations of tracheobronchitis include fever, cough, wheezing, hemoptysis, or dyspnea. These infections can also be asymptomatic and noted during routine surveillance bronchoscopy in lung transplant recipients. Airway involvement can lead to airway stenosis and, in lung transplant recipients, to suture line dehiscences and to fatal erosion into the adjacent pulmonary artery [11,58]. It can progress to or be associated with invasive pulmonary aspergillosis. Diagnosis is made by bronchoscopy, with which the plugs and ulcerations are clearly seen. Airway lesions may not be removed easily because of local invasion. In lung transplant recipients, an increased risk of subsequent bronchial stenosis or bronchomalacia has been noted, related either to the infection or to the underlying ischemic injury that led to its development.

Invasive sinusitis caused by *Aspergillus* is also a concern in HSCT patients, particularly when associated with neutropenia [59,60]. This condition is less common in solid organ transplant recipients. It carries a high mortality, particularly with invasion of bone and spread to the orbit and brain [1,59,60]. In transplant recipients who have invasive *Aspergillus* sinusitis, a chest CT should be done to exclude pulmonary involvement.

Diagnosis

A definite diagnosis of IPA requires both histopathologic evidence of acute-angle branching and

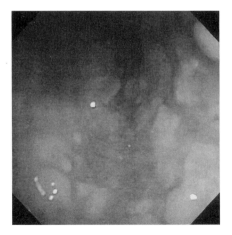

Fig. 5. *Aspergillus* bronchitis. Bronchoscopy showed extensive white endobronchial patches that could not be removed by washing in this patient who had received HSCT.

septated nonpigmented hyphae and a culture yielding *Aspergillus* in specimens obtained by biopsy of involved organs. As discussed later, some criteria also allow use of Galactomannan (GM) antigen to be used as evidence of invasive disease [61]. A definite diagnosis often is not possible in clinical practice, and treatment frequently is given for a presumptive diagnosis based on radiographic and clinical features or recovery of the organism in respiratory secretions.

Cultures of respiratory tract secretions have had limited success, and interpretation is complicated by the potential for the organism to be a colonizer. *Aspergillus* is recovered in sputum specimens in approximately 25% of cases of invasive disease [9]. Bronchoscopy, including washings and BAL, has a yield of 45% to 62%, with only a few cases found by transbronchial biopsy [9,62–64]. The positive predictive value of recovery of *Aspergillus* in respiratory secretion in HSCT recipients is as high as 80% to 90%, and most isolates require treatment [62]. In solid organ transplant recipients, however, the false-positive rates associated with recovery of *Aspergillus* are variable, as previously discussed. The highest rate of airway colonization is seen after lung transplantation, and clinical judgment must be used in interpretation of positive cultures in this setting [9–11,62]. When fine-needle aspirates of focal lesions can be obtained safely, they have a yield of 50% to 67% [52,64,65].

GM is a cell wall component of *Aspergillus* species that is released when there is tissue invasion by the fungus and can be detected in blood, cerebrospinal fluid, and bronchial fluid. Recently the double-sandwich enzyme-linked immunosorbent assay, which can detect low levels of GM antigen, has become commercially available in the United States. Studies have shown that the sensitivity and specificity of this test depends on the cutoff value used for positive findings, which has ranged from 0.5 to 1.5 ng/mL [66–74]. The Food and Drug Administration approved the serum-based assay for use in the United States with a positive result defined with a cutoff index of 0.5 ng/mL. Several prospective studies of the GM antigen assay, mainly in HSCT recipients, showed a sensitivity of 89% to 94% for invasive *Aspergillus* and a specificity of 94% to 99% [66–69]. In these studies, the test was used to screen serum samples of high-risk patients twice weekly. A positive value was defined as two consecutive results greater than 0.5 ng/mL. In one report of 100 allogeneic HSCT recipients, of whom 18 had proven invasive aspergillosis, antigenemia was detected before or with the development of fever in 6 of 11 patients; in another seven patients who remained afebrile

during their entire course, antigenemia was the earliest indicator of infection [67]. A positive antigen preceded the development of radiographic abnormalities in 80% of patients, by a median of 8 days before findings on chest radiographs and by a median of 6 days before CT findings. This early detection of IPA by GM testing before its clinical and radiographic appearance raised hope that the course of the infection might be altered by earlier presumptive therapy. Unfortunately, other studies in different settings have found much less promising results [70–74]. In a group of patients who had hematologic malignancy or HSCT with neutropenic fever or suspected *Aspergillus* infection, GM detection had a sensitivity of only 29% using a threshold of greater than 1.5 ng/mg; sensitivity improved to 50% with a cutoff of 0.7 ng/mL [70]. GM antigen was the first positive test in only 3 of 153 cases. Several other studies found that the assay missed many, if not all, cases of definite invasive *Aspergillus* [71,72]. Few studies of GM testing are available in the solid organ transplant population. One report in lung transplant recipients found a sensitivity of 30%, and GM antigen did not detect any of the cases of endobronchial aspergillosis [73]. The specificity, however, was 95%, and there were no positive findings in patients believed to be only colonized. In liver transplant recipients for whom archived sera were tested, the sensitivity of the test was 55.6%, and specificity was 93.9% [74]. Another prospective study in liver transplant recipients also found a high specificity of 98.5% [75].

Some studies have looked at detection of GM antigen in BAL fluid [76–80]. Levels of the antigen may be higher closer to the source of the infection, and the test may be more sensitive. A recent study retrospectively analyzed BAL specimens from 49 patients being evaluated for HSCT or after transplantation who underwent bronchoscopy and were believed to have proven or probable IPA and from 50 control patients without the diagnosis [76]. The study looked at a variety of cutoff points for positivity. The sensitivity and specificity were 76% and 94%, respectively, with the optimal cutoff of 0.5 ng/mL. When the BAL was culture-negative for *Aspergillus*, the sensitivity of the GM antigen was 59%, suggesting that adjunctive use of this test in addition to culture may enhance the yield of BAL [76–81]. The clinical impact in this study was that 11 of 13 open biopsies might have been avoided. False-positive results that could have led to an incorrect diagnosis were obtained for four control patients, however.

There are several confounding factors in interpreting GM levels. Patients receiving antifungal agents may have a false-negative test. It is postulated that treatment lowers the level by decreasing the fungal load. Autoreactive antibodies, which may be seen in GVHD or in patients who have autoimmune disease or are receiving piperacillin-tazobactam, can result in false-positive levels [1,81]. The effect of renal failure and dialysis are uncertain, because GM is cleared in the urine. Conflicting data must be resolved with further studies to determine the exact role of GM testing in various clinical situations, such as screening serum for early detection, diagnosis of infection in serum or BAL, and after response to treatment. At present, GM testing should be considered an adjuvant test, and each value must be assessed independently in light of the clinical circumstances.

Several polymerase chain-reaction protocols have been developed using different formats and have been studied as a means of detecting *Aspergillus* in blood and BAL fluid [78–80,82,83]. None are standardized or commercially available. Polymerase chain reaction is substantially more sensitive than culture and GM assay but has a low positive predictive value [82]. A negative test may be most useful, suggesting a low chance of infection.

Management

The mainstay of treatment has been drug therapy supplemented when indicated or feasible by reversal of underlying immunosuppression, surgery and, rarely, immune modulation. The drugs currently available that are effective against *Aspergillus* species are amphotericin (including liposomal forms), itraconazole, voriconazole, and caspofungin. Posaconazole may soon become available. *Aspergillus* may occasionally be resistant to some of these drugs; for example, *A terreus* has a high incidence of resistance to amphotericin. In most cases, however, failure of these drugs is caused not by drug resistance but by the immune status of the patient. Length of therapy is not standardized, but many courses continue for 10 to 12 weeks or several weeks after clinical and radiographic resolution.

Drugs

Amphotericin B has been the main antifungal drug in use for *Aspergillus* infection, but voriconazole is now considered a first-line therapy and is being used increasingly. In a randomized, prospective trial comparing voriconazole with conventional amphotericin B in 277 immunocompromised patients (including 79 HSCT and 14 solid organ transplant recipients) with confirmed or probable invasive aspergillosis, the use of voriconazole was associated with a greater likelihood of complete or partial response at 12 weeks, lower mortality, and less likelihood of needing other drugs [83]. A few other reports in small numbers of transplant recipients indicate that voriconazole seems to be equivalent to amphotericin [84,85], and both amphotericin and voriconazole are widely used for treatment in the transplant setting. The currently available lipid preparations of amphotericin B are amphotericin B lipid complex, liposomal amphotericin, and amphotericin B colloidal dispersion. A dose of 5 mg/kg/d is given as initial treatment. High doses may be more effective in some select situations, but superior efficacy has not been proven. There are conflicting data in the transplant population on whether lipid preparations are superior in efficacy to amphotericin B. One retrospective study in 41 liver transplant recipients showed a mortality rate of 33% in those receiving lipid forms of amphotericin versus 83% in those who received conventional amphotericin [86]. In contrast, another study in immunocompromised patients, including some who had received stem cell and organ transplants, showed equivalent efficacy for the two preparations [87]. Liposomal preparations do seem to be associated with a more favorable side-effect profile than standard amphotericin B, particularly with respect to the risk of nephrotoxicity.

Voriconazole use in transplant patients leads to increased levels of cyclosporine, tacrolimus, or sirolimus secondary to inhibition of the P-450 cytochrome system. The interaction is most severe with sirolimus, and this combination is discouraged. Intravenous voriconazole is contraindicated in patients whose creatinine clearance is less than 50 mL/min because of accumulation of the renally excreted carrier. Itraconazole is also useful, but its oral absorption is less reliable. Posaconazole is a new triazole with significant activity against *Aspergillus*.

Caspofungin is a member of the new echinocandin family of drugs with activity on the fungal cell wall rather than the cell membrane. It is approved as second-line therapy for refractory aspergillosis. Studies that have included HSCT and organ transplant recipients and leukemic patients have showed a favorable response in approximately 45% of patients who were not responding to or were intolerant of amphotericin [88,89]. The drug was well tolerated in all studies. Concurrent administration of caspofungin and cyclosporin resulted in increased concentration of caspofungin but no change in cyclosporine level. Administration with tacrolimus has resulted in slightly reduced tacrolimus levels, and the level of tacrolimus needs to be monitored. Elevations of liver enzymes can occur, but significant hepatotoxicity is rare.

Combination therapy

There had been concern about combining azoles and amphotericin because some animal studies showed antagonism [90–92]. This antagonism was assumed to be caused by alterations of the sterol composition induced by the azoles that made amphotericin less effective. With echinocandins, antagonism would not be anticipated. Some animal studies of echinocandins combined with either amphotericin or caspofungin have been promising [93,94]. There are limited clinical studies, but one report of 30 patients who had leukemia and IPA who had an inadequate response to amphotericin found the combination of amphotericin and caspofungin gave a 60% response rate [95]. Another study of the combination found a 54% response rate when combination therapy was used as the primary treatment but a response rate of only 35% when used as salvage therapy [96]. Another salvage study of 47 patients who did not respond to therapy with amphotericin and who received either voriconazole or combination of voriconazole and caspofungin as salvage showed improved survival in the combination group [97].

Therapy for tracheobronchitis

There are no good studies reporting results of strategies for treating *Aspergillus* tracheobronchitis. A common practice at some centers is to use aerosolized amphotericin combined with some systemic antifungal therapy, typically intravenous amphotericin or an oral azole [1,2]. Anecdotal reports of success with single drug or various combination drug regimens have been described [57,98,99]. Stents may need to be placed for postinfectious bronchial stenosis.

Immunotherapy

There are anecdotal reports of success with use of granulocyte transfusion from donors stimulated with granulocyte colony-stimulating factor during treatment of IPA, with five of nine patients in one study responding [100,101]. Adjunctive immunotherapy with gamma interferon has also been reported in chronic granulomatous disease but has been of concern in the setting of HSCT because of the risk of exacerbation of GVHD. A recent article from the MD Anderson Cancer Center reported on 32 patients who received interferon-gamma-1b for invasive fungal infections after HSCT [102]. During therapy, fever was common, but therapy did not precipitate or exacerbate acute or chronic GVHD. The primary endpoint in this study was safety, but the authors were encouraged that three of five patients who had disseminated disease survived, higher than the usual survival rate for this presentation.

Surgery

Surgery has been used to salvage patients who have focally persisting IPA resistant to medical therapy, particularly if they are then to undergo transplantation or other cytotoxic therapy [103–108]. Surgery is also used for control of massive hemoptysis if the cause is focal disease. It has also been suggested that, for patients who have one or two focal lesions, surgery with resection added to primary medical therapy may improve outcome [105,106]. The theory is that radical surgical removal of necrotic and poorly perfused lung tissue will clear IPA more quickly. This approach is used more commonly in infections caused by *Mucor* than in those caused by *Aspergillus*. Multiple studies have shown that resection can be performed with acceptable mortality, but the exact setting in which surgery should be performed is unclear [103–108]. A recent study of 41 patients who had hematologic disease and suspected IPA who underwent resection (lobectomy in 23, wedge resection in 16, nonpulmonary resection in 2), documented major complications in 10% of cases, with one death related to surgery. Mortality within 30 days was 10%. Infection was cleared in 87% of cases, although relapse occurred in 10% [107]. The authors were unable to find any characteristic that could distinguish between survivor and nonsurvivors. The 30-day mortality for resection of *Aspergillus* has ranged from 0% to 30% in various series [103–108].

Prophylaxis

Hematopoietic stem cell transplantation

Traditionally, prophylaxis in HSCT recipients focused on the first 100 days after transplantation, when the risk of *Aspergillus* infections was highest. Because the timing of these infections has changed, prophylactic strategies must also switch, and the appropriate time period may be different for each patient. There are no clear-cut guidelines. Low-dose amphotericin has been used most commonly, although it is not proven to be of benefit and is associated with significant renal toxicity [109]. Liposomal amphotericin at a dose of 2 mg/kg three times per week is well tolerated, but its efficacy has not been proven definitively [110]. Aerosolized amphotericin has not been shown to be consistently beneficial [111,112]. Itraconazole has been found to decrease fungal infection in most studies but is associated with gastrointestinal side effects [113–115]. No studies are available to assess the role of voriconazole at present. One concern in more widespread use of azoles in prophylaxis is the occurrence of breakthrough Zygomycetes infection [116].

Solid organ transplantation

Lung transplant recipients frequently receive prophylaxis despite the lack of controlled trials. In a survey of 37 lung transplant centers in the United States, fungal surveillance before transplantation, predominantly using sputum cultures, was performed by 81% of the centers [117]. Seventy-two per cent received antifungal treatment if *Aspergillus* species were isolated before transplantation; itraconazole was the preferred agent. After transplantation, 76% of centers administered antifungal prophylaxis, although some did so only in selected patients. Agents used were inhaled amphotericin B (61%), itraconazole (46%), parenteral amphotericin (25%), and fluconazole (21%), with some using more than one agent. Because many of the infections in lung transplant recipients are tracheobronchial, the aerosolized approach would seem to be beneficial, particularly because achievable concentrations in the airways are likely to be higher than with systemic administration. Several studies of aerosolized amphotericin preparations show safety and suggest possible benefit [118,119]. One study of 381 treatments of aerosolized liposomal amphotericin administered to 51 patients found it to be well tolerated, with only one patient unable to continue therapy [118]. Nausea and vomiting, which can be related to oral deposition, occurred in less than 2% cases. No clinically significant bronchospasm was apparent, and only 5% of treatments were associated with 20% decline in the ratio of forced expiratory volume in 1 second/forced vital capacity. Biopsies performed for surveillance in these patients showed no evidence of lipoid pneumonia or other apparent tissue toxicity. A few reports suggest that itraconazole may be an effective antifungal prophylactic agent in colonized patients [120–122].

In liver transplants recipients, prophylaxis is generally used only for those patients at high risk for developing *Aspergillus* infections. The lipid formulations of amphotericin B in dose of 1 to 5 mg/kg/d in selected populations seem to be beneficial [123,124]. Use of oral itraconazole has been limited because of potential hepatotoxicity as well as concerns about gastrointestinal absorption in critically ill liver transplant recipients who unable to eat and have altered gastric acidity. Routine prophylaxis is not given to all heart transplant patients but only to those deemed to be at high risk.

Summary

Aspergillus remains a challenging infection in the transplant population. As the epidemiology and treatment options change, clinicians must continue to use all the tools at their disposal to develop effective prophylactic strategies, diagnose infections as early as possible, and determine optimal treatment regimens.

References

[1] Singh N, Paterson DL. Aspergillus infections in transplant recipients. Clin Micro Rev 2005;44:1–56.

[2] Kotloff RM, Ahya VN, Crawford SW. Pulmonary complications of solid organ and hematopoietic stem cell transplantation. Am J Respir Crit Care Med 2004; 170:22–78.

[3] Wald A, Leisenring W, van Burik JA, et al. Epidemiology of *Aspergillus* infections in a large cohort of patients undergoing bone marrow transplantation. J Infect Dis 1997;175:1459–66.

[4] Fukuda TM, Boeckh M, Carter RA, et al. Risks and outcomes of invasive fungal infections in recipients of allogeneic hematopoietic stem cell transplants after non myeloablative conditioning. Blood 2003;102: 827–33.

[5] Wingard JR, Beals SU, Santos GW. *Aspergillus* infection in bone marrow transplant recipients. Bone Marrow Transplant 1987;2:175–80.

[6] Marr KA, Carter RA, Crippa F, et al. Epidemiology and outcome of mould infections in hematopoietic stem cell transplant recipients. Clin Infect Dis 2002; 34:909–17.

[7] Wald A, Leisenring W, van Burik JA, et al. Epidemiology of *Aspergillus* infections in a large cohort of patients undergoing bone marrow transplantation. J Infect Dis 1997;175:1459–66.

[8] Singh N, Wagener NM, Marino IR, et al. Trends in invasive fungal infections in liver transplant recipi-

ents: correlation with evolution in transplantation practices. Transplantation 2002;73:63–7.

[9] Paterson DL, Singh N. Invasive aspergillosis in transplant recipients. Medicine 1999;78:123–38.

[10] Munoz P, Alcala L, Sanchez Conde M, et al. The isolation of *Aspergillus fumigatus* from respiratory tract specimens in heart transplant recipients is highly predictive of invasive aspergillosis. Transplantation 2003;75:326–9.

[11] Mehrad B, Paciocco G, Martinez FJ, et al. Spectrum of *Aspergillus* infection in lung transplant recipients: case series and review of the literature. Chest 2001; 119:169–75.

[12] Westney GE, Kesten S, De Hoyos A, et al. *Aspergillus* infection in single and double lung transplant recipients. Transplantation 1996;61:915–9.

[13] Fortun JP, Martin-Davila P, Moreno S, et al. Risk factors for invasive aspergillosis in liver transplant recipients. Liver Transplant 2002;8:1065–70.

[14] Baddley JW, Stroud TP, Salzman D, et al. Invasive mold infections in allogeneic bone marrow transplant recipients. Clin Infect Dis 2001;32:1319–24.

[15] Schaffner A, Douglas H, Braud A. Selective protection against conidia by mononuclear and against mycelia by polymorphonuclear phagocytes in resistance to *Aspergillus*: observations on these two lines of defense *in vitro* with human and mouse phagocytes. J Clin Invest 1982;69:617–31.

[16] Roilides E, Dimitriadou-Georgiadou A, Sein T, et al. Tumor necrosis factor alpha enhances antifungal activities of polymorphonuclear and mononuclear phagocytes against *Aspergillus fumigatus*. Infect Immun 1998;66:5999–6003.

[17] Waldorf AR, Levitz S, Diamond RD. In vivo bronchoalveolar macrophage defense against *Rhizopus oryzae* and *Aspergillus fumigatus*. J Infect Dis 1984;150:752–60.

[18] Lionakis MS, Kontoyiannis DA. Glucocorticoids and invasive fungal infections. Lancet 2003;362:1828–38.

[19] Cenci E, Mencacci A, Bacci A, et al. T cell vaccination in mice with invasive pulmonary aspergillosis. J Immunol 2000;165:381–8.

[20] Cenci E, Mencacci A, Del Sero G, et al. Interleukin-4 causes susceptibility to invasive pulmonary aspergillosis through suppression of protective type I responses. J Infect Dis 1999;180:1957–68.

[21] Clemons KV, Grunig G, Sobel A, et al. Role of IL-10 in invasive aspergillosis: increased resistance of IL-10 gene knockout mice to lethal systemic aspergillosis. Clin Exp Immunol 2000;122:186–91.

[22] Mehrad B, Striete RM, Standiford TJ. Role of TNF-α in pulmonary host defense in murine invasive aspergillosis. J Immunol 1999;162:1633–40.

[23] Parkin J, Cohen B. An overview of the immune system. Lancet 2001;357:1777–89.

[24] Roilides E, Dimitriadou A, Kadiltsoglou I, et al. IL-10 exerts suppressive and enhancing effects on antifungal activity of mononuclear phagocytes against *Aspergillus fumigatus*. J Immunol 1997;158:322–9.

[25] Netea MG, Warris A, Van der Meer WM, et al. *Aspergillus fumigatus* evades immune recognition during germination through loss of Toll-like receptor-4-mediated signal transduction. J Infect Dis 2003; 188:320–6.

[26] Marr KA, Carter RA, Boeckh M, et al. Invasive aspergillosis in allogeneic stem cell transplant recipients: changes in epidemiology and risk factors. Blood 2002;00:4358–66.

[27] Bensinger WI. Blood or marrow? Lancet 2000;355: 1199–200.

[28] Nachbaur D, Fink FM, Nussbaumer W, et al. CD34 + -selected autologous peripheral blood stem cell transplantation (PBSCT) in patients with poor-risk hematological malignancies and solid tumors. A single-centre experience. Bone Marrow Transplant 1997;20:827–34.

[29] O'Donnell MR, Schmidt GM, Tegtmeier BR, et al. Prediction of systemic fungal infection in allogeneic marrow recipients: impact of amphotericin prophylaxis in high-risk patients. J Clin Oncol 1994;12: 827–34.

[30] Marty FM, Lee SJ, Alyes EP, et al. Infliximab use in patients with severe graft-versus-host disease and other emerging risk factors of non-*Candida* invasive fungal infections in allogeneic hematopoietic stem cell transplant recipients: a cohort study. Blood 2003; 102:2768–76.

[31] Singh N, Heitman J. Antifungal attributes of immunosuppressive agents: new paradigms in management and elucidating the pathophysiologic basis of opportunistic mycoses in organ transplant recipients. Transplantation 2004;77:795–800.

[32] High KP, Washburn RG. Invasive aspergillosis in mice immunosuppressed with cyclosporin A, tacrolimus (FK506), or sirolimus (rapamycin). J Infect Dis 1997; 175:222–5.

[33] Singh N, Husain S. *Aspergillus* infections after lung transplantation: clinical differences in type of transplant and implications for management. J Heart Lung Transplant 2003;21:258–66.

[34] Hadjiliadis DH, Howell DN, Davis RD, et al. Anastomotic infections in lung transplant recipients. Ann Transplant 2000;3:13–9.

[35] Husni RN, Gordon SM, Longworth DL, et al. Cytomegalovirus infection is a risk factor for invasive aspergillosis in lung transplant recipients. Clin Infect Dis 1998;26:753–5.

[36] Flume PA, Egan TM, Paradowski LJ, et al. Infectious complications of lung transplantation. Impact of cystic fibrosis. Am J Respir Crit Care Med 1994;149: 1601–7.

[37] Cahill BC, Hibbs JR, Savik K, et al. Aspergillus airway colonization and invasive disease after lung transplantation. Chest 1997;112:1160–4.

[38] Grossi P, Farina C, Fiocchi R, et al. Prevalence and outcome of invasive fungal infections in 1,963 thoracic organ transplant recipients. Transplantation 2000;70:112–6.

[39] Lenner R, Padilla ML, Teirstein AS, et al. Pulmonary complications in cardiac transplant recipients. Chest 2001;120:508–13.

[40] Cisneros JM, Munoz P, Torre-Cisneros J, et al. Spanish Transplantation Infection Study Group. Pneumonia after heart transplantation: a multi-institutional study. Clin Infect Dis 1998;27:324–31.

[41] Munoz P, Rodriguez C, Bouza E, et al. Risk factors of invasive aspergillosis after heart transplantation: protective role of oral itraconazole prophylaxis. Am J Transplant 2004;4:636–43.

[42] Singh N, Arnow PM, Bonham A, et al. Invasive aspergillosis in liver transplant recipients in the 1990s. Transplantation 1997;64:716–20.

[43] Torre-Cisneros J, Lopez OL, Kusne S, et al. CNS aspergillosis in organ transplantation: a clinicopathologic study. J Neurol Neurosurg Psychiatr 1993;56: 188–93.

[44] Bonham CA, Dominguez EA, Fukui MB, et al. Central nervous system lesions in liver transplant recipients: prospective assessment of indications for biopsy and implications for management. Transplantation 1998;66:1596–604.

[45] Singh N, Avery RK, Munoz P, et al. Trends in risk profiles for and mortality associated with invasive aspergillosis among liver transplant recipients. Clin Infect Dis 2003;36:46–52.

[46] Husain S, Tollemar J, Dominguez EA, et al. Changes in the spectrum and risk factors for invasive candidiasis in liver transplant recipients: prospective, multicenter, case-controlled study. Transplantation 2003;75:2023–9.

[47] Altiparmak MR, Apaydin S, Trablus S, et al. Systemic fungal infections after renal transplantation. Scand J Infect 2002;Dis. 34:284–8.

[48] Gallis HA, Berman RA, Cate TR, et al. Fungal infection following renal transplantation. Arch Intern Med 1975;135:1163–72.

[49] Gustafson TL, Schaffner W, Lavely GB, et al. Invasive aspergillosis in renal transplant recipients: correlation with corticosteroid therapy. J Infect Dis 1983;148:230–8.

[50] Panackal AA, Dahlman A, Keil KT, et al. Outbreak of invasive aspergillosis among renal transplant recipients. Transplantation 2003;15:1050–3.

[51] Jantunen E, Ruutu P, Niskanen L, et al. Incidence and risk factors for invasive fungal infections in allogeneic BMT recipients. Bone Marrow Transplant 1997;19:801–8.

[52] Jantunen E, Piilonen A, Volin L, et al. Diagnostic aspects of invasive *Aspergillus* infections in allogeneic BMT recipients. Bone Marrow Transplant 2000; 25:867–71.

[53] Kim MJ, Lee KS, Kim J, et al. Crescent sign in invasive pulmonary aspergillosis: frequency and related CT and clinical factors. J Comput Assist Tomogr 2001;25:305–10.

[54] Caillot D, Casasnovas O, Bernard A, et al. Improved management of invasive pulmonary aspergillosis in neutropenic patients using early thoracic computed tomographic scan and surgery. J Clin Oncol 1997; 15:139–47.

[55] Hines DW, Haber MH, Yaremko L. Pseudomembranous tracheobronchitis caused by *Aspergillus*. Am Rev Respir Dis 1991;143:1408–11.

[56] Kemper CA, Hostetler JS, Follansbee SE, et al. Ulcerative and plaque-like tracheobronchitis due to infection with *Aspergillus* in patients with AIDS. Clin Infect Dis 1993;17:344–52.

[57] Kramer MR, Denning DW, Marshall SE, et al. Ulcerative tracheobronchitis after lung transplantation: a new form of invasive aspergillosis. Am Rev Respir Dis 1991;144(3 pt 1):552–6.

[58] Kessler R, Massard G, Warter A, et al. Bronchial–pulmonary artery fistula after unilateral lung transplantation: a case report. J Heart Lung Transplant 1997;16:674–7.

[59] Sterman BM. Sinus surgery in bone marrow transplantation patients. Am J Rhinol 1999;13:315–7.

[60] Iwen P, Reed E, Armitage JO, et al. Nosocomial invasive aspergillosis in lymphoma patients treated with bone or peripheral stem cell transplants. Infect Control Hosp Epidemiol 1993;14:131–9.

[61] Ascioglu S, Rex JH, de Pauw B, et al. Defining opportunistic invasive fungal infections in immunocompromised patients with cancer and hematopoietic stem cell transplants: an international consensus. Clin Infect Dis 2002;34:7–14.

[62] Horvath JA, Dummer S. The use of respiratory tract cultures in the diagnosis of invasive pulmonary aspergillosis. Am J Med 1996;100:171–8.

[63] Levy HD, Horak DA, Tegtmeier BR, et al. The value of bronchoalveolar lavage and bronchial washings in the diagnosis of invasive pulmonary aspergillosis. Respir Med 1992;86:243–8.

[64] Crawford SW, Hackman RC, Clark JG. Biopsy diagnosis and clinical outcome of persistent focal pulmonary lesions after marrow transplantation. Transplantation 1989;48:266–71.

[65] Jantunen E, Piilonen A, Violin L, et al. Radiologically guided fine needle lung biopsies in the evaluation of focal pulmonary lesions in allogeneic stem cell transplant recipients. Bone Marrow Transplant 2002; 29:353–6.

[66] Maertens J, Verhaegen J, Lagrou K, et al. Screening for circulating galactomannan as a non invasive diagnostic tool for invasive aspergillosis in prolonged neutropenic patients and stem cell transplantation; a prospective validation. Blood 2001;97:1604–10.

[67] Maertens J, Verhaegen J, Lagrou K, et al. Use of circulating galactomannan screening for early diagnosis of invasive aspergillosis in allogeneic stem cell transplant recipients. J Infect Dis 2002;186: 1297–306.

[68] Maertens JJ, Verhaegan J, Demuynck H, et al. Autopsy-controlled prospective evaluation of serial screening for circulating galactomannan by a sandwich enzyme-linked immunosorbent assay for hema-

tological patients at risk for invasive Aspergillosis. J Clin Microbiol 1999;37:3223–8.

[69] Sulahian A, Boutboul F, Ribaud P, et al. Value of antigen detection using an enzyme immunoassay in the diagnosis and prediction of invasive aspergillosis in two adult an pediatric hematology units during a 4-year prospective study. Cancer 2001;91:311–8.

[70] Herbrecht R, Letscher-Bru V, Oprea C, et al. Aspergillus galactomannan detection in the diagnosis of invasive aspergillosis in cancer patients. J Clin Oncol 2002;20:1898–906.

[71] Pinel C, Fricker-Hidalgo H, Lebeau B, et al. Detection of circulating Aspergillus fumigatus galactomannan; value and limits of the Platelia test for diagnosing invasive aspergillosis. J Clin Microbiol 2003;41:2184–6.

[72] Ferns RB, Fletcher H, Bradley S, et al. The prospective evaluation of a nested polymerase chain reaction assay for the early detection of Aspergillus infection in patients with leukemia or undergoing allograft treatment. Br J Haematol 2002;119:720–5.

[73] Husain S, Kwak E, Obman A, et al. Prospective assessment of Platelia Aspergillus galactomannan antigen for the diagnosis of invasive aspergillosis in lung transplant recipients. Am J Transplant 2004;4: 796–802.

[74] Fortun J, Martin-Davila P, Alvarez ME, et al. Aspergillus antigenemia sandwich enzyme immunoassay test as a serodiagnostic method for invasive aspergillosis in liver transplant recipients. Transplantation 2001;71:145–9.

[75] Kwak E, Husain S, Obman A, et al. Efficacy of galactomannan antigen using Platelia Aspergillus enzyme immunoassay for the diagnosis of invasive aspergillosis in liver transplant recipients. J Clin Microbiol 2004;42:435–8.

[76] Musher B, Fredricks D, Leisenring W, et al. Aspergillus galactomannan enzyme immunoassay and quantitative PCR for diagnosis of invasive aspergillosis with bronchoalveolar fluid. J Clin Microbiol 2004;42:5517–22.

[77] Becker MJ, Lugtenburg EJ, Cornelissen JJ, et al. Galactomannan detection in computerized tomography-based broncho-alveolar lavage fluid and serum in hematological patients at risk for invasive pulmonary aspergillosis. Br J Haematol 2003;121:448–57.

[78] Buchheidt D, Baust C, Skladny H, et al. Detection of Aspergillus species in blood and bronchoalveolar lavage samples from immunocompromised patients by means of 2-step polymerase chain reaction: clinical results. Clin Infect Dis 2001;33:428–35.

[79] Sanguinetti M, Posteraro B, Pagano L, et al. Comparison of real-time PCR, conventional PCR, and galactomannan antigen detection by enzyme-linked immunosorbent assay using bronchoalveolar lavage fluid samples from hematology patients for diagnosis of invasive pulmonary aspergillosis. J Clin Microbiol 2003;41:3922–5.

[80] Verweij PE, Latge JP, Rijs AJ, et al. Comparison of antigen detection and PCR assay using bronchoalveolar lavage fluid for diagnosing invasive pulmonary aspergillosis in patients receiving treatment for hematological malignancies. J Clin Microbiol 1995; 33:3150–3.

[81] Singh N, Obman A, Husain S, et al. Reactivity of Platelia Aspergillus galactomannan antigen with piperacillin-tazobactam: clinical implications based on achievable serum concentrations. Antimicrob Agents Chemother 2004;48:1989–92.

[82] Loeffler J, Kloepfer K, Hebart H, et al. Polymerase chain reaction detection of Aspergillus DNA in experimental models of invasive aspergillosis. J Infect Dis 2002;158:1203–6.

[83] Herbrecht R, Denning DW, Patterson TF, et al. Voriconazole versus amphotericin B for primary therapy of invasive aspergillosis. N Engl J Med 2002;347: 408–15.

[84] Denning DW, Ribaud P, Milpied N, et al. Efficacy and safety of voriconazole in the treatment of acute invasive aspergillosis. Clin Infect Dis 2002; 34:563–71.

[85] Mattei D, Mordani N, Lo Nigro C, et al. Voriconazole in the management of invasive aspergillosis in two patients with acute myeloid leukemia undergoing stem cell transplantation. Bone Marrow Transplant 2002;30:967–70.

[86] Linden P, Cole K, Kramer D, et al. Invasive aspergillosis in liver transplant recipients: comparison of outcome with amphotericin B lipid complex and conventional amphotericin B therapy. Transplantation 1999;67:S232.

[87] Bowden R, Chandrasekar P, White MH, et al. A double-blind, randomized, controlled trial of amphotericin B colloidal dispersion versus amphotericin B for treatment of invasive aspergillosis in immunocompromised patients. Clin Infect Dis 2002;35: 359–66.

[88] Kartsonis NA, Saah AJ, Lipka J, et al. Salvage therapy with caspofungin for invasive aspergillosis; results from the caspofungin compassionate use study. J Infect 2005;50:196–205.

[89] Maertens J, Raad I, Petrikkos G, et al. Efficacy and safety of caspofungin for treatment of invasive aspergillosis in patients refractory to or intolerant of conventional antifungal therapy. Clin Infect Dis 2004; 39:1563–71.

[90] Aliff TB, Maslak PG, Jurcic JG, et al. Refractory Aspergillus pneumonia in patients with acute leukemia: successful therapy with combination caspofungin and liposomal amphotericin. Cancer 2003;97: 1025–32.

[91] Schaffner A, Frick PG. The effect of ketoconazole on amphotericin B in a model of disseminated aspergillosis. J Infect Dis 1985;151:901–10.

[92] Polak A. Combination therapy of experimental candidiasis, cryptococcosis, aspergillosis and wangiellosis in mice. Chemotherapy 1987;33:381–95.

[93] Polak A, Scholer HJ, Wall M. Combination therapy

of experimental candidiasis, cryptococcosis and aspergillosis in mice. Chemotherapy 1982;28:461–79.

[94] Graybill JR, Bocanegra R, Gonzalez GM, et al. Combination antifungal therapy of murine aspergillosis: liposomal amphotericin B and micafungin. J Antimicrob Chemother 2003;52:656–62.

[95] Perea S, Gonzalez G, Fothergill AW, et al. In vitro interaction of caspofungin acetate with voriconazole against clinical isolates of *Aspergillus* spp. Antimicrob Agents Chemother 2002;46:3039–41.

[96] Kontoyiannis DPR, Hachem R, Lewis RE, et al. Efficacy and toxicity of caspofungin in combination with liposomal amphotericin B as primary or salvage treatment of invasive aspergillosis in patients with hematologic malignancies. Cancer 2003;98:292–9.

[97] Marr KA, Boeckh M, Carter RA, et al. Combination antifungal therapy for invasive aspergillosis. Clin Infect Dis 2004;39:797–802.

[98] Westney GE, Kesten S, De Hoyos A, et al. *Aspergillus* infection in single and double lung transplant recipients. Transplantation 1996;61:915–9.

[99] Monforte V, Roman A, Gavalda J, et al. Nebulized amphotericin B prophylaxis for *Aspergillus* infection in lung transplantation study of risk factors. J Heart Lung Transplant 2001;20:1274–81.

[100] Dignani MD, Anaissie EJ, Hester JP, et al. Treatment of neutropenia-related fungal infections with granulocyte colony-stimulating factor-elicited white blood cell transfusions: a pilot study. Leukemia 1997;11:1621–30.

[101] Catalano L, Fontane R, Scarpato N, et al. Combined treatment with amphotericin B and granulocyte infusion from G-CSF stimulated donors in an aplastic patient with invasive aspergillosis undergoing bone marrow transplantation. Haematologica 1997;82:71–2.

[102] Safdar A, Rodriquez G, Ohmagari N, et al. The safety of interferon-γ-1b therapy for invasive fungal infections after hematopoietic stem cell transplantation. Cancer 2005;103:731–9.

[103] Pidhorecky I, Urschel J, Anderson T. Resection of invasive pulmonary aspergillosis in immunocompromised patients. Ann Surg Oncol 2000;7:312–7.

[104] Gossot D, Validire P, Vaillancourt R, et al. Full thoracoscopic approach for surgical management of invasive pulmonary aspergillosis. Ann Thorac Surg 2002;73:240–4.

[105] Habicht JM, Reichenberger F, Gratwohl A, et al. Surgical aspects of resection for suspected invasive pulmonary fungal infection in neutropenic patients. Ann Thorac Surg 1999;68:321–5.

[106] Gow KW, Hayes-Jordan AA, Billups CA, et al. Benefit of surgical resection of invasive pulmonary aspergillosis in pediatric patients undergoing treatment for malignancies and immunodeficiency syndromes. J Pediatr Surg 2003;38:1354–60.

[107] Matt P, Bernet F, Habicht J, et al. Predicting outcome after lung resection for invasive pulmonary aspergillosis in patients with neutropenia. Chest 2004;126:1783–8.

[108] Habicht JM, Matt P, Passweg JR, et al. Invasive pulmonary fungal infection in hematologic patients; is resection effective? Hematol J 2001;2:250–6.

[109] Wolff SN, Fay J, Stevens D, et al. Fluconazole vs. low-dose amphotericin B for the prevention of fungal infections in patients undergoing bone marrow transplantation: a study of the North American Marrow Transplant Group. Bone Marrow Transplant 2000;25:853–9.

[110] Kelsey SM, Goldman JM, McCann S, et al. Liposomal amphotericin (AmBisome) in the prophylaxis of fungal infections in neutropenic patients: a randomized, double-blind placebo-controlled study. Bone Marrow Transplant 1999;23:163–8.

[111] Conneally E, Cafferkey MT, Daly PA, et al. Nebulized amphotericin B as prophylaxis against invasive aspergillosis in granulocytic patients. Bone Marrow Transplant 1990;5:403–6.

[112] Behre GF, Schwartz S, Lenz K, et al. Aerosol amphotericin B inhalations for prevention of invasive pulmonary aspergillosis in neutropenic cancer patients. Ann Hematol 1995;71:287–91.

[113] Harousseau L, Dekker AW, Stamatoullas-Bastard A, et al. Itraconazole oral solution for primary prophylaxis of fungal infections in patients with hematological malignancy and profound neutropenia: a randomized, double-blind, double-placebo multicenter trial comparing itraconazole and amphotericin B. Antimicrob Agents Chemother 2000;44:1887–93.

[114] Morgentern GR, Prentice AG, Prentice HG, et al. A randomized controlled trial of itraconazole versus fluconazole for the prevention of fungal infections in patients with hematological malignancies. Br J Haematol 1999;105:901–11.

[115] Marr KA, Crippa F, Leisenring W, et al. Itraconazole versus fluconazole for prevention of fungal infections in patients receiving allogeneic stem cell transplants. Blood 2004;103:1527–33.

[116] Imhof A, Balajee A, Fredricks DN, et al. Breakthrough fungal infections in stem cell transplant recipients receiving voriconazole. Clin Infect Dis 2004;39:743–6.

[117] Dummer JS, Lazariashvilli N, Barnes J, et al. A survey of anti-fungal management in lung transplantation. J Heart Lung Transpl 2004;23:1376–81.

[118] Palmer S, Drew RH, Whitehouse JD, et al. Safety of aerosolized amphotericin B lipid complex in lung transplant recipients. Transplantation 2001;72:545–8.

[119] Minari A, Husni R, Avery RK, et al. The incidence of invasive aspergillosis among solid organ transplant recipients and implications for prophylaxis in lung transplants. Transpl Infect Dis 2002;4:195–200.

[120] Drew RH, Dodds A, Benjamin DK, et al. Comparative safety of amphotericin B lipid complex and amphotericin B deoxycholate as aerosolized antifungal prophylaxis in lung-transplant recipients. Transplantation 2004;77:232–7.

[121] Hamacher J, Spiliopoulos A, Kurt A-M, et al for the Geneva Lung Transplantation Group. Pre-emptive therapy with azoles in lung transplant patients. Eur Respir J 1999;13:180–6.

[122] Calvo V, Borro JM, Morales P, et al. Antifungal prophylaxis during the early postoperative period of lung transplantation. Chest 1999;115:1301–4.

[123] Singh N, Paterson DL, Gayowski T, et al. Preemptive prophylaxis with a lipid preparation of amphotericin B for invasive fungal infections in liver transplant recipients requiring replacement therapy. Transplantation 2001;71:910–3.

[124] Singhal S, Ellis RW, Jones SG, et al. Targeted prophylaxis with amphotericin B lipid complex in liver transplantation. Liver Transplant 2000;6: 588–95.

ELSEVIER
SAUNDERS

Clin Chest Med 26 (2005) 675 – 690

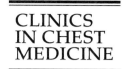

Non-*Aspergillus* Fungal Pneumonia in Transplant Recipients

Sylvia F. Costa, MD[a], Barbara D. Alexander, MD[b],*

[a]*Division of Pulmonary, Allergy, and Critical Care, Department of Medicine, Duke University Medical Center,
Room 7453 Hospital North, Erwin Road, Durham, NC 27710, USA*
[b]*Division of Infectious Diseases and International Health, Department of Medicine, Box 3035, 1116 G CARL Building,
Research Drive, Duke University Medical Center, Durham, NC 27710, USA*

The number of validly described fungal species is estimated to be between 100,000 to 200,000, and new species are continuing to be discovered. To date, approximately 270 different species have been recognized as human pathogens. Although species of *Aspergillus* and *Candida* account for most deeply invasive and life-threatening fungal infections [3], the past decades have seen a rise in the immunocompromised population. With this increase, additional fungi have emerged as important agents of morbidity and mortality [1,4–6]. These opportunistic fungi are characterized by their ubiquitous presence in the environment, their ability to cause disease in immunosuppressed patients, and their diminished susceptibility to the currently available antifungal agents. Pneumonia, one aspect of a myriad of clinical manifestations caused by these fungal pathogens, is discussed in this article.

Factors predisposing to fungal pneumonia

The risk of fungal infection in transplant recipients can be determined by a combination of factors distilled into two conditions: the intensity of the epidemiologic exposure and the net state of immunosuppression [7]. Exposures to potential pathogens occur in both the community and the hospital setting.

Exposure to fungi in the community may be recent or remote, and nosocomial exposures may occur within the patient care unit or during patient transport. Multiple factors interact to form the net state of immunosuppression, the most important of which are the immunosuppressive regimen, immunomodulating viruses, and the aftermath of surgical procedures [7]. Factors unique to the individual organs transplanted further influence the development and manifestation of fungal disease. For example, neutropenia and graft-versus-host disease (GVHD) have been linked with the development of fungal infection in hematopoietic stem cell transplant (HSCT) recipients. On the other hand, in lung transplant recipients, direct environmental communication of the transplanted graft and continuous exposure to potential pathogens together with diminished cough reflex, decreased mucociliary clearance, and poor lymphatic drainage are key. It is most likely these unique risks that lead to the different rates and clinical manifestations of invasive fungal infection (IFI) in the different transplant populations.

Types of non-*Aspergillus* fungi

In the early 1990s, fungi other than *Aspergillus* accounted for approximately 2% of mycelial infections in solid organ transplant (SOT) recipients [3,8,9]. A recent study, however, reported non-*Aspergillus* molds as the causative agent in 27% of mycelial fungal infections [10]. A similar trend was

---

* Corresponding author.
E-mail address: alexa011@mc.duke.edu
(B.D. Alexander).

noted among HSCT recipients with a noticeable increase in infections caused by *Fusarium* and the Zygomycetes [11]. In support of these observations, an overview from the Centers for Disease Control–sponsored TRANSNET surveillance program for IFIs in recipients of HSCT and SOT between March 2001 and December 2003 reported non-*Aspergillus* molds were responsible for 14% of IFI, whereas *Cryptococcus* constituted 4%, endemic fungi 3%, and pneumocystosis 2% [12]. The non-*Aspergillus* fungal category is a diverse group of organisms. For purposes of this discussion, the non-*Aspergillus* fungi associated with pulmonary disease in transplant populations are categorized by taxonomic characteristics and are discussed individually (Table 1).

Hyaline Hyphomycetes

Molds that comprise the Hyphomycetes group of fungi include *Aspergillus*, *Fusarium*, *Scedosporium*, *Acremonium*, *Paecilomyces*, *Trichoderma,* and *Penicillium* species, among others [1,4,5,10,11,14]. The non-*Aspergillus* hyalohyphomycetes resemble *Asper-*

gillus on histologic examination, with septate, hyaline hyphae, and vessel invasion. Several of these organisms differ from *Aspergillus* in their ability to produce adventitial forms that facilitate angioinvasion and in vivo sporulation, which probably is responsible for the relative frequency of positive blood cultures and dissemination encountered with theses pathogens [2,15–17]. Culture is the only means of distinguishing among these organisms, which is crucial because many have high minimal inhibitory concentrations for currently employed antifungals.

Fusarium

Members of the genus *Fusarium* are found as soil saprophytes and plant pathogens; *F solani*, *oxysporum,* and *moniliforme* are the species most frequently isolated from clinical specimens. Human infection begins with entry of the fungal microconidia through inhalation into the alveolar spaces, through breaks in the integrity of the skin, or through the gastrointestinal tract. Regardless of the site of initial inoculation, the infection frequently involves the lung [1,4,5,13,16]. In one center, *Fusarium* infection involved the lung in 81% of cases and was disseminated in 74% of the cases [11].

It seems that fusariosis may have different manifestations in SOT and HSCT recipients. In SOT recipients, the infection tends to be localized, fungemia is uncommon, onset of infection occurs during the late posttransplantation period, and mortality is around 33% [18]. In HSCT recipients, infection is disseminated, fungemia occurs in 20% to 70% of cases, onset of infection occurs early in the posttransplantation period, and mortality is high (70%–100%) [18]. Symptoms in SOT recipients with *Fusarium* pneumonia may include productive cough, dyspnea, pleuritic chest pain, and fever. Although the lung examination may be unremarkable, imaging of the lungs may reveal thin-walled cavities, which are visualized better with CT scan [19,20]. In HSCT recipients, fever refractory to antibiotics and antifungal agents is the usual presenting symptom. Nodular or cavitary lesions may be seen on lung imaging. Most *Fusarium* infections in HSCT patients occur in allogeneic recipients who are either neutropenic or who have acute GVHD [15,17].

Scedosporium

Species of the genus *Scedosporium* are frequently encountered in soil, manure of cattle and fowl, polluted waters and sewage, and occasionally in the air in hospitals during construction [1,4,5,14]. Infections are caused by two species, *S apiospermum* (the asexual state of *Pseudallescheria boydii)* and *S pro-*

Table 1
Non-*Aspergillus* etiologies of fungal pneumonia in transplant recipients

Pathogen	Representative case reports and summaries
Hyaline Hyphomycetes	
Fusarium	[11,13,15,16,18–20,70]
Scedosporium	[22–29]
Paecilomyces	[31]
Trichoderma	[34]
Scopulariopsis	[36,38]
Dematiaceous Hyphomycetes	
Alternaria	[70,72]
Fonsecaea	[62]
Dactylaria	[73–75]
Zygomycetes	
Mucor	[51,53,60]
Rhizopus	[51,52,54,56,57,59,60]
Cunninghamella	[46–49,54]
Absidia	[58]
Endemic fungi	
Histoplasma capsulatum	[76–78]
Blastomyces dermatitidis	[79,80]
Coccidioides immitis	[82–86,88,90]
Penicillium marneffei	[91,92]
Paracoccidioides brasiliensis	[95,96,98]
Yeasts	
Cryptococcus neoformans	[100–103]
Trichosporon	[106]
Pneumocystis	
Pneumocystis jiroveci	[114,117–122]

lificans. Importantly, *S apiospermum* tends to be resistant or to have erratic susceptibility to polyenes, whereas *S prolificans* is largely resistant to all currently available antifungal agents, including amphotericin B and the newer azoles [21,22].

The portal of entry seems to be the respiratory tract through inhalation, although entry may occur through the skin through intravenous catheters [22,23]. From the lungs, widespread dissemination to other organs ensues through the bloodstream [1,2]. Although disseminated infection seems to predominate in the immunocompromised population, localized pneumonia caused by *S prolificans* and *S apiospermum* has been reported in SOT recipients [10,24–26] as well as in HSCT recipients [11,24, 27,28]. A recent literature review of 80 cases of *Scedosporium* infection in the transplant population occurring between 1985 and 2003 found the majority of infections were caused by *S apiospermum*, but, importantly, 19% of the infections in SOT recipients and 39% in HSCT recipients were caused by *S prolificans*. Predictably, *S prolificans* was associated with a higher mortality (78%) in both populations. The median onset of *Scedosporium* infection after transplantation was 4 months for SOT recipients and 1.2 months for HSCT recipients. Forty-three percent of the *Scedosporium* infections in SOT recipients were pulmonary, and 46% were disseminated [24]. In HSCT recipients, 41% of *Scedosporium* infections were pulmonary, and 69% were disseminated. HSCT recipients were more likely to have fungemia than SOT recipients [24].

Infection involving the lung may present as fever refractory to antibiotics and amphotericin B or as productive cough and malaise. Imaging of the lungs may reveal interstitial infiltrates, effusion, nodular or cavitary lesion, or formation of an air-crescent sign [25,26]. In a case series from Australia, pulmonary scedosporiosis was reported in lung transplant recipients noted to have structurally abnormal airways caused by either ischemic stenosis or bronchiolitis obliterans syndrome and prior itraconazole therapy [29].

Acremonium

Members of the genus *Acremonium* are found as saprobes in the soil and decaying vegetation and can be pathogens of plants, insects, and humans. Human infection has been reported with *A alabamensis*, *A falciforme*, *A kiliense*, *A rose-griseum*, *A strictum*, *A potroni*, and *A recifei*. The apparent portal of entry is inoculation through a penetrating injury, the respiratory tract, or possibly the gastrointestinal tract, given that the organism has been cultured from stool [30]. Cases of localized and disseminated infection with *Acremonium* have been described in transplant recipients, and lung infection has been described in leukemic patients undergoing conventional chemotherapy. Pneumonia has not been reported as an isolated clinical presentation in the transplant population, although it is likely that cases of pulmonary disease in the transplant population will occur eventually [30].

Paecilomyces

Paecilomyces species are often implicated in decay of food and cosmetics. The two most common species are *P lilacinus* and *P variotii*, both of which can be pathogenic for humans. The portal of entry seems to be breaks in the integument, such as after trauma or caused by intravascular catheters [31,32]. As with *Fusarium*, *Scedosporium*, and *Acremonium*, blood cultures may be positive [2], and although infection with *Paecilomyces* tends to be confined to the skin or ocular structures, fungemia and subsequent involvement of the lung have been described in the HSCT population [31]. *P variotii* has also been isolated after lung transplantation from the airway of a pediatric patient who had cystic fibrosis [33]; however, as with *Aspergillus*, isolation of the organism from the airway may reflect transient colonization rather than invasive disease.

Trichoderma

Trichoderma was historically considered a soil saprophyte, isolated from plant and decaying wood with low pathogenicity for humans [4,6,34]. It now seems that human infection does occur. Although several species comprise the genus, most cases in humans are caused by *T longibrachiatum*. Reports of infection in SOT recipients (two cases) and HSCT recipients (one case) have described infection of the lungs, usually discovered as pulmonary abscesses at autopsy [34,35]. This organism has increased minimum inhibitory concentrations and diminished clinical response to conventional antifungal agents [35].

Scopulariopsis

Scopulariopsis is found in soil, and the two species most commonly isolated from clinical samples are *S brevicaulis* and *S brumptii*. These organisms rarely cause human infection, although cases have been described in both immunocompetent and immunocompromised patients. Hypersensitivity pneumonitis has been reported in immunosuppressed patients after chemotherapy [36,37], and lung infections have been reported in HSCT and SOT recipients [38–40]. Most patients present with fever refractory to antibiotics; those with lung involvement have persistent or increasing pulmonary infiltrates on chest radiograph. *Microascus trigonosporus,* the asexual state of *S trigonospora,* has been reported to cause fatal pneumonia in an allogeneic HSCT recipient with GVHD [38]. Persistent fever, cough, dyspnea, and severe hypoxemia associated with diffuse bilateral opacities on chest radiograph eventually progressed to respiratory failure and multiorgan failure.

Penicillium

Penicillium is a ubiquitous saprophyte with more than 900 known species, most of which are found in soil, decaying vegetation, seeds, and grains [14,41]. Other than *P marneffei* (discussed later as an endemic mycosis), *Penicillium* species often are recovered from clinical specimens as culture contaminants or transient colonizers [42] and only rarely cause disease in humans [43,44]. A case report of *P brevicompactum* causing necrotizing lung infection in a HSCT recipient has been published [41]. The patient presented with fever, cough, pleuritic chest pain, and a small, round lesion on chest imaging that progressed to cavitation.

Zygomycetes

The agents of zygomycosis are members of the orders Entomophthorales and Mucorales. These organisms are characterized by sparsely septate hyphae in tissue. The hyphae are broad, variable in diameter with irregular branching, and, in the case of the Mucorales, invade blood vessels resulting in thrombosis, tissue infarction, and necrosis [4–6,14]. Members of the order Mucorales are found in a wide geographic distribution and cause the bulk of pulmonary Zygomycete infections in transplant populations [45]. When compared with *Fusarium* or *Scedosporium,* Zygomycete infection is less often disseminated outside the sinopulmonary tree. Although *Rhizopus* and *Mucor* remain the most frequently isolated Zygomycetes, cases of *Cunninghamella* infection are being increasingly reported in both HSCT [46,47] and SOT recipients [48,49]. Pulmonary infection with *Absidia corymbifera* has also been reported [50].

Inhalation of spores is the mechanism of entry for pulmonary disease, and in one center 55% of HCST patients who had zygomycosis had disease involving the lungs. Presentation of pulmonary zygomycosis varies, with fever, nonproductive cough, pleuritic chest pain, and hemoptysis possible. Radiographic

images are also heterogeneous and have included infiltrates, nodules, cavities, fungal balls, and pleural effusions. Reports to date suggest HSCT patients who have zygomycosis are predominantly allogeneic recipients with severe neutropenia or undergoing treatment for GVHD [11,51–53]. Two centers reported severe iron overload in their transplant recipients who had zygomycosis [51]. Although most infections with Zygomycetes occur late (> 100 days) after HSCT transplantation, a few infections have been diagnosed within 90 days of transplantation [52]. Mortality in this population is generally high (75%–80%) [11,51,52].

The incidence of zygomycosis in the HSCT population varies between 0.5% and 1.9% [11, 51–53], although data from several large transplant centers shows an apparent increase in the number of Zygomycete infections in HSCT recipients since the mid-1990s [11,45]. More recently, breakthrough infections with Zygomycetes have been reported in HSCT recipients receiving voriconazole [54–56]. Of the 14 total cases reported from three centers, 12 involved the lung, and all 14 of these patients had GVHD. Whether these cases represent the selective pressure of voriconazole therapy or simply a continued increase in the previously documented trend is speculative.

Cases of isolated pulmonary zygomycosis in SOT populations have also been reported [57–59]. Patients typically present with cough, hemoptysis, pleuritic chest pain, and worsening pulmonary function. Radiographic studies are varied, with cavities, infiltrates and pleural effusion noted. Among liver and heart transplant recipients, Zygomycetes constituted 5.7% of 53 invasive mycelial infections [10]. In liver and kidney-pancreas recipients, an incidence of 0.7% (5/763 patients) has been reported [60].

Dematiaceous Hyphomycetes

The dematiaceous fungi are a heterogeneous group of organisms that have a darkly pigmented cell wall containing dihydroxynapthalene melanin. When isolated in culture, dematiaceous molds often are considered colonizers or contaminants. The species most often implicated in human infections include members of the *Bipolaris, Cladophialophora, Dactylaria, Alternaria, Exophiala, Phialophora,* and *Curvularia* genuses. In immunosuppressed patients, dematiaceous molds can cause pneumonia, and some species have an increased ability to disseminate to the central nervous system (CNS) [1,4,5,61–69]. Infections have been reported in both HSCT and SOT recipients.

In one series of HSCT recipients, *Alternaria* species involving the respiratory tract accounted for 5% of 123 non-*Candida* fungal infections in 1186 patients [70]. *Fonsecaea pedrosoi* was diagnosed in a HSCT recipient who had two densities on chest radiograph; lavage fluid grew the organism, as did open lung biopsy. The patient subsequently became lethargic, with new lesions on head CT that on biopsy yielded *Emericella nidulans* [62]. This case highlights the possibility that more than one mold may simultaneously infect a patient and stresses the need for an aggressive approach toward diagnosis when a patient has progression of known lesions or develops new lesions while receiving therapy.

In liver and heart transplant recipients with invasive mycelial infection, 9.4% of infections were caused by dematiaceous molds, 40% of which involved the lungs [10]. In a separate review of dematiaceous mold infections in 34 SOT recipients, two distinct clinical presentations were noted: (1) skin or soft tissue infection (excluding visceral organs) in 79% of the patients, mostly caused by *Exophiala*, and (2) systemic invasive infections in 21% of the patients, with *Dactylaria* species predominating [71]. Median time to onset after transplantation was 22 months. Overall, the mortality is high, with the worst prognosis seen in patients who have systemic infection rather than in those with skin, soft tissue, or joint infection. The SOT patients who have dematiaceous mold pulmonary infections may be asymptomatic or have fever and cough as presenting symptoms. Patients who have pulmonary disease disseminated to the CNS may also have neurologic deficits. Radiographic studies can show a nodule, cavitary lesion, or diffuse pulmonary infiltrates [72–75].

Endemic mycoses

The endemic mycoses are thermally dimorphic fungi growing in mycelial form in the environment (25°C) but as yeast or yeast-like form in the body (37°C). The major causative agents of endemic mycoses are *Histoplasma capsulatum*, *Coccidioides immitis*, *Blastomyces dermatitidis*, *Paracoccidioides brasiliensis*, *Sporothrix schenkii,* and *Penicillium marneffei*, each of which has a distinct geographic distribution. These fungi are usually present in the soil, and inhalation of conidia leads to infection. Manifestation of disease may occur during primary exposure or through reactivation. An overview of the TRANSNET database reported 886 IFIs in 20,000 HSCT and SOT recipients; endemic fungi accounted for 3% of infections [12]. The endemic mycoses are seen primarily in SOT rather than in HSCT patients.

Histoplasma capsulatum

Two varieties of *Histoplasma* may cause disease in humans, *H capsulatum* var. *capsulatum* (endemic in Ohio, Mississippi, the St. Lawrence River valley, the eastern half of the United States, and most of Latin America) and *H capsulatum* var. *duboisii* (found in tropical Africa). Most cases remain asymptomatic; however, immunocompromised patients may develop symptoms after primary infection. Acute self-limited pulmonary histoplasmosis, progressive pulmonary histoplasmosis, and progressive disseminated histoplasmosis are among the clinical presentations. Also of note, transmission of *H capsulatum* with a donor organ has also been reported [76,77]. In one case from Japan, disseminated histoplasmosis including cavitary pulmonary disease was diagnosed 4 years after transplantation of a kidney harvested from a resident of Texas.

Series of SOT recipients as well as HSCT recipients in both nonendemic and endemic areas have been published. Five cases of disseminated histoplasmosis occurred in approximately 1300 renal transplant recipients during a 4-year period in Minneapolis, a nonendemic area, for an estimated incidence of 0.4% [78]. Most presented as nonspecific febrile illness, with one patient presenting with cough and dyspnea. Most cases were judged to be caused by endogenous reactivation. In endemic regions, in the absence of an outbreak, the incidence of disease in the transplant population seems to be similar (0.5%) to the incidence of disease in the transplant population in non-endemic regions. However, the origin of most infections in endemic areas seems to be primary acquisition. Almost all patients with primary acquisition have pulmonary involvement, and the rate of dissemination is high.

Blastomyces dermatitidis

In the United States, *B dermatitidis* is found in the south central and southeastern states, those bordering the Mississippi and Ohio River basins, the Canadian provinces, and the Great Lakes, and areas of Canada and New York along the St. Lawrence River. It is also endemic in Africa [14]. Clinical presentation of pulmonary blastomycosis is varied and includes flulike illness, acute pneumonia, subacute or chronic respiratory illness, and fulminant acute respiratory distress syndrome [14]. Cases of blastomycosis have been reported in SOT recipients, although the numbers are small [79,80]. A Medline review from 1966 to 1991 revealed only one case series of blastomycosis in transplant recipients [79]. Four of the five patients identified were renal transplant recipients. Time to onset of infection was variable (3 weeks to 4 years after transplantation), and blastomycosis was not associated with any particular immunosuppressive regimen. Infection most often originated in the lung and frequently disseminated, with skin lesions present in two patients [81]. Symptoms include persistent fever or nonproductive cough and radiographic imaging revealing interstitial infiltrates, reticulonodular infiltrates, nodules, and cavitary lung lesions [79,80].

Coccidioides immitis

C immitis is found in the soil in the southwestern United States, Mexico, and Central and South America [14,82] After transplantation, coccidioidomycosis may occur as a primary infection or through reactivation of latent infection. Infections in SOT recipients have been reported, with an incidence of approximately 4% to 9% in highly endemic areas, most occurring in the first year after transplantation [82–89]. A recent series of liver transplant recipients in a highly endemic area reported an incidence of only 0.6% to 1.4% [87]. The clinical presentation in SOT recipients is variable; those with pulmonary involvement may have an acute illness with fever, cough, and dyspnea, whereas some progress to respiratory distress, altered sensorium, and even disseminated intravascular coagulation with multiorgan failure [85,86,88,90]. Dissemination to the CNS is common. Radiographic evaluation may reveal diffuse bilateral infiltrates or lobar, nodular, alveolar, or cavitary lesions, but no one pattern predominates.

In SOT recipients, antirejection therapy was associated with an increased risk of coccidioidomycosis [82]. The risk after transplantation also is increased if there is a prior history of coccidioidomycosis or if there is a positive serologic assay in the period just before transplantation. In highly endemic areas, some centers test for *C immitis* and prophylactically treat patients who have a positive result or prior history of coccidioidomycosis before transplantation [87]. Transmission through the donated organ also occurs, and reports of such transmission frequently describe fulminant infection occurring early in the posttransplantation period, usually within 2 to 3 weeks [85,86,88].

Penicillium marneffei

P marneffei, the only *Penicillium* species that is dimorphic, is endemic in Southeast Asia. Reports of infection in Europe, Australia, and the United States have been limited primarily to HIV-infected travelers returning home [1,4,6,14]. Four cases of *P marneffei* have been reported in renal transplant recipients [91–93], one of which presented with disseminated

disease and pneumonia 9 months after transplantation [93].

Paracoccidioides brasiliensis

P brasiliensis is endemic in Latin America [14]. Most primary infections are self-limited, but the organism has the ability to remain dormant for long periods and cause clinical disease at a time when host defenses are impaired [94]. Infections in SOT patients have been reported, all from areas in which the fungus is endemic [95–98]. Of 102 autopsies performed on renal transplant recipients receiving care at an endemic medical center, 71 (69.6%) revealed an infectious cause of death. Fungi represented 27.5% of infections, and *P brasiliensis* accounted for 4.5% of the IFIs [98]. In three additional case reports, renal transplant recipients with pulmonary paracoccidioidomycosis presented 11 to 14 years after their transplantation. Presenting symptoms included fever, cough, malaise, anorexia, and weight loss. Radiographic images predominantly showed multiple nodules [95–97]. No report of *P brasiliensis* lung infection in an HSCT recipient has been published.

Yeasts

Invasive pulmonary infections caused by yeast are relatively uncommon in the transplant populations. *Cryptococcosis* is the most common yeast infection encountered. Cases of pulmonary infection caused by *Trichosporon*, *Blastoschizomyces,* and *Malassezia* are rare but have been reported.

Cryptococcus

C neoformans is an encapsulated yeast that causes disease after inhalation of yeast cells. Although not considered an endemic mycosis, the risk of developing cryptococcosis among immunocompromised patients may be influenced by geographic region. A higher frequency of cryptococcosis in individuals infected with the HIV has been reported in the eastern part of the United States than in the western part [99]. This geographic distribution may also affect the rates of cryptococcosis in SOT recipients. So far, limited epidemiologic information suggests the majority of cases in SOT are caused by *C neoformans* var. *grubii* (serotype A). Within the transplant population, the infection is seen almost exclusively in recipients of solid organs, with the majority of infections developing late (>6 months) in the posttransplantation period [7]. Isolated cryptococcal pneumonia has not been reported in a HSCT recipient.

Several retrospective reviews of cryptococcosis in adult SOT recipients have been performed. The average incidence of cryptococcocal disease is 2.8% [100]. The lung and CNS are the most common sites of involvement, although disseminated disease is not rare [101]. In patients who have symptomatic pulmonary infection, the most frequent radiographic signs are unilateral, nodular, or cavitary infiltrates [100]. Asymptomatic pulmonary cryptococcosis has also been reported [102], typically discovered as an incidental finding on radiographic imaging (ground-glass infiltrates, multiple nodules, or mass with cavitation). Transmission of cryptococcosis through a transplanted lung allograft has been reported [103].

Trichosporon

Trichosporon species are pathogenic yeasts that cause infection in immunocompromised patients [1,4,5]. The cases of isolated pulmonary disease caused by *Trichosporon* have been in patients who have hematologic malignancy [104,105]. Only one case of invasive pulmonary disease and fungemia caused by *T cutaneum* has been reported in the HSCT population [106]. This patient had severe respiratory distress with hypoxemia despite a clear chest radiograph. In SOT recipients, there have been case reports of pulmonary infection caused by *Trichosporon* resulting from dissemination from another primary site of infection [107,108], but no cases of isolated pulmonary involvement in this population have been published.

Blastoschizomyces

Blastoschizomyces capitatus, formerly known as *Trichosporon capitatus*, produces infections in neutropenic patients or those receiving corticosteroid therapy [1,4]. In a review of immunocompromised patients with leukemia, cases of pulmonary involvement with cavity formation and liver involvement, similar to hepatosplenic candidiasis, were described [109]. In some leukemic patients who have cavitary lung lesions, spontaneous pneumothorax ensued [110]. No cases of pulmonary disease have been reported in either the HSCT or SOT populations to date.

Pneumocystis

Pneumocystis pneumonia (PCP) is an important cause of morbidity and mortality in the immunocompromised host. Although the genus *Pneumocystis* has been known for years, taxonomic assignment of *Pneumocystis* has placed it with either fungi or protozoa; phylogenetic data and characteristics support its place in either group [111]. Recent molecular analysis has revealed genomic diversity of the

organism in different host species; *P carinii* was shown to infect rodents, and the species that infects humans was renamed *P jiroveci* [112,113]. The term PCP, however, is retained as it may be used to refer to *Pneumocystis* pneumonia.

Acquisition seems to be through inhalation of aerosolized organisms, and primary exposure and reactivation of latent infection have been proposed as mechanisms of disease. In both the SOT and HSCT populations, the period associated with the greatest risk for PCP is the first 6 months after transplantation [7,114]. The incidence of PCP in HSCT was 5% to 15% before prophylaxis, with virtual elimination after institution of prophylaxis with trimethoprim-sulfamethoxazole (TMP/SMX) administered for 6 months after transplantation [115]. Recent data from the TRANSNET surveillance program reported that pneumocystosis accounts for 2% of IFI in the transplant population [12].

The typical presentation of PCP includes increasing dyspnea, nonproductive cough, fever, and occasionally chest pain. In seriously ill patients, hypoxemia is often present, and elevated lactate dehydrogenase levels reflect the extent of tissue injury. Radiographic imaging reveals bilateral interstitial infiltrates, although atypical images such as unilateral infiltrates, alveolar infiltrates, nodules, and cavities have been seen [116]. Asymptomatic infection has also been reported in lung transplant recipients [117], as have unusual presentations, such as granulomatous pneumocystosis [118,119].

As noted previously, widespread use of prophylaxis for PCP has decreased rates of infection and improved survival. Breakthrough infections in patients receiving TMP/SMX with adequate systemic absorption are rare, but when they do occur the clinical presentation is often atypical, and diagnosis may require lung biopsy. Breakthrough infection with PCP has been reported in liver transplant recipients receiving low-dose daily TMP/SMX [120], in bone marrow and heart transplant patients receiving low-dose atovaquone [121], and in HSCT recipients receiving aerosolized pentamidine [122].

Diagnosis

Diagnosis of IFIs requires a multifaceted approach. A set of standard definitions for IFIs in HSCT and SOT recipients has been developed [123]. These criteria, however, frequently cannot be applied in the clinical setting, where the condition of the patient may limit the extent of a diagnostic work-up. All the clinician may have at his disposal is a high index of suspicion and preliminary information.

Diagnostic evaluation of pulmonary infiltrates in transplant recipients often starts with radiographic imaging [115]. When the chest radiograph is negative or shows only minimal changes, chest CT is useful for defining the location, extent, and configuration of pulmonary lesions. Fiberoptic bronchoscopy with bronchoalveolar lavage is frequently the first step in the direct evaluation of lesions in transplant recipients; transbronchial biopsy is an option in non-thrombocytopenic patients [124,125]. Unfortunately, the diagnostic yield is variable, especially for HSCT recipients, and a negative bronchoscopy result does not exclude fungal infection. Although open lung biopsy is a more invasive method for obtaining tissue, it is used in patients who can tolerate the procedure and for whom the bronchoscopic approach was non-diagnostic [126].

Laboratory methods available for the diagnosis of IFI in the transplant population involve culture of the organism from clinical specimens, detection of antigens with serologic tests, or histopathologic inspection of tissue [127]. In addition to routine fungal cultures, blood cultures may also be of diagnostic value for yeast and those molds that produce adventitial forms in vivo (*Fusarium*, *Scedosporium*, *Paecilomyces*, *Acremonium*) [1,2]. Serologic tests may detect circulating antigen released during invasive infection. (1-3)-β-D-glucan, a cell wall component of yeasts and filamentous molds, is detectable at high levels in the blood during infection with *Aspergillus*, *Candida*, *Fusarium*, *Trichosporon*, *Saccharomyces*, and *Acremonium* and has recently been approved by the US Food and Drug Administration for this purpose [127,128]. PCR assays for the detection of IFIs are not yet commercially available. Histopathology allows the morphologic detection of fungi and demonstrates the pattern and degree of host response. Histopathology alone, however, does not suffice to distinguish among fungal pathogens such as between *Aspergillus* and other hyalohyphomycetes, and definitive diagnosis requires fungal culture [14]. Thus, histopathology and microbiology are complementary methods in the diagnosis of IFIs.

Therapy

The challenge of treating transplant recipients with non-*Aspergillus* pulmonary infection is multidimensional. The therapeutic armamentarium against fungi includes agents from different antifungal classes with diverse mechanisms of action (Table 2). The number of agents is limited [14], however, and many of the emerging fungal pathogens have intrinsic or variable resistance to the available drugs [129]. In the transplant recipient, choice of antifungal therapy is influenced further by the individual patient's comorbid conditions and concomitant medications. Finally, interventions to enhance clinical response such as aggressive surgical debulking and drainage may not be possible.

Key to successful therapy is knowing the infecting pathogen (Table 3) [130]. *Fusarium* and *Scedosporium* are the most commonly isolated non-*Aspergillus* hyaline hyphomycetes [4,10,11]. Voriconazole has emerged as the leading currently available antifungal agent for these organisms. Sixty-three percent (15/24) of *S apiospermum* infections and 43% (9/21) of *Fusarium* infections reported in the voriconazole package insert responded to therapy [131]. Voriconazole was also evaluated as salvage therapy in patients refractory to or intolerant of standard antifungal therapy and was effective in 46% of *Fusarium* but only 30% of *Scedosporium* (2/6 *S apiospermum* and 1/4 *S prolificans*) infections [132]. The relative lack of response in the salvage study was primarily caused by *S prolificans*, which is known to be resistant to all available agents [21,22]. Use of an azole and terbinafine in combination has demonstrated in vitro synergy against *Scedosporium* [133], and successful control of disseminated *S prolificans* was documented in an HSCT recipient treated with a combination of voriconazole and terbinafine plus aggressive surgical débridement [134].

When treating *Paecilomyces*, it is important to distinguish between *P variotii* and *P lilacinus*, because these two organisms differ in their susceptibility patterns. Although the former is susceptible to amphotericin B, the latter tends to be resistant to this agent but shows some in vitro susceptibility to voriconazole [21]. *Trichoderma* has been reported to have decreased susceptibility to amphotericin B and azoles, [21,34], and most cases have had a fatal outcome despite aggressive therapy [34,35,135].

The mainstay of therapy for invasive zygomycosis consists of aggressive surgical débridement and high-dose amphotericin B products [4,45,136]. When disease has been localized, recovery of neutrophil count, discontinuation of corticosteroids, and reversal of metabolic abnormalities aid in outcome. The only azole with activity against the Zygomycetes is posaconazole, for which Food and Drug Administration approval is being sought for use in the United States. Sixteen of 23 Zygomycete infections treated through a compassionate release study responded

Table 2
Antifungal agents for management of pulmonary fungal disease

Class	Mechanism of action	Drugs within class
Polyenes	Binds to ergosterol in the fungal cell membrane causing osmotic disruption; interferes with membrane-associated oxidative enzyme function	Amphotericin B desoxycholate Amphotericin B lipid complex Liposomal amphotericin B Amphotercin B colloidal dispersion
Azoles	Inhibits cytochrome p-450–dependent 14-α-demethylase; blocks conversion of lanosterol to ergosterol in the fungal cell membrane leading to loss of membrane integrity and impaired activity of membrane oxidative enzymes	Fluconazole (no activity against molds) Itraconazole Voriconazole Posaconazole[a]
Pyrimidine analogue	Disrupts pyrimidine metabolism; interferes with synthesis of DNA, RNA, and proteins in the fungal cell	5-Flucytosine (5-FC)
Echinocandins	Inhibits $(1-3)$-β-D-glucan synthase; disrupts cell wall synthesis	Caspofungin Micafungin Anidulafungin[a]
Allylamine	Inhibits squalene epoxidase, enzyme involved in the synthesis of ergosterol in the fungal cell membrane; causes osmotic disruption	Terbinafine

[a] Currently in investigational trials.

to posaconazole, a percentage comparable with the 72% (46/64) response rate reported for amphotericin B lipid complex.

Treatment of dematiaceous fungi involves surgical intervention along with antifungal therapy as management. High-dose amphotericin B preparations historically have been used against dematiaceous molds [4]. In vitro studies demonstrate activity of triazoles (itraconazole, voriconazole, and posaconazole) against these fungi as well [137], and in the voriconazole salvage study, five of five patients who had phaeohyphomycosis responded to therapy [132]. For disease limited to the lung, most experts would agree that a triazole is first-line therapy.

Amphotericin B products are effective against the dimorphic fungi [4] and should be used, at least as induction therapy, for life-threatening disease. After a period of induction therapy and stabilization, patients can be switched to an azole, historically itraconazole for all dimorphic fungi except *Coccidioides*, for which fluconazole may also be used [91,92].

Much of the data on treatment for *Cryptococcus* in transplant patients is derived from patients who have AIDS and cryptococcal meningitis [138]. Current guidelines from the Infectious Disease Society of America published in 2000 recommend that immunocompromised hosts (including transplant recipients) with non-CNS disease should be treated in the same fashion as those with CNS disease, regardless of the site of involvement. Based on these guidelines, treatment should include an amphotericin B product together with flucytosine for a 2-week induction with subsequent switch to fluconazole to complete a

minimum of 10 weeks of therapy. Assuming resolution of disease, chronic suppressive doses of fluconazole should be continued for 6 to 12 months [139]. Fluconazole monotherapy for mild to moderate pulmonary cryptococcosis in the transplant recipient has also been used with good response, although the actual clinical data to support this treatment are limited [140,141]. Use of fluconazole monotherapy to treat asymptomatic pulmonary cryptococcosis in three SOT patients also has been reported, but two of these patients received adjunctive surgical resection. The third patient was treated for 9 months without subsequent evidence of recurrence [102].

Trichosporon is susceptible to fluconazole [142] and voriconazole in vitro [143,144]. Fluconazole has been used alone [145] or in combination with amphotericin B in the critically ill [106,145]. *Blastoschizomyces* has been treated with amphotericin B, with or without flucytosine, in immunocompromised patients [109]. Fluconazole has also been used in a case report; although it stabilized the infection, response was not complete [146]. In vitro studies suggest that voriconazole may be an alternative agent for this pathogen [143].

The agent of choice for treatment for *Pneumocystis* is TMP/SMX [147]. Treatment with this drug typically results in complete recovery in the transplant patient [148]. Unfortunately, for a variety of reasons, some patients do not tolerate this antimicrobial combination. Alternative agents, as outlined in Table 3, are available as second-line therapy. Each of these agents has a unique adverse-effect profile. Early diagnosis and reduction in immunosuppres-

Table 3
Antifungal drugs for consideration in the treatment of fungal pneumonia by pathogen

Pathogen	Antifungal agent	Comment
Hyaline hyphomycetes		
Fusarium	Voriconazole	
	Amphotericin B product	
Scedosporium	Voriconazole	*S apiospermum* may be treated with voriconazole; *S prolificans* is highly resistant: consider azole + terbinafine[a] [133]
Acremonium	Amphotericin B product	Surgical debulking when possible; only in vitro data available for voriconazole [130]
	Voriconazole[a]	
Paecilomyces	Amphotericin B product	*P lilacinus* is more resistant than P *variotii* [21]; surgical debulking when possible
	Voriconazole[a]	
Trichoderma	Amphotericin B product	Highly resistant to most agents
Dematiaceous hyphomycetes		
Alternaria	Itraconazole	
Bipolaris	Voriconazole[a]	
Curvularia	Posaconazole[a,b]	
Dactylaria	Amphotericin B product	
Exophiala		
Cladophialophora		
Ramichloridium		
Zygomycetes		
Mucor	Amphotericin B product	Surgical debulking when possible; response to posaconazole may be dependent on the infecting genus
Rhizopus	Posaconazole[b]	
Cunninghamella		
Absidia		
Endemic fungi[c]		
H capsulatum	Itraconazole	
	Amphotericin B product	
C immitis	Fluconazole	
	Itraconazole	
	Amphotericin B product	
B dermatitidis	Amphotericin B product	Amphotericin B induction followed by itraconazole
	Itraconazole	
P brasiliensis	Itraconazole	
	Amphotericin B product	
P marneffei	Amphotericin B product	Amphotericin B induction followed by itraconazole
	Itraconazole	
Yeasts		
Cryptococcus	Amphotericin B + flucytosine	Amphotericin B + flucytosine as induction therapy in CNS disease; fluconazole in isolated pulmonary disease or as consolidation therapy
	Fluconazole	
Trichosporon	Amphotericin B product	Only in vitro data supports voriconazole use [143,144]
	Fluconazole	
	Voriconazole[a]	
Pneumocystis		
P jiroveci	TMP/SMX	TMP/SMX if first-line therapy; all other drugs are considered second-line agents
	Pentamidine, intravenous	
	Dapsone + trimethoprim	
	Atovaquone	
	Trimetrexate	
	Clindamycin + primaquine	
	Pyrimethamine + sulfadiazine	

[a] Based on in vitro data.

[b] Currently in investigational trials.

[c] Amphotericin B should be used initially in severe or life-threatening disease.

sion, when feasible, usually portend an excellent response to therapy.

Immunotherapy for invasive fungal infection

Efforts to evaluate augmentation of the host immune response during IFI are ongoing [149,150]. Granulocyte infusions have been used in an attempt to bolster neutrophil counts and activity. Studies to date, however, do not suggest a strong benefit for granulocyte transfusions for patients who have IFI, especially when molds are involved [149,150]. In vitro and animal data suggest that growth factors, granulocyte colony-stimulating factor, granulocyte macrophage colony-stimulating factor, and mcrophage colony-stimulating factor, increase the activity of effector cells against many pathogens, although this action is dependent on the pathogenic organism and the cytokine tested. In humans, growth factors are important for shortening the period of neutropenia, but their role in the treatment of IFI remains unclear [149].

There are abundant in vitro and animal model data on the proinflammatory cytokines, interferon-gamma (IFN-γ) and interleukin-12, regarding activity of macrophages and other mediators of Th-1 response. In vivo data have demonstrated increased survival, decreased tissue fungal burden, and enhanced anticryptococcal activity in experimentally infected animals. In humans, recombinant IFN-γ has been used in children with chronic granulomatous disease to prevent bacterial and fungal infection. Studies of IFN-γ in HIV-positive patients who have *C neoformans* meningitis are ongoing, with one published study showing a trend toward more rapid clearance of *C neoformans* from cerebrospinal fluid in IFN-γ recipients compared with placebo recipients. A placebo-controlled trial of IFN-γ in conjunction with voriconazole in immunocompromised patients who have invasive aspergillosis has been initiated recently. Whether IFN-γ may be useful for patients who have IFI is still controversial; most of the data have been obtained from animal models, and it remains to be seen if clinical data support their use. Further, and particularly relevant for the transplant recipient, is whether these agents might promote rejection of the allograft [149,150].

Passive immunotherapy has been advocated as a potential adjunct to antifungal therapy in IFI. Although animal data have been promising, use of intravenous immunoglobulin prophylaxis in high-risk patients has yielded conflicting results [149,150]. Monoclonal antibodies, specifically anticryptococcal antibodies, have demonstrated increased fungal killing, enhanced granuloma formation, and prolonged survival in animal models. Clinical benefit in humans is still unproven, although studies are ongoing [149,150].

Summary

As more patients undergo transplantation, the population of immunocompromised patients will continue to expand. Most of these patients will do quite well; however, a portion of patients will be haunted by the specter of rejection or GVHD, prolonged high doses of immunosuppression, and increased vulnerability to infection. IFIs are likely to continue to cause a significant number of pneumonias, and, as has been the trend in the past decade, increasing numbers of infections caused by non-*Aspergillus* fungal pathogens should be expected. The challenge to clinicians and researchers alike is multifold: to develop methods for earlier diagnosis, to identify effective prevention programs, to develop new antifungal agents, to perform clinical trials to assess combination therapy, and to investigate new and innovative immunomodulatory regimens that can regulate the degree of immunosuppression more precisely.

References

[1] Perfect JR, Schell WA. The new fungal opportunists are coming. Clin Infect Dis 1996;22(Suppl 2): S112–8.

[2] Schell WA. New aspects of emerging fungal pathogens. A multifaceted challenge. Clin Lab Med 1995; 15(2):365–87.

[3] Paya CV. Fungal infections in solid-organ transplantation. Clin Infect Dis 1993;16(5):677–88.

[4] Groll AH, Walsh TJ. Uncommon opportunistic fungi: new nosocomial threats. Clin Microbiol Infect 2001; 7(Suppl 2):8–24.

[5] Jahagirdar BN, Morrison VA. Emerging fungal pathogens in patients with hematologic malignancies and marrow/stem-cell transplant recipients. Semin Respir Infect 2002;17(2):113–20.

[6] Walsh TJ, Groll A, Hiemenz J, et al. Infections due to emerging and uncommon medically important fungal pathogens. Clin Microbiol Infect 2004;10(Suppl 1): 48–66.

[7] Fishman JA, Rubin RH. Infection in organ-transplant recipients. N Engl J Med 1998;338(24):1741–51.

[8] Briegel J, Forst H, Spill B, et al. Risk factors for systemic fungal infections in liver transplant recipients. Eur J Clin Microbiol Infect Dis 1995;14(5): 375–82.

[9] Singh N, Gayowski T, Wagener MM, et al. Invasive fungal infections in liver transplant recipients receiving tacrolimus as the primary immunosuppressive agent. Clin Infect Dis 1997;24(2):179–84.

[10] Husain S, Alexander BD, Munoz P, et al. Opportunistic mycelial fungal infections in organ transplant recipients: emerging importance of non-Aspergillus mycelial fungi. Clin Infect Dis 2003;37(2):221–9.

[11] Marr KA, Carter RA, Crippa F, et al. Epidemiology and outcome of mould infections in hematopoietic stem cell transplant recipients. Clin Infect Dis 2002; 34(7):909–17.

[12] Pappas PG, Alexander B, Marr KA, et al. Invasive fungal infections (IFIs) in hematopoietic stem cell (HSCTs) and organ transplant recipients (OTRs): overview of the TRANSNET database. In: Proceedings of the 42nd Annual Meeting of the Infectious Disease Society of America. Boston: Infectious Diseases Society of America; 2004. p. 174.

[13] Bigley VH, Duarte RF, Gosling RD, et al. Fusarium dimerum infection in a stem cell transplant recipient treated successfully with voriconazole. Bone Marrow Transplant 2004;34(9):815–7.

[14] Anaissie EJ, McGinnis MR, Pfaller MA. Clinical mycology. 1st edition. Philadelphia: Churchill Livingstone; 2003.

[15] Nucci M, Marr KA, Queiroz-Telles F, et al. Fusarium infection in hematopoietic stem cell transplant recipients. Clin Infect Dis 2004;38(9):1237–42.

[16] Martino P, Gastaldi R, Raccah R, et al. Clinical patterns of Fusarium infections in immunocompromised patients. J Infect 1994;28(Suppl 1):7–15.

[17] Boutati EI, Anaissie EJ. Fusarium, a significant emerging pathogen in patients with hematologic malignancy: ten years' experience at a cancer center and implications for management. Blood 1997;90(3): 999–1008.

[18] Sampathkumar P, Paya CV. Fusarium infection after solid-organ transplantation. Clin Infect Dis 2001; 32(8):1237–40.

[19] Arney KL, Tiernan R, Judson MA. Primary pulmonary involvement of Fusarium solani in a lung transplant recipient. Chest 1997;112(4):1128–30.

[20] Herbrecht R, Kessler R, Kravanja C, et al. Successful treatment of Fusarium proliferatum pneumonia with posaconazole in a lung transplant recipient. J Heart Lung Transplant 2004;23(12):1451–4.

[21] Espinel-Ingroff A. In vitro fungicidal activities of voriconazole, itraconazole, and amphotericin B against opportunistic moniliaceous and dematiaceous fungi. J Clin Microbiol 2001;39(3):954–8.

[22] Berenguer J, Rodriguez-Tudela JL, Richard C, et al. Deep infections caused by Scedosporium prolificans. A report on 16 cases in Spain and a review of the literature. Scedosporium Prolificans Spanish Study Group. Medicine (Baltimore) 1997; 76(4):256–65.

[23] Idigoras P, Perez-Trallero E, Pineiro L, et al. Disseminated infection and colonization by Scedosporium prolificans: a review of 18 cases, 1990–1999. Clin Infect Dis 2001;32(11):E158–65.

[24] Husain S, Munoz P, Forrest G, et al. Infections due to Scedosporium apiospermum and Scedosporium prolificans in transplant recipients: clinical characteristics and impact of antifungal agent therapy on outcome. Clin Infect Dis 2005;40(1):89–99.

[25] Castiglioni B, Sutton DA, Rinaldi MG, et al. Pseudallescheria boydii (Anamorph Scedosporium apiospermum). Infection in solid organ transplant recipients in a tertiary medical center and review of the literature. Medicine (Baltimore) 2002;81(5): 333–48.

[26] Perlroth MG, Miller J. Pseudoallescheria boydii pneumonia and empyema: a rare complication of heart transplantation cured with voriconazole. J Heart Lung Transplant 2004;23(5):647–9.

[27] Garcia-Arata MI, Otero MJ, Zomeno M, de la Figuera MA, et al. Scedosporium apiospermum pneumonia after autologous bone marrow transplantation. Eur J Clin Microbiol Infect Dis 1996;15(7):600–3.

[28] Klopfenstein KJ, Rosselet R, Termuhlen A, et al. Successful treatment of Scedosporium pneumonia with voriconazole during AML therapy and bone marrow transplantation. Med Pediatr Oncol 2003; 41(5):494–5.

[29] Tamm M, Malouf M, Glanville A. Pulmonary scedosporium infection following lung transplantation. Transpl Infect Dis 2001;3(4):189–94.

[30] Schell WA, Perfect JR. Fatal, disseminated Acremonium strictum infection in a neutropenic host. J Clin Microbiol 1996;34(5):1333–6.

[31] Chan-Tack KM, Thio CL, Miller NS, et al. Paecilomyces lilacinus fungemia in an adult bone marrow transplant recipient. Med Mycol 1999;37(1):57–60.

[32] Shing MM, Ip M, Li CK, et al. Paecilomyces varioti fungemia in a bone marrow transplant patient. Bone Marrow Transplant 1996;17(2):281–3.

[33] Das A, MacLaughlin EF, Ross LA, et al. Paecilomyces variotii in a pediatric patient with lung transplantation. Pediatr Transplant 2000;4(4):328–32.

[34] Chouaki T, Lavarde V, Lachaud L, et al. Invasive infections due to Trichoderma species: report of 2 cases, findings of in vitro susceptibility testing, and review of the literature. Clin Infect Dis 2002; 35(11):1360–7.

[35] Richter S, Cormican MG, Pfaller MA, et al. Fatal disseminated Trichoderma longibrachiatum infection in an adult bone marrow transplant patient: species identification and review of the literature. J Clin Microbiol 1999;37(4):1154–60.

[36] Neglia JP, Hurd DD, Ferrieri P, et al. Invasive Scopulariopsis in the immunocompromised host. Am J Med 1987;83(6):1163–6.

[37] Wheat LJ, Bartlett M, Ciccarelli M, et al. Opportunistic Scopulariopsis pneumonia in an immunocompromised host. South Med J 1984;77(12):1608–9.

[38] Mohammedi I, Piens MA, Audigier-Valette C, et al. Fatal Microascus trigonosporus (anamorph Scopulari-

opsis) pneumonia in a bone marrow transplant recipient. Eur J Clin Microbiol Infect Dis 2004; 23(3):215–7.

[39] Patel R, Gustaferro CA, Krom RA, et al. Phaeo-hyphomycosis due to Scopulariopsis brumptii in a liver transplant recipient. Clin Infect Dis 1994; 19(1):198–200.

[40] Steinbach WJ, Schell WA, Miller JL, et al. Fatal Scopulariopsis brevicaulis infection in a paediatric stem-cell transplant patient treated with voriconazole and caspofungin and a review of Scopulariopsis infections in immunocompromised patients. J Infect 2004;48(1):112–6.

[41] de la Camara R, Pinilla I, Munoz E, et al. Penicillium brevicompactum as the cause of a necrotic lung ball in an allogeneic bone marrow transplant recipient. Bone Marrow Transplant 1996;18(6): 1189–93.

[42] Yuen KY, Woo PC, Ip MS, et al. Stage-specific manifestation of mold infections in bone marrow transplant recipients: risk factors and clinical significance of positive concentrated smears. Clin Infect Dis 1997;25(1):37–42.

[43] Morrison VA, Haake RJ, Weisdorf DJ. The spectrum of non-Candida fungal infections following bone marrow transplantation. Medicine (Baltimore) 1993; 72(2):78–89.

[44] Breton P, Germaud P, Morin O, et al. [Rare pulmonary mycoses in patients with hematologic diseases]. Rev Pneumol Clin 1998;54(5):253–7 [in French].

[45] Kontoyiannis DP, Wessel VC, Bodey GP, et al. Zygomycosis in the 1990s in a tertiary-care cancer center. Clin Infect Dis 2000;30(6):851–6.

[46] Darrisaw L, Hanson G, Vesole DH, et al. Cunninghamella infection post bone marrow transplant: case report and review of the literature. Bone Marrow Transplant 2000;25(11):1213–6.

[47] Garey KW, Pendland SL, Huynh VT, et al. Cunninghamella bertholletiae infection in a bone marrow transplant patient: amphotericin lung penetration, MIC determinations, and review of the literature. Pharmacotherapy 2001;21(7):855–60.

[48] Kolbeck PC, Makhoul RG, Bollinger RR, et al. Widely disseminated Cunninghamella mucormycosis in an adult renal transplant patient: case report and review of the literature. Am J Clin Pathol 1985;83(6): 747–53.

[49] Nimmo GR, Whiting RF, Strong RW. Disseminated mucormycosis due to Cunninghamella bertholletiae in a liver transplant recipient. Postgrad Med J 1988; 64(747):82–4.

[50] Leleu X, Sendid B, Fruit J, et al. Combined antifungal therapy and surgical resection as treatment of pulmonary zygomycosis in allogeneic bone marrow transplantation. Bone Marrow Transplant 1999;24(4): 417–20.

[51] Gaziev D, Baronciani D, Galimberti M, et al. Mucormycosis after bone marrow transplantation: report of four cases in thalassemia and review of the literature. Bone Marrow Transplant 1996;17(3): 409–14.

[52] Maertens J, Demuynck H, Verbeken EK, et al. Mucormycosis in allogeneic bone marrow transplant recipients: report of five cases and review of the role of iron overload in the pathogenesis. Bone Marrow Transplant 1999;24(3):307–12.

[53] Morrison VA, McGlave PB. Mucormycosis in the BMT population. Bone Marrow Transplant 1993; 11(5):383–8.

[54] Imhof A, Balajee SA, Fredricks DN, et al. Breakthrough fungal infections in stem cell transplant recipients receiving voriconazole. Clin Infect Dis 2004;39(5):743–6.

[55] Marty FM, Cosimi LA, Baden LR. Breakthrough zygomycosis after voriconazole treatment in recipients of hematopoietic stem-cell transplants. N Engl J Med 2004;350(9):950–2.

[56] Siwek GT, Dodgson KJ, de Magalhaes-Silverman M, et al. Invasive zygomycosis in hematopoietic stem cell transplant recipients receiving voriconazole prophylaxis. Clin Infect Dis 2004;39(4):584–7.

[57] Demirag A, Elkhammas EA, Henry ML, et al. Pulmonary Rhizopus infection in a diabetic renal transplant recipient. Clin Transplant 2000;14(1):8–10.

[58] Mattner F, Weissbrodt H, Strueber M. Two case reports: fatal Absidia corymbifera pulmonary tract infection in the first postoperative phase of a lung transplant patient receiving voriconazole prophylaxis, and transient bronchial Absidia corymbifera colonization in a lung transplant patient. Scand J Infect Dis 2004;36(4):312–4.

[59] Tobon AM, Arango M, Fernandez D, et al. Mucormycosis (zygomycosis) in a heart-kidney transplant recipient: recovery after posaconazole therapy. Clin Infect Dis 2003;36(11):1488–91.

[60] Jimenez C, Lumbreras C, Aguado JM, et al. Successful treatment of mucor infection after liver or pancreas-kidney transplantation. Transplantation 2002;73(3):476–80.

[61] Revankar SG, Sutton DA, Rinaldi MG. Primary central nervous system phaeohyphomycosis: a review of 101 cases. Clin Infect Dis 2004;38(2):206–16.

[62] Morris A, Schell WA, McDonagh D, et al. Pneumonia due to Fonsecaea pedrosoi and cerebral abscesses due to Emericella nidulans in a bone marrow transplant recipient. Clin Infect Dis 1995;21(5):1346–8.

[63] Sutton DA, Slifkin M, Yakulis R, et al. US case report of cerebral phaeohyphomycosis caused by Ramichloridium obovoideum (R. mackenziei): criteria for identification, therapy, and review of other known dematiaceous neurotropic taxa. J Clin Microbiol 1998;36(3):708–15.

[64] Levin TP, Baty DE, Fekete T, et al. Cladophialophora bantiana brain abscess in a solid-organ transplant recipient: case report and review of the literature. J Clin Microbiol 2004;42(9):4374–8.

[65] Salama AD, Rogers T, Lord GM, et al. Multiple Cladosporium brain abscesses in a renal transplant

patient: aggressive management improves outcome. Transplantation 1997;63(1):160–2.

[66] Emmens RK, Richardson D, Thomas W, et al. Necrotizing cerebritis in an allogeneic bone marrow transplant recipient due to Cladophialophora bantiana. J Clin Microbiol 1996;34(5):1330–2.

[67] Lundstrom TS, Fairfax MR, Dugan MC, et al. Phialophora verrucosa infection in a BMT patient. Bone Marrow Transplant 1997;20(9):789–91.

[68] Khan ZU, Lamdhade SJ, Johny M, et al. Additional case of Ramichloridium mackenziei cerebral phaeohyphomycosis from the Middle East. Med Mycol 2002;40(4):429–33.

[69] Kanj SS, Amr SS, Roberts GD. Ramichloridium mackenziei brain abscess: report of two cases and review of the literature. Med Mycol 2001;39(1):97–102.

[70] Morrison VA, Haake RJ, Weisdorf DJ. Non-Candida fungal infections after bone marrow transplantation: risk factors and outcome. Am J Med 1994;96(6):497–503.

[71] Singh N, Chang FY, Gayowski T, et al. Infections due to dematiaceous fungi in organ transplant recipients: case report and review. Clin Infect Dis 1997;24(3):369–74.

[72] Halaby T, Boots H, Vermeulen A, et al. Phaeohyphomycosis caused by Alternaria infectoria in a renal transplant recipient. J Clin Microbiol 2001;39(5):1952–5.

[73] Burns KE, Ohori NP, Iacono AT. Dactylaria gallopava infection presenting as a pulmonary nodule in a single-lung transplant recipient. J Heart Lung Transplant 2000;19(9):900–2.

[74] Mancini MC, McGinnis MR. Dactylaria infection of a human being: pulmonary disease in a heart transplant recipient. J Heart Lung Transplant 1992;11(4 Pt 1):827–30.

[75] Jenney A, Maslen M, Bergin P, et al. Pulmonary infection due to Ochroconis gallopavum treated successfully after orthotopic heart transplantation. Clin Infect Dis 1998;26(1):236–7.

[76] Limaye AP, Connolly PA, Sagar M, et al. Transmission of Histoplasma capsulatum by organ transplantation. N Engl J Med 2000;343(16):1163–6.

[77] Watanabe M, Hotchi M, Nagasaki M. An autopsy case of disseminated histoplasmosis probably due to infection from a renal allograft. Acta Pathol Jpn 1988;38(6):769–80.

[78] Davies SF, Sarosi GA, Peterson PK, et al. Disseminated histoplasmosis in renal transplant recipients. Am J Surg 1979;137(5):686–91.

[79] Serody JS, Mill MR, Detterbeck FC, et al. Blastomycosis in transplant recipients: report of a case and review. Clin Infect Dis 1993;16(1):54–8.

[80] Winkler S, Stanek G, Hubsch P, et al. Pneumonia due to Blastomyces dermatitidis in a European renal transplant recipient. Nephrol Dial Transplant 1996;11(7):1376–9.

[81] Butka BJ, Bennett SR, Johnson AC. Disseminated inoculation blastomycosis in a renal trans-

plant recipient. Am Rev Respir Dis 1984;130(6):1180–3.

[82] Blair JE, Logan JL. Coccidioidomycosis in solid organ transplantation. Clin Infect Dis 2001;33(9):1536–44.

[83] Blair JE. Coccidioidal pneumonia, arthritis, and soft-tissue infection after kidney transplantation. Transpl Infect Dis 2004;6(2):74–6.

[84] Logan JL, Blair JE, Galgiani JN. Coccidioidomycosis complicating solid organ transplantation. Semin Respir Infect 2001;16(4):251–6.

[85] Wright PW, Pappagianis D, Wilson M, et al. Donor-related coccidioidomycosis in organ transplant recipients. Clin Infect Dis 2003;37(9):1265–9.

[86] Tripathy U, Yung GL, Kriett JM, et al. Donor transfer of pulmonary coccidioidomycosis in lung transplantation. Ann Thorac Surg 2002;73(1):306–8.

[87] Blair JE, Douglas DD, Mulligan DC. Early results of targeted prophylaxis for coccidioidomycosis in patients undergoing orthotopic liver transplantation within an endemic area. Transpl Infect Dis 2003;5(1):3–8.

[88] Miller MB, Hendren R, Gilligan PH. Posttransplantation disseminated coccidioidomycosis acquired from donor lungs. J Clin Microbiol 2004;42(5):2347–9.

[89] Hall KA, Sethi GK, Rosado LJ, et al. Coccidioidomycosis and heart transplantation. J Heart Lung Transplant 1993;12(3):525–6.

[90] Cha JM, Jung S, Bahng HS, et al. Multi-organ failure caused by reactivated coccidioidomycosis without dissemination in a patient with renal transplantation. Respirology 2000;5(1):87–90.

[91] Wang JL, Hung CC, Chang SC, et al. Disseminated Penicillium marneffei infection in a renal-transplant recipient successfully treated with liposomal amphotericin B. Transplantation 2003;76(7):1136–7.

[92] Chan YH, Wong KM, Lee KC, et al. Pneumonia and mesenteric lymphadenopathy caused by disseminated Penicillium marneffei infection in a cadaveric renal transplant recipient. Transpl Infect Dis 2004;6(1):28–32.

[93] Hung CC, Hsueh PR, Chen MY, et al. Invasive infection caused by Penicillium marneffei: an emerging pathogen in Taiwan. Clin Infect Dis 1998;26(1):202–3.

[94] dos Santos JW, Debiasi RB, Miletho JN, et al. Asymptomatic presentation of chronic pulmonary paracoccidioidomycosis: case report and review. Mycopathologia 2004;157(1):53–7.

[95] Shikanai-Yasuda MA, Duarte MI, Nunes DF, et al. Paracoccidioidomycosis in a renal transplant recipient. J Med Vet Mycol 1995;33(6):411–4.

[96] Zavascki AP, Bienardt JC, Severo LC. Paracoccidioidomycosis in organ transplant recipient: case report. Rev Inst Med Trop Sao Paulo 2004;46(5):279–81.

[97] Sugar AM, Restrepo A, Stevens DA. Paracoccidioidomycosis in the immunosuppressed host: report of a case and review of the literature. Am Rev Respir Dis 1984;129(2):340–2.

[98] Reis MA, Costa RS, Ferraz AS. Causes of death in renal transplant recipients: a study of 102 autopsies from 1968 to 1991. J R Soc Med 1995;88(1):24–7.

[99] Hajjeh RA, Conn LA, Stephens DS, et al. Cryptococcosis: population-based multistate active surveillance and risk factors in human immunodeficiency virus-infected persons. Cryptococcal Active Surveillance Group. J Infect Dis 1999;179(2):449–54.

[100] Husain S, Wagener MM, Singh N. Cryptococcus neoformans infection in organ transplant recipients: variables influencing clinical characteristics and outcome. Emerg Infect Dis 2001;7(3):375–81.

[101] Pappas PG, Patel R, Hadley S, et al. Cryptococcosis in transplant recipients: an analysis of 102 subjects. In: Proceedings of the 42nd Annual Meeting of the Infectious Disease Society of America. Boston: Infectious Diseases Society of America; 2004.

[102] Mueller NJ, Fishman JA. Asymptomatic pulmonary cryptococcosis in solid organ transplantation: report of four cases and review of the literature. Transpl Infect Dis 2003;5(3):140–3.

[103] Kanj SS, Welty-Wolf K, Madden J, et al. Fungal infections in lung and heart-lung transplant recipients. Report of 9 cases and review of the literature. Medicine (Baltimore) 1996;75(3):142–56.

[104] Tashiro T, Nagai H, Nagaoka H, et al. Trichosporon beigelii pneumonia in patients with hematologic malignancies. Chest 1995;108(1):190–5.

[105] Onishi T, Fujita J, Ikeda K, et al. [Two cases of Trichosporon beigelii pneumonia in immunocompromised hosts]. Nihon Kyobu Shikkan Gakkai Zasshi 1991;29(3):365–71 [in Japanese].

[106] Lowenthal RM, Atkinson K, Challis DR, et al. Invasive Trichosporon cutaneum infection: an increasing problem in immunosuppressed patients. Bone Marrow Transplant 1987;2(3):321–7.

[107] Grossi P, Farina C, Fiocchi R, et al. Prevalence and outcome of invasive fungal infections in 1,963 thoracic organ transplant recipients: a multicenter retrospective study. Italian Study Group of Fungal Infections in Thoracic Organ Transplant Recipients. Transplantation 2000;70(1):112–6.

[108] Saul SH, Khachatoorian T, Poorsattar A, et al. Opportunistic Trichosporon pneumonia. Association with invasive aspergillosis. Arch Pathol Lab Med 1981;105(9):456–9.

[109] Martino P, Venditti M, Micozzi A, et al. Blastoschizomyces capitatus: an emerging cause of invasive fungal disease in leukemia patients. Rev Infect Dis 1990;12(4):570–82.

[110] Martino P, Girmenia C, Venditti M, et al. Spontaneous pneumothorax complicating pulmonary mycetoma in patients with acute leukemia. Rev Infect Dis 1990;12(4):611–7.

[111] Fishman JA. Prevention of infection due to Pneumocystis carinii. Antimicrob Agents Chemother 1998; 42(5):995–1004.

[112] Frenkel JK. Pneumocystis jiroveci n. sp. from man: morphology, physiology, and immunology in relation to pathology. Natl Cancer Inst Monogr 1976;43: 13–30.

[113] Stringer JR, Beard CB, Miller RF, et al. A new name (Pneumocystis jiroveci) for Pneumocystis from humans. Emerg Infect Dis 2002;8(9):891–6.

[114] Yoo JH, Lee DG, Choi SM, et al. Infectious complications and outcomes after allogeneic hematopoietic stem cell transplantation in Korea. Bone Marrow Transplant 2004;34(6):497–504.

[115] Yen KT, Lee AS, Krowka MJ, et al. Pulmonary complications in bone marrow transplantation: a practical approach to diagnosis and treatment. Clin Chest Med 2004;25(1):189–201.

[116] Walzer PD. Pneumocystis carinii. In: Mandell GL, Bennett JE, Dolin R, editors. Principles and practice of infectious diseases. 5th edition. Philadelphia: Churchill Livingstone; 2000. p. 2781–95.

[117] Gryzan S, Paradis IL, Zeevi A, et al. Unexpectedly high incidence of Pneumocystis carinii infection after lung-heart transplantation. Implications for lung defense and allograft survival. Am Rev Respir Dis 1988;137(6):1268–74.

[118] Leroy X, Copin MC, Ramon P, et al. Nodular granulomatous Pneumocystis carinii pneumonia in a bone marrow transplant recipient. Case report. APMIS 2000;108(5):363–6.

[119] Hazzan M, Copin MC, Pruvot FR, et al. Lung granulomatous pneumocystosis after kidney transplantation: an uncommon complication. Transplant Proc 1997;29(5):2409.

[120] Torre-Cisneros J, De la Mata M, Pozo JC, et al. Randomized trial of weekly sulfadoxine/pyrimethamine vs. daily low-dose trimethoprim-sulfamethoxazole for the prophylaxis of Pneumocystis carinii pneumonia after liver transplantation. Clin Infect Dis 1999;29(4): 771–4.

[121] Rodriguez M, Sifri CD, Fishman JA. Failure of low-dose atovaquone prophylaxis against Pneumocystis jiroveci infection in transplant recipients. Clin Infect Dis 2004;38(8):e76–8.

[122] Marras TK, Sanders K, Lipton JH, et al. Aerosolized pentamidine prophylaxis for Pneumocystis carinii pneumonia after allogeneic marrow transplantation. Transpl Infect Dis 2002;4(2):66–74.

[123] Ascioglu S, Rex JH, de Pauw B, et al. Defining opportunistic invasive fungal infections in immunocompromised patients with cancer and hematopoietic stem cell transplants: an international consensus. Clin Infect Dis 2002;34(1):7–14.

[124] Dunagan DP, Baker AM, Hurd DD, et al. Bronchoscopic evaluation of pulmonary infiltrates following bone marrow transplantation. Chest 1997;111(1): 135–41.

[125] Cordonnier C, Bernaudin JF, Bierling P, et al. Pulmonary complications occurring after allogeneic bone marrow transplantation. A study of 130 consecutive transplanted patients. Cancer 1986;58(5): 1047–54.

[126] Weill D, McGiffin DC, Zorn Jr GL, et al. The utility

of open lung biopsy following lung transplantation. J Heart Lung Transplant 2000;19(9):852–7.

[127] Alexander BD. Diagnosis of fungal infection: new technologies for the mycology laboratory. Transpl Infect Dis 2002;4(Suppl 3):32–7.

[128] Yoshida M, Obayashi T, Iwama A, et al. Detection of plasma (1 → 3)-beta-D-glucan in patients with Fusarium, Trichosporon, Saccharomyces and Acremonium fungaemias. J Med Vet Mycol 1997;35(5): 371–4.

[129] Pfaller MA, Messer SA, Hollis RJ, et al. Antifungal activities of posaconazole, ravuconazole, and voriconazole compared to those of itraconazole and amphotericin B against 239 clinical isolates of Aspergillus spp. and other filamentous fungi: report from SENTRY Antimicrobial Surveillance Program, 2000. Antimicrob Agents Chemother 2002;46(4): 1032–7.

[130] Saldarreaga A, Garcia MP, Ruiz AJ, et al. [Antifungal susceptibility of Acremonium species using E-test and Sensititre]. Rev Esp Quimioter 2004;17(1):44–7 [in Spanish].

[131] Voriconazole package insert. New York: Pfizer, Inc.; 2005. p. 1–41.

[132] Perfect JR, Marr KA, Walsh TJ, et al. Voriconazole treatment for less-common, emerging, or refractory fungal infections. Clin Infect Dis 2003;36(9): 1122–31.

[133] Gosbell IB, Toumasatos V, Yong J, et al. Cure of orthopaedic infection with Scedosporium prolificans, using voriconazole plus terbinafine, without the need for radical surgery. Mycoses 2003;46(5–6): 233–6.

[134] Howden BP, Slavin MA, Schwarer AP, et al. Successful control of disseminated Scedosporium prolificans infection with a combination of voriconazole and terbinafine. Eur J Clin Microbiol Infect Dis 2003; 22(2):111–3.

[135] Gautheret A, Dromer F, Bourhis JH, et al. Trichoderma pseudokoningii as a cause of fatal infection in a bone marrow transplant recipient. Clin Infect Dis 1995;20(4):1063–4.

[136] Herbrecht R, Letscher-Bru V, Bowden RA, et al. Treatment of 21 cases of invasive mucormycosis with amphotericin B colloidal dispersion. Eur J Clin Microbiol Infect Dis 2001;20(7):460–6.

[137] McGinnis MR, Pasarell L. In vitro testing of susceptibilities of filamentous ascomycetes to voriconazole, itraconazole, and amphotericin B, with consideration of phylogenetic implications. J Clin Microbiol 1998;36(8):2353–5.

[138] Perfect JR, Casadevall A. Cryptococcosis. Infect Dis Clin North Am 2002;16(4):837–74, v–vi.

[139] Saag MS, Graybill RJ, Larsen RA, et al. Practice guidelines for the management of cryptococcal disease. Infectious Diseases Society of America. Clin Infect Dis 2000;30(4):710–8.

[140] Vilchez RA, Irish W, Lacomis J, et al. The clinical epidemiology of pulmonary cryptococcosis in non-AIDS patients at a tertiary care medical center. Medicine (Baltimore) 2001;80(5):308–12.

[141] Dromer F, Mathoulin S, DuPont B, et al. Comparison of the efficacy of amphotericin B and fluconazole in the treatment of cryptococcosis in human immunodeficiency virus-negative patients: retrospective analysis of 83 cases. French Cryptococcosis Study Group. Clin Infect Dis 1996;22(Suppl 2): S154–60.

[142] Anaissie EJ, Hachem R, Karyotakis NC, et al. Comparative efficacies of amphotericin B, triazoles, and combination of both as experimental therapy for murine trichosporonosis. Antimicrob Agents Chemother 1994;38(11):2541–4.

[143] Espinel-Ingroff A. In vitro activity of the new triazole voriconazole (UK-109,496) against opportunistic filamentous and dimorphic fungi and common and emerging yeast pathogens. J Clin Microbiol 1998; 36(1):198–202.

[144] McGinnis MR, Pasarell L, Sutton DA, et al. In vitro activity of voriconazole against selected fungi. Med Mycol 1998;36(4):239–42.

[145] Nettles RE, Nichols LS, Bell-McGuinn K, et al. Successful treatment of Trichosporon mucoides infection with fluconazole in a heart and kidney transplant recipient. Clin Infect Dis 2003;36(4):E63–6.

[146] Girmenia C, Micozzi A, Venditti M, et al. Fluconazole treatment of Blastoschizomyces capitatus meningitis in an allogeneic bone marrow recipient. Eur J Clin Microbiol Infect Dis 1991;10(9):752–6.

[147] Fishman JA. Treatment of infection due to Pneumocystis carinii. Antimicrob Agents Chemother 1998; 42(6):1309–14.

[148] Grossi P, Ippoliti GB, Goggi C, et al. Pneumocystis carinii pneumonia in heart transplant recipients. Infection 1993;21(2):75–9.

[149] Pappas PG. Immunotherapy for invasive fungal infections: from bench to bedside. Drug Resist Updat 2004;7(1):3–10.

[150] Casadevall A, Pirofski LA. Adjunctive immune therapy for fungal infections. Clin Infect Dis 2001;33(7): 1048–56.

ELSEVIER
SAUNDERS

Clin Chest Med 26 (2005) 691 – 705

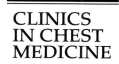

Cytomegalovirus Pneumonia in Transplant Recipients

Michael G. Ison, MD, MS[a], Jay A. Fishman, MD[a,b,*]

[a]Transplant Infectious Disease and Compromised Host Program, Infectious Disease Division, Massachusetts General Hospital, 55 Fruit Street, GRJ 504, Boston, MA 02114, USA
[b]Harvard Medical School, Boston, MA, USA

Cytomegalovirus (CMV) pneumonia is uncommon in patients who have intact immune systems other than as an occasional complication of cardiopulmonary bypass [1]. Most affected patients have immune deficits including AIDS, malignancy, or congenital immune deficiencies or are receiving immunosuppressive therapies. The spectrum of CMV pneumonia has changed with the introduction of routine antiviral prophylaxis. CMV pneumonia is most common after hematopoietic stem cell transplantation (HSCT; 10%–30%) and in lung and heart-lung transplant recipients (15%–55%) [2]. In these populations, CMV pneumonia is associated with high mortality (often caused by superinfection); mortality in other groups depends on the nature of invasive CMV disease (Table 1) [3,4]. Diagnosis often is confounded by viral secretion in patients who do not have invasive disease and must be considered with an appreciation of the host's immune deficits and clinical syndromes consistent with this infection. Therapy is most effective when started early, before the development of significant respiratory compromise. Antiviral resistance is emerging in patients who have chronic exposure to antiviral agents.

Virology and pathogenesis

CMV is a β-herpesvirus and, with a 230-million dalton linear double-stranded DNA molecule that encodes 230 proteins, is the largest known virus to infect humans. The infectious virion is composed of the DNA wrapped in nucleoprotein and surrounded by matrix proteins. The major matrix protein is the pp65 "early antigen," the target of antigenemia assays for the diagnosis of CMV infection. The virion is enveloped in a lipid membrane with numerous viral glycoproteins essential for viral entry. The receptor for CMV is unclear; attachment to the cell membrane results in endocytosis of the virus. Once within the cell, the viral genome is uncoated, and the DNA protein core is transported to the nucleus. CMV replication occurs in the nucleus after the UL54 protein (DNA polymerase) and UL44 protein (an accessory protein for DNA polymerase) are synthesized. The distinctive nuclear "owl's-eye" inclusions seen in CMV-infected cells represent new viral particles [5].

Human CMV establishes latency in cell types including vascular endothelial cells, monocytes and macrophages, polymorphonuclear neutrophils, and renal and pulmonary epithelial cells. A discrete set of viral genes is expressed during latency as opposed to productive or nonproductive infections. Multiple viral genes are involved in viral replication and in the establishment of latent infection in hematopoietic and endothelial cells. The nature of latency and the genes expressed in latent infection may determine risk for viral reactivation or dissemination. In some tissues (eg, lung, kidney), low-level viral replication is common; it is unclear whether this prevalence reflects persistence or reactivation of latent infection. CMV replication increases in the setting of immune deficiency or in response to a variety of stimuli including inflammation (eg, with fever and expression of tumor necrosis factor-α [TNF-α] and nuclear

* Corresponding author. Transplant Infectious Disease and Compromised Host Program, Infectious Disease Division, Massachusetts General Hospital, 55 Fruit Street, GRJ 504, Boston, MA 02114.
E-mail address: jfishman@partners.org (J.A. Fishman).

0272-5231/05/$ – see front matter © 2005 Elsevier Inc. All rights reserved.
doi:10.1016/j.ccm.2005.06.013

Table 1
Incidence of cytomegalovirus pneumonia by transplant populations

Transplant populations	Incidence (%)
HSCT	
Allogeneic [43]	10–30
Autologous [53]	1–9
SOT	
Lung [2]	15–55
Heart-lung [64]	71
Heart [11]	0.8–6.6
Renal [2,66]	<1–53
Liver [69]	0–9.2

Incidence has been reduced by routine use of antiviral prophylaxis. See text for details.

Abbreviations: HSCT, hematopoietic stem cell transplantation; SOT, solid organ transplantation.

factor κB [NFκB]), alloimmune responses, and other infections [6–8].

The mechanisms controlling latency and progression to lytic infection are not understood completely (Fig. 1). TNF-α contributes to activation of latent virus through activation of protein kinase C and NFκB. NFκB, in turn, binds to a promoter region in the virus to activate expression of the immediate-early genes and initiates replication [6,8]. CMV does not immortalize cells but seems to contribute indirectly to oncogenesis (eg, through immune suppression and promoting other viral infections). Some viral proteins contribute to evasion of the immune system. Two such proteins, US 2 and US 11, promote degradation of HLA-1 molecules. As a result, presentation of complexes of HLA-1 and CMV glycoproteins as targets for activation of cellular immunity may be altered [9].

The pathogenesis of CMV pneumonitis is complex and incompletely understood. CMV causes cy-

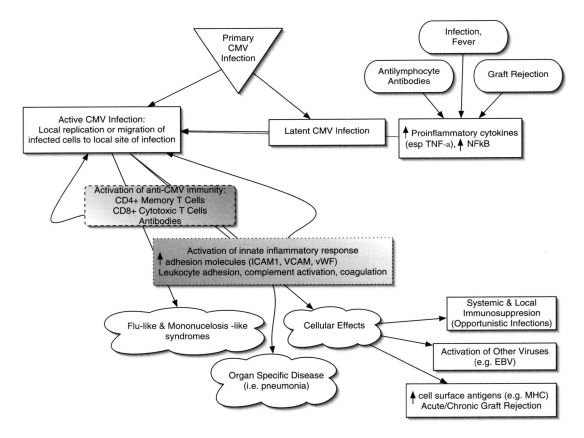

Fig. 1. The direct and indirect effects of cytomegalovirus. The activation of latent CMV alters many aspects of the innate and adaptive immune response. The indirect effects include predisposition to opportunistic infections, activation of other latent viruses, and graft rejection or graft-versus-host disease.

topathic effects in the lower airways after activation in epithelial cells, vascular endothelia, or resident macrophages [10]. In addition, infected endothelial cells from other sites may migrate to the lungs [11]. CMV replication may activate endothelial cells, contributing to the increased expression of intercellular adhesion molecule 1, vascular adhesion molecule 1, or von Willebrand's factor on the surface of endothelial cells [12–16]. As a result, CMV infection may be associated with leukocyte margination, complement activation, and intravascular coagulation with microvascular compromise [17,18].

The importance of host responses in the manifestations of CMV pneumonia is demonstrated by studies in mice and patients that correlate CD8$^+$ CMV-specific cytotoxic T-lymphocyte responses with protection from development of CMV pneumonia [19–21]. CD4$^+$ CMV-specific T-helper (Th1) responses correlate less well with clinical outcomes but have a major role in the maintenance of protective cellular immunity [22]. CD8$^+$ and CD4$^+$ T-lymphocytes may also contribute to damage to tissues manifesting viral antigen expression. The relative contributions of infection and host response vary with the nature of the infection (viral strain, quantity, site of infection) and the intensity of the host response (prior immunity, immune deficits).

Diagnosis of cytomegalovirus infection and disease

It is essential to distinguish between CMV infection and invasive disease [23]. CMV infection is defined as isolation of the CMV virus or detection of viral proteins or nucleic acids in any bodily fluid or tissue specimen. The multiple methods for the microbiologic diagnosis of CMV have varying degrees of sensitivity and specificity. Detection of CMV in the blood is defined by the test used for detection. Thus, CMV viremia is defined as the isolation of CMV from the blood by culture that involves the use of either standard or shell vial techniques. Antigenemia is defined as the detection of CMV pp65 in leukocytes. DNAemia and RNAemia are defined as the detection of CMV DNA or RNA in samples of plasma, whole blood, and isolated peripheral blood leukocytes or in buffy-coat specimens.

The diagnosis of CMV pneumonia is defined appropriately by the presence of signs or symptoms of pulmonary disease combined with the detection of CMV in lung tissue samples. Secretion of CMV into lung fluids may result in detection of CMV in bronchoalveolar lavage (BAL) or sputum specimens in the absence of invasive disease, thereby confound-

ing the diagnosis. Molecular or protein-based assays (ELISA) may be overly sensitive for use with BAL samples. Thus, although it may be useful to initiate therapy on the identification of CMV in respiratory tract secretions (eg, see reference [23]), the definition of CMV pneumonia should include virus isolation or histopathologic or immunohistochemical evidence of the presence of CMV in the lung parenchyma in the setting of a clinically compatible syndrome. Dual infections are common (eg, CMV with *Aspergillus* or *Pneumocystis*), and the relative contributions of each pathogen must be considered in such patients, with the awareness that CMV is a major promoter of other invasive infections and often merits therapy in such situations.

Radiology

In addition to appropriate clinical symptoms, radiologic evaluation is a component of the diagnosis of CMV pneumonia. Plain films demonstrate abnormalities in many patients who have documented CMV pneumonia. The most common radiographic findings include interstitial patterns with parenchymal consolidation and multiple nodules, usually less than 5 mm. Up to 9% of individuals with CMV pneumonia have radiographs without focal findings [24–26]. CT is more sensitive in detecting pulmonary abnormalities and demonstrates patchy or diffuse ground-glass attenuation. Focal consolidations, reticular opacities, thickened interlobular septa, and tree-in-bud abnormalities are also seen. Pleural effusions are present in up to 20% of patients.

Pathologic diagnosis

Because no radiologic finding is pathognomonic for CMV pneumonia, invasive techniques may be needed to document invasive infection. The criterion standard for the diagnosis of CMV pneumonia is biopsy, with highly characteristic intranuclear inclusions within epithelial cells. Additional, nonspecific findings include thickening of the alveolar interstitium with cellular infiltrates and edema, diffuse alveolar damage, and hemorrhage. Immunostaining may enhance the sensitivity of detecting CMV within cells.

Bronchoscopic studies

Cytologic examination of BAL samples may be useful in diagnosing CMV pneumonia by demonstrating viral inclusions within cells recovered from the lower respiratory tract. Cytology is highly specific for the diagnosis of CMV pneumonitis but lacks sensitivity. Immunohistochemical staining, employing various anti-CMV antibodies, may provide enhanced sensitivity in detecting infected BAL cells without sacrificing specificity. In 442 immunocompromised patients, the sensitivity, specificity, and positive and negative predictive values of BAL immunostaining for the diagnosis of CMV pneumonia were 88.9%, 98.6%, 72.7%, and 99.5%, respectively [27]. Rapid culture of BAL fluid, employing the shell vial technique, is highly sensitive in detecting virus but cannot differentiate viral shedding into the respiratory tract from tissue invasion (ie, pneumonia). The performance characteristics of the various BAL modalities in diagnosing CMV pneumonia are summarized in Table 2.

Laboratory diagnosis

Serologic testing generally is not useful in the diagnosis of CMV pneumonia in immunocompromised individuals. In immunocompetent patients, antibodies to CMV develop over the first 4 to 7 weeks after infection [28]; a fourfold rise between acute and convalescent titers is required for diagnosis. In immunocompromised hosts, serologic conversion is delayed (often beyond 6 months in solid organ transplant [SOT] recipients) and may be absent. Thus, such tests are not useful in acute infections.

Viral culture has been the criterion for identification of CMV. Most laboratories use human fibroblastoid cell lines, such as MRC-5 cells, to grow the virus. Growth takes 1 to 4 weeks (usually 7 to 12 days), depending on the strain and titer of virus. Infected cells can be identified readily by the presence of large, round, ground-glass inclusions within the nucleus or in plaque assays. Use of immunofluorescence or similar techniques, often in association with shell vial techniques, may allow more rapid detection of CMV. Virus can be isolated from multiple sites, including urine, oral swabs, blood, buffy coat, cervical tissue, or infected tissues. Asymptomatic shedding from the throat, urine, and respiratory secretions is common and cannot be used in the diagnosis of invasive disease.

More recently, additional methods have become available for the detection of viral replication in the peripheral blood: pp65 antigenemia, CMV quantitative viral load testing, hybrid capture assays, and the pp67 mRNA assay. In the pp65 antigenemia assay, neutrophils are stained for the presence CMV pp65 antigen that correlates semiquantitatively with viral replication [29–32]. The pp65 antigenemia assay is limited by the need for an adequate neutrophil count (>1000/mL). The pp65 antigenemia value often rises in the first week of appropriate therapy. In CMV quantitative viral load testing, DNA is extracted from whole blood, plasma, or peripheral blood leukocytes, and CMV-specific primers expand and quantify the number of CMV DNA copies present [33,34]. One commercial assay (COBAS Amplicor CMV Monitor; Roche Diagnostics, Indianapolis, Indiana) uses primers directed at a 365-bp region of the CMV polymerase gene and has a linear range of 400 to 50,000 copies/mL [35]. Many in-house assays have also been developed with varying degrees of standardization [35]. PCR viral load assays involve significant cost and training time for laboratory staff. The hybrid capture method (Hybrid Capture System CMV DNA test; Diagen Corp, Gaithersburg, Maryland) uses an RNA probe and a labeled antibody for signal amplification from RNA-DNA hybrids. This test has a linear range of 1400 to 560,000 copies/mL and requires whole cells, limiting its use in neutropenic patients [36]. Qualitative RNA amplification (NucliSens CMV test, bioMérieux, Durham, NC) detects pp67 mRNA, which is produced during active replication but not by latently infected cells [37]. Viral load monitoring may become positive sooner in infection and remains positive longer during therapy than the antigenemia assay [36]. The sensitivity of these tests is similar, however, and they are equally effective in monitoring CMV infection and disease [38].

Viral loads have been shown to correlate with risk for invasive disease. Quantitative viral loads in blood above 1000 to 1200 copies/μg DNA have been associated with CMV pneumonia, although elevation of the viral load is not specific for pneumonia. Viremia precedes clinical signs of CMV pneumonia by up to 3 weeks [39–42]. Quantitative assays should be used to monitor response to therapy. If a response to appropriate intravenous therapy (eg, ganciclovir) is not demonstrated within 2 weeks, antiviral resistance

Table 2
Performance characteristics of bronchoalveolar lavage diagnostic modalities

Method	Sensitivity (%)	Specificity (%)
Shell vial culture	99	67–83
Cytology	25–73	100
In situ hybridization	55	94
Immunohistochemistry	73–89	77–99
Pulmonary cytomegalovirus viral load	100	91–99

Data from Refs. [27,33,41,116–118].

must be considered, and molecular resistance testing must be obtained.

An emerging technique for diagnosing CMV pneumonia is quantitative CMV viral load testing of BAL fluid. Two studies have documented that 100 or more copies/μg DNA in BAL fluid is suggestive of CMV pneumonia, with higher levels increasingly associated with disease; false-positive results have been noted with this threshold [42].

Epidemiology and clinical syndromes

Although infection with CMV is common in all societies, with prevalence rates of 70% in the United States and approximately 100% in African populations, CMV pneumonia typically occurs in individuals with cellular immune deficits. CMV pneumonia presents with a rapid onset of fever, nonproductive cough, dyspnea, and hypoxia. Pleurisy is common. Chest radiographs have evidence of diffuse interstitial pneumonia with or without nodules. The differential diagnosis of this clinical and radiologic presentation includes radiation pneumonitis, chemotherapy or other drug-induced pulmonary injury, pulmonary edema, pulmonary hemorrhage, metastatic cancer, and other infections including community respiratory viruses, and *Pneumocystis* pneumonia. Early therapy is associated with improved outcomes.

Hematopoietic stem cell transplant recipients

The development of CMV infection after HSCT is driven by a number of factors: the nature of preparative chemotherapy, the duration of leukopenia (notably the T-cell deficiency), antiviral prophylaxis, the presence of graft-versus-host disease (GVHD), other intercurrent infections (notably viral), and the presence or absence of specific immunity in donor and host. Traditional times of onset for CMV infection have shifted because nonmyeloablative transplants or chimeric mini-transplants have gained in popularity and engraftment occurs earlier. In the past, CMV was described as occurring during the pre-engraftment (<30 days after bone marrow transplantation), postengraftment (30–99 after bone marrow transplantation), or late (≥100 days after bone marrow transplantation) period. In contrast with CMV viremia that may occur at any time while patients are neutropenic, symptomatic disease often is detected with immune reconstitution (in patients who do not have GVHD) from engraftment until approximately 100 days afterward. GVHD and immunosuppressive treatment may provoke CMV pneumonia

after the first 100 days [43]. Use of CMV prophylaxis can delay or prevent development of CMV pneumonia. Late disease can be seen in up to 17.8% of HSCT recipients (median, 169 days after engraftment) [44]. Late CMV disease is associated with a lower mortality rate (46%) and recurrence in nearly 40% of patients.

The risk of CMV pneumonia is greatest in the allogeneic HSCT population, with incidences between 10% and 30%. The median time to occurrence of CMV pneumonia in the preprophylaxis era was 44 days, but onset can be delayed (49–188 days) by prophylaxis [43]. Allogeneic recipients at greatest risk are seropositive before transplantation, older (relative risk, 1.4 per decade), have received total-body irradiation, have depleted antithymocyte globulins, have received T-cell–depleted stem cell transplants, or have viuria or viremia [45]. T-cell depletion of transplanted stem cells may also be associated with earlier onset of CMV disease [46,47]. The most severe disease occurs in the seropositive recipient (R$^+$) of seronegative grafts (D$^-$); the recipient activates CMV in the lungs during leukopenia, and the immunologically naive graft generates an immune response against infected lung cells. This immune response serves to enhance viral replication; pneumonitis often persists even after abrogation of viral replication by antiviral agents [48]. GVHD and its treatment are associated with impaired CMV-specific cytotoxic T-lymphocyte responses, increasing the risk of CMV disease and pneumonia [19,49]. Historically, the mortality in these patients has been 80% to 100% without therapy, although mortality has fallen to less than 50% in the era of effective antiviral therapy. A clinical scoring system initially developed for renal transplant recipients has been found to be predictive of survival in HSCT recipients (Table 3) [50]. A clinical severity score of 8 or higher was strongly correlated with death (sensitivity 100%; specificity 91%). This scoring system does not include GVHD and may underestimate risk in these patients.

In autologous HSCT recipients, the frequency of CMV infection is similar to that in allogeneic recipients, but tissue-invasive disease is significantly less common and less severe [51,52]. In particular, the incidence of CMV pneumonia generally has been reported in the range of only 1% to 9% [53]. The most significant risk factor for CMV pneumonia in autologous HSCT recipients is CMV seropositivity before transplantation and hematologic malignancy as the indication for transplantation. Some studies have identified CD34 selection as a risk factor for disease, with incidence of disease as high as 23% [54], but others have not documented this association

Table 3
Risk assessment system for predicting outcomes from cytomegalovirus pneumonia after allogeneic hematopoietic stem cell transplantation

Risk factor	Attributable points
Fever >38.3°C	
2–20 days	1
>21 days	3
Leucopenia (≤4 × 10⁹/L)	1
Thrombocytopenia (≤4 × 10⁹/L)	1
Hepatitis	
Liver function tests ≥2 times upper limit of normal	1
Jaundice	3
Degree of pulmonary disease	
Infiltrate without symptoms	1
Infiltrate with symptoms	2
Mechanical ventilation	3
Any evidence of CMV involvement of the gastrointestinal tract	3
Central nervous syttem status	
Lethargy	1
Stupor	2
Coma	3
Renal status	
Creatinine 2–4 times the best posttransplantation value	3
Creatinine >4 times the best posttransplantation value	
Nephrectomy with permanent dialysis	3
Arthritis or muscle wasting	2
Any superinfection	3
Death	4

Abbreviation: CMV, cytomegalovirus.
Adapted from Gentile G, Donati PP, Capobianchi A, et al. Evaluation of a score system for the severity and outcome of cytomegalovirus interstitial pneumonia in allogeneic bone marrow recipients. J Infect 1997;35:117–23; with permission.

[53]. In autologous HSCT recipients, there is a bimodal distribution in the time of onset of symptoms: 69% occur early after transplantation (median, 17 days; range, 5–26 days; 55% before engraftment), and 31% occur late (median, 209 days; range, 138–329 days) [53]. Most patients present with fever (94%), cough (63%), hypoxia (63%), and dyspnea (50%). Most of these patients have radiologic infiltrates, which typically are bilateral and diffuse. Pleural effusions are seen in almost half of patients. Concurrent infection with bacteria, community respiratory viruses, or *Pneumocystis* is common, occurring in approximately one third of cases. Extrapulmonary disease is rare. Morality ranges from 31% to 100% with mortality increased in early

posttransplantation infections and with delayed antiviral therapy.

Lung transplantation

Among all SOT recipients, CMV pneumonia is most common in lung transplant recipients, with an incidence that ranges from 15% to 55% with routine antiviral prophylaxis [2]. The rate of CMV pneumonitis without antiviral prophylaxis is high in CMV R⁺ recipients (up to 75%) and in CMV D⁺/R⁻ recipients (86%–100%) [55–58]. The high risk for disease may reflect, in part, the viral burden in the graft and resident macrophages or the chronic stimulation of the lungs by the environment and by graft rejection. Many cases (10%–15%) of CMV pneumonia are asymptomatic and are detected only on protocol biopsies [59]. CMV pneumonia was associated with a high mortality (54%–100%) in some series [3] but is less common in the era of widespread prophylaxis and effective treatment. CMV pneumonitis has been identified as a risk factor for bronchiolitis obliterans syndrome (BOS) [60,61].

Without prophylaxis, most patients develop CMV pneumonia between day 16 and 60; with prophylaxis, CMV disease may develop later, depending on the duration of antiviral use and the nature of the immune deficits [62]. Symptomatic patients generally present with one of two clinical syndromes. In the first, mild or moderate illness, characterized by cough, fever, and impaired oxygenation not requiring ventilatory support, is accompanied by interstitial infiltrates on chest radiographs; this syndrome is most common in seropositive (partially immune) patients. Clinical symptoms develop over several days and respond to antiviral therapy over 4 to 7 days. In the second syndrome, usually seen in D⁺/R⁻ recipients, rapid onset and progression of hypoxia with marked changes on chest radiography are present. Mortality is high, because the response to therapy tends to be slower. These patients may develop coinfection with other pathogens, including bacteria and fungi. Universal prophylaxis of D⁺/R⁻ recipients has successfully attenuated the severity of CMV pneumonitis in most cases, so this more explosive course of disease is now relatively rare.

Heart-lung transplantation

Patients who receive heart-lung transplants are also at significant risk for CMV pneumonia, particularly with primary CMV infection (D⁺/R⁻ recipients) and thymocyte depletion for transplantation [63]. As in lung transplant recipients, there is increased risk of CMV pneumonia in CMV D^+/R^- and D^+/R^+ recipients; the true rate of invasive disease is hard to ascertain, although the rate of CMV isolation (~71%) is roughly equivalent in all groups [64]. CMV pneumonia usually occurs during the first 3 months after transplantation or after the cessation of prophylaxis and frequently coexists with other infections, notably *Pseudomonas aeruginosa* or *Staphylococcus aureus* pneumonia. CMV pneumonia is associated with high mortality (32%), and survivors may have persistently abnormal lung function [64,65]. The clinical presentation is similar to that in lung transplant recipients.

Heart transplantation

Heart transplant recipients who have CMV pneumonia tend to present with a gradual onset of symptoms and may first notice a dry cough or hypoxemia. The incidence of CMV pneumonia in heart transplant recipients is 0.8% to 6.6% [11]. This incidence may be exacerbated by activation of CMV infection during cardiopulmonary bypass.

Renal transplantation

The incidence of CMV pneumonia in renal transplant recipients is estimated to be less than 1% [2]; a significant incidence of pulmonary involvement (53%) may occur during extrapulmonary CMV disease [66]. As in other SOT populations, antilymphocyte induction and D^+/R^- status are the greatest risk factors for CMV pneumonia. Tacrolimus and mycophenolate mofetil regimens (ie, intensity of immune suppression) may contribute to risk for CMV pneumonia in renal transplant recipients [67].

Liver transplantation

CMV pneumonia occurs in up to 9.2% of liver recipients and generally presents concurrently with CMV hepatitis at a median of 38 days (range, 29–316 days) [2,68,69]. One-year mortality is substantially higher after CMV pneumonia, with one series documenting an 84.6% mortality rate (67.4% directly attributable to CMV), versus 17.2% mortality among recipients who did not have pneumonia [69]. D^+/R^- CMV serologic status, the presence of CMV viremia, abdominal re-exploration after transplantation, and invasive fungal disease seem to be risk factors for CMV pneumonia in this population [69].

Available agents with activity against cytomegalovirus

Drugs with activity against CMV approved by the Food and Drug Administration include acyclovir and its valine prodrug, valacyclovir; ganciclovir and its valine prodrug, valganciclovir; cidofivir; and foscarnet. Leflunomide is not approved for this indication but has some useful antiviral activity. In addition, CMV immune globulin (CMVIG) is approved for the prevention of CMV infection and disease. Features of these agents are summarized in Table 4.

Ganciclovir is a nucleoside analogue of guanosine that is a potent inhibitor of CMV DNA polymerase. Activation of ganciclovir requires phosphorylation to the monophosphate form by the CMV-encoded UL97 kinase and subsequent phosphorylation by host cellular enzymes. In oral form, this drug had 4% to 6% bioavailability. To improve bioavailability, a valine ester prodrug, valganciclovir, was developed with approximately 60% bioavailability. Intestinal and hepatic esterases rapidly remove the valine, releasing ganciclovir into the bloodstream. In patients who have normal renal function, a 900-mg oral dose produces drug exposure similar to that obtained with 5 mg/kg ganciclovir given intravenously [70]. Standard doses of ganciclovir and valganciclovir are listed in Table 5.

Cidofivir is a nucleotide analogue that inhibits the viral DNA polymerase. Because it is already monophosphorylated, it requires cellular kinases to become active and does not require CMV-encoded UL97. Cidofivir has a long half-life in vivo and may require weekly or less frequent dosing. Hydration and coadministration with probenecid are used to reduce nephrotoxicity, which remains common, notably in patients receiving concomitant therapy with other nephrotoxic agents (eg, calcineurin inhibitors). Foscarnet is a competitor of pyrophosphate that inhibits DNA polymerase and does not require metabolic activation. Leflunomide is an isoxazole protein kinase and pyrimidine synthase inhibitor that is approved for the treatment of rheumatoid arthritis. The drug is an immunosuppressant that has activity against a number of viruses including CMV and BK polyomavirus. The antiviral mechanism is unclear; leflunomide interferes with virion assembly [71–73]. Leflunomide is metabolized by the gastrointestinal tract and liver to an active metabolite, A77 1726. Optimal regimens for use as an antiviral agent remain undefined [74].

CMVIG is an IgG preparation from pooled adult human plasma that contains a standardized amount of antibody to CMV. Although CMVIg generally is well

Table 4
Key characteristics of agents with activity against cytomegalovirus

Drug	IC$_{50}$	Resistance[a]	Bioavailability	Excretion	Major adverse effects
Ganciclovir	0.02–3.48 μg/mL	≥ 6 μM suggest UL97 mutations	Poor (6%)	Renal	Leukopenia, anemia, and less commonly thrombocytopenia, abnormal liver function tests, fever, rash (2%), and central nervous system adverse effects (5%)
Valganciclovir	0.0–3.48 μg/mL	≥ 32 μM suggest presence of UL54 mutations	Good (60%)	Renal	Leukopenia, anemia, and less commonly thrombocytopenia, abnormal liver function tests, fever, rash (2%), and central nervous system adverse effects (5%)
Cidofivir	0.5–2.8 μM	≥ 2 μM	Poor	Renal (secreted by the proximal renal tubules)	Nephrotoxicity (Fanconi-like syndrome: proteinuria, glucosuria, and bicarbonate wasting), neutropenia, acute iritis, and ocular hypotonia. Contraindicated with patients with creatinine levels >1.5 mg/dL or ≥ 2 mg/dL and proteinuria
Foscarnet	50–800 μM (mean, 269 μM)	≥ 400 μM	Poor	Renal	Nephrotoxicity, anemia, electrolyte imbalances, nausea, vomiting, genital ulcerations, and seizures
Leflunomide	40–60 μM[b]			Renal	Cytopenia, hepatotoxicity, rashes including Stevens-Johnson syndrome, immunosuppression, and malignancy; not approved by the Food and Drug Administration

Abbreviation: IC$_{50}$, concentration that inhibits 50% of cytomegalovirus.
[a] Value listed is standardized cutoff for in vitro susceptibility testing.
[b] Activity is preserved in a strain resistant to ganciclovir, cidofivir, and foscarnet [72].

tolerated, low-grade fevers may occur during administration, as may uncommon side effects including volume overload, pulmonary edema, flushing, chills, muscle cramps, back pain, nausea, vomiting, arthralgia, or wheezing. Rarely, as with any blood product, transfusion-related acute lung injury, hypotension, acute renal failure, Stevens-Johnson syndrome, erythema multiforme, hemolysis, angioneurotic edema, and anaphylactic shock can occur.

Prevention of cytomegalovirus disease

The best strategy for prevention of CMV infection depends on resources (time, personnel, and cost) as well as efficacy. Pre-emptive prophylaxis initiates antiviral therapy after a microbiologic assay has documented viral replication. This approach carries lower drug costs but higher personnel expenses and requires constant communication between medical staff and patients and meticulous viral testing and reporting of viral assay data. Universal prophylaxis gives antiviral therapy to all at-risk patients for a fixed period. Prophylaxis is subject to the inherent toxicities of the agents used and higher intrinsic medication costs but fewer breakthrough infections. If opportunistic infections, graft dysfunction and rejection, and cancer are believed to be indirect effects of viral infections, routine prophylaxis is the preferred method of prevention.

Among CMV-naive recipients, prevention of CMV disease usually can be achieved by use of CMV-negative donor organs and blood products. The use of leukocyte-reduced blood products provides incomplete protection, with an incidence of CMV infection of around 2% to 4% [75–77]. For CMV R$^+$ recipients and for R$^-$/D$^+$ recipients, strategies for prophylaxis include passive immunization with immunoglobulin and use of antiviral agents. Passive

Table 5
Dosage of anti-cytomegalovirus antiviral agents

Drug	Indication	Creatinine clearance	Route	Dose	Frequency
Ganciclovir	Therapy	≥ 70 mL/min	IV	5 mg/kg	q12h
		50–69 mL/min		2.5 mg/kg	q12h
		25–49 mL/min		2.5 mg/kg	q24h
		10–24 mL/min		1.25 mg/kg	q24h
		<10 mL/min		1.25 mg/kg	After hemodialysis, tiw
	Prevention	≥70 mL/min	IV	5 mg/kg	q24h
		50–69 mL/min		2.5 mg/kg	q24h
		25–49 mL/min		1.25 mg/kg	q24h
		10–24 mL/min		0.625 mg/kg	q24h
		<10 mL/min		0.625 mg/kg	After hemodialysis, tiw
Valganciclovir[a]	Therapy	≥ 60 mL/min	po	900 mg	bid
		40–59 mL/min		450 mg	bid
		25–39 mL/min		450 mg	qd
		10–24 mL/min		450 mg	q48h
	Prevention[b]	≥ 60 mL/min		900 mg	qd
		40–59 mL/min		450 mg	qd
		25–39 mL/min		450 mg	q48h
		10–24 mL/min		450 mg	biw
Cidofivir[c]		Normal (≥ 60)	IV	5 mg/kg	qw
Foscarnet[c]	Induction	Normal	IV	180 mg/kg	Divided q12h
		1–1.4 mL/kg/min		140 mg/kg	Divided q12h
		0.8–1 mL/kg/min		100 mg/kg	Divided q12h
		0.6–0.8 mL/kg/min		80 mg/kg	Divided q12h
		0.5–0.6 mL/kg/min		60 mg/kg	qd
		0.4–0.5 mL/kg/min		50 mg/kg	qd
		<0.4 mL/kg/min		Not available	
	Maintenance	Normal	IV	90–120 mg/kg	qd
		1–1.4 mL/kg/min		70–90 mg/kg	qd
		0.8–1 mL/kg/min		50–65 mg/kg	qd
		0.6–0.8 mL/kg/min		80–105 mg/kg	q48h
		0.5–0.6 mL/kg/min		60–80 mg/kg	q48h
		0.4–0.5 mL/kg/min		50–65 mg/kg	q48h
		<0.4 mL/kg/min			
Leflunomide[d]				100 mg qd for 3 days then 20 mg qd	

Agents are not approved by the Food and Drug Administration (FDA) for all indications.

[a] Valganciclovir dosing in practice is started at 900 mg per dose (therapy: bid; prevention: qd) although most renal transplant recipients require 450 mg qd.

[b] Not approved for use in liver transplantation.

[c] Cidofovir and Foscarnet have significant toxicities in renal impairment.

[d] Dose adjustments for leflunomide for renal and hepatic dysfunction have not been studied. This agent is not FDA approved for this indication.

Data from Refs. [90–94].

immunization, using IVIG or CMVIG, is effective in preventing CMV disease and pneumonia in renal (4%, versus 17% in controls), liver (7%, versus 18% in controls), pancreas, and heart transplant recipients [78,79]. Prophylaxis with CMVIG alone is less effective than when it is used in combination with antiviral agents, especially in lung transplant recipients [80]. In the HSCT population, IVIG is beneficial against GVHD but generally does not reduce the incidence of CMV infection or disease [80–82].

In the HSCT population, acyclovir, famciclovir, and valacyclovir delay reactivation of virus and reduce CMV infection, disease, and mortality [83]. Prophylaxis generally is given during the first 100 days after transplantation. Valacyclovir results in fewer episodes of CMV infection than acyclovir, possibly because of the improved bioavailability of the prodrug [84]. Acyclovir administered before engraftment followed by ganciclovir after engraftment significantly decreases the incidence of CMV disease and pneumonitis [85–88]. No prospective comparative studies of valganciclovir have been completed in this population. Foscarnet and cidofvir have significant toxicities that make their use in prophylaxis impractical. Thus, valacyclovir and famciclovir may be preferred for prophylaxis in HSCT recipients, given the hematopoietic toxicity of ganciclovir. In renal transplant recipients, valacyclovir administered for 90 days reduced the incidence and delayed the onset of CMV disease as well as reducing the rate of rejection during the first 6 months after transplantation [89]. A number of different prophylactic regimens, including intravenous ganciclovir for up to 90 days, induction with intravenous followed by oral ganciclovir, or oral ganciclovir alone, have been documented to be effective in preventing CMV disease in all SOT groups [90,91]. The optimal regimens for ganciclovir prophylaxis in lung transplant recipients have not been defined; current regimens are associated with a high rate of disease (42% in one series) [4,92]. Ganciclovir therapy alone or in combination with CMVIG is associated with reduction of the incidence of BOS in lung transplant recipients [58,93,94]. In a recent prospective, randomized trial of valganciclovir versus oral ganciclovir prophylaxis in high-risk (D$^+$/R$^-$) heart, liver, kidney, and kidney-pancreas recipients, valganciclovir was associated with a significantly lower frequency of viremia during the treatment phase and with delayed time-to-onset of viremia and CMV disease [95]. The overall incidence of CMV disease was equivalent at 6 and 12 months, however. Drug-induced neutropenia may be slightly more pronounced in association with valganciclovir [95,96]. Given its superior bioavailability and therapeutic equivalence, valganciclovir is generally preferred for prophylaxis in SOT recipients.

Current practice in most lung transplant centers has extended prophylaxis to a minimum of 6 months and often to 1 year after transplantation. In general, a combination of intravenous ganciclovir during hospitalization followed by oral valganciclovir (900 mg/day) is used in combination with CMVIG. Combination prophylaxis decreases the frequency of acute rejection episodes and development of BOS and reduces mortality after lung transplantation [97,98]. Combination therapy also reduces the rate of coronary allograft vasculopathy, the incidence of CMV disease, acute rejection, and mortality in cardiac transplant recipients. The role of CMVIG with anti-viral agents for prophylaxis in other SOT populations, although effective in reducing the incidence of CMV disease, is less certain. Combined prophylaxis has not been studied prospectively in the HSCT population. In addition to the proven prophylactic strategies, adoptive cellular immunotherapies using ex vivo expanded donor T cells and CMV vaccines are under study.

Therapy

In the HSCT population, ganciclovir has been used as a single agent or in combination with foscarnet or CMVIG for CMV pneumonia [99,100]. Cidofovir and foscarnet are considered second-line therapies because of toxicities. Monotherapy with IVIG or CMVIG has not demonstrated consistent benefit [101,102]. The combination of foscarnet plus ganciclovir may provide antiviral synergy but requires careful monitoring [103]. Uncontrolled series using ganciclovir with CMVIG or IGIV document a survival benefit (mortality, 0%–47%) when therapy is initiated before respiratory compromise.

Antiviral therapy is generally more effective in SOT populations than in the HSCT population. Ganciclovir has been shown to benefit renal, heart, heart-lung, and lung transplant recipients who have CMV disease and pneumonia [104–107]. There is less experience with cidofvir and foscarnet. Cidofvir is poorly tolerated in SOT because of its nephrotoxicity in combination with calcineurin inhibitors, whereas foscarnet requires careful attention to hydration and magnesium wasting. The combination of ganciclovir plus IGIV or CMVIG is associated with increased survival in SOT populations, especially in lung transplant recipients [4,97,108]. Ganciclovir is considered the first-line therapy for all SOT recipients who have CMV pneumonia, except for lung transplant recipients, for whom combination therapy may be preferred. Other immunologic modalities, such as donor lymphocyte infusion or primed cytotoxic lymphocyte infusions, are under investigation.

Resistance

Resistance to approved anti-CMV therapies has been recognized both in vitro and in vivo. Resistance may be characterized as clinical (rising viral load and persistent symptoms during therapy) or genotypic (documented mutations in viral genes). In vitro phenotypic susceptibility testing, although useful, is labor intensive and is oo slow to be used routinely in patient management. Most resistant CMV variants have been documented in immunocompromised patients who have high viral loads and prior exposure to antiviral agents. Lung transplant recipients, particularly D^+/R^- recipients, are considered to have the highest risk of developing ganciclovir-resistant CMV disease [109]. The rate of resistant CMV remains low (~5% in most centers) [110].

In most cases, resistance is attributed to a series of mutations in either the *UL97 kinase* or the *UL54 DNA polymerase* genes. *UL97* encodes a phosphotransferase that is responsible for converting ganciclovir into ganciclovir monophosphate [111]. Mutations in the *UL97* gene, usually 1 of 11 frequent gene alterations in the codon regions from 460 to 607, impair or eliminate this first step in ganciclovir activation. The second mechanism relates to mutations in the UL54 DNA polymerase. Most viruses with *UL54* mutations have concurrent *UL97* mutations [111]. The location of the *UL54* mutation determines the degree of resistance: mutations in the region of 395–540 confer resistance to ganciclovir and cidofivir; mutations in the 696–845 region confer resistance to foscarnet; mutations in the 756–809 confer resistance to ganciclovir and foscarnet; and mutations in the 978–988 region confer cross-resistance to all three antiviral agents [110,112,113].

Resistance should be suspected when the patient fails to respond clinically or with a decline in quantitative viral load within 2 weeks of therapy. Phenotypic or genotypic resistance testing can document the presence of resistant variants. Phenotypic methods assess the 50% inhibitory concentration of the drugs by plaque reduction assay; unfortunately, the test requires the growth of virus and therefore is slow (10–21 days). Genotypic assays, in which the *UL97* and *UL54* genes are sequenced or probed, can be performed rapidly but depend on detection of previously documented mutations associated with resistance. Many patients who have resistant virus have multiple viral subpopulations with differing susceptibility patterns.

Management of resistant CMV depends on knowing the mechanism of resistance. If the virus is known to have only *UL97* mutations, either foscarnet or cidofivir should have activity. Ganciclovir-resistant virus may be controlled effectively by the combination of ganciclovir and foscarnet [114,115]. The combination of approximately half-dose foscarnet (escalated to 125 mg/kg/day intravenously) and ganciclovir (2.5 mg/kg two times per day) may be considered in cases of resistant CMV pneumonia [115].

Summary

The incidence of CMV pneumonia has been reduced by routine antiviral prophylaxis in susceptible populations. Many of the complications of this infection are caused by indirect effects of the virus, including acute and chronic graft rejection, GVHD, and superinfection by other viruses, bacteria, and fungi. Distinction must be made between viral secretion and invasion. Invasive procedures are often required for the optimal management of such infections. The use of sensitive and quantitative assays has greatly improved the outcomes of CMV infection.

References

[1] Kantor GL, Johnson BLJ. Cytomegalovirus infection associated with cardiopulmonary bypass. Arch Intern Med 1970;125:488–92.

[2] Kotloff RM, Ahya VN, Crawford SW. Pulmonary complications of solid organ and hematopoietic stem cell transplantation. Am J Respir Crit Care Med 2004; 170:22–48.

[3] Duncan AJ, Dummer JS, Paradis IL, et al. Cytomegalovirus infection and survival in lung transplant recipients. J Heart Lung Transplant 1991;10: 638–44 [discussion: 645–6].

[4] Zamora MR. Cytomegalovirus and lung transplantation. Am J Transplant 2004;4:1219–26.

[5] Mocarski ES, Courcell CT. Cytomegalovirus and their replication. In: Knipe DM, Howley PM, editors. Field's virology. 4th edition. Philadephia: Lippincott, Williams, & Wilkins; 2003. p. 2629–74.

[6] Stein J, Volk HD, Liebenthal C, et al. Tumour necrosis factor alpha stimulates the activity of the human cytomegalovirus major immediate early enhancer/promoter in immature monocytic cells. J Gen Virol 1993;74(Pt 11):2333–8.

[7] Reinke P, Fietze E, Ode-Hakim S, et al. Late-acute renal allograft rejection and symptomless cytomegalovirus infection. Lancet 1994;344:1737–8.

[8] Prosch S, Wuttke R, Kruger DH, et al. NF-kappaB – a potential therapeutic target for inhibition of human cytomegalovirus (re)activation? Biol Chem 2002; 383:1601–9.

[9] Beersma MF, Bizlemaker MJ, Ploegh HL. Human cytomegalovirus down regulates HLA class I expression by reducing the stability of class I H chains. J Immunol 1993;151:4455–64.

[10] Crumpacker CS. Cytomegalovirus. In: Mandell GL, Bennett JE, Dolin R, editors. Principles and practices of infectious diseases. 5th edition. Philadelphia: Churchill Livingstone; 2000. p. 1586–98.

[11] de Maar EF, Verschuuren EA, Harmsen MC. Pulmonary involvement during cytomegalovirus infection

in immunosuppressed patients. Transpl Infect Dis 2003;5:112–20.

[12] Kas-Deelen AM, de Maar EF, Harmsen MC, et al. Uninfected and cytomegalic endothelial cells in blood during cytomegalovirus infection: effect of acute rejection. J Infect Dis 2000;181:721–4.

[13] Koskinen PK. The association of the induction of vascular cell adhesion molecule-1 with cytomegalovirus antigenemia in human heart allografts. Transplantation 1993;56:1103–8.

[14] Waldman WJ, Knight DA. Cytokine-mediated induction of endothelial adhesion molecule and histocompatibility leukocyte antigen expression by cytomegalovirus-activated T cells. Am J Pathol 1996;148:105–19.

[15] Sedmak DD, Guglielmo AM, Knight DA, et al. Cytomegalovirus inhibits major histocompatibility class II expression on infected endothelial cells. Am J Pathol 1994;144:683–92.

[16] Persoons MC, Stals FS, van dam Mieras MC, et al. Multiple organ involvement during experimental infection is associated with disseminated vascular pathology. J Pathol 1998;184:103–9.

[17] Span AH, van dam Mieras MC, Mullers W, et al. The effect of virus infection on the adherence of leukocytes or platelets to endothelial cells. Eur J Clin Invest 1991;21:331–8.

[18] van Son WJ, Tegzess AM, Hauw The T, et al. Pulmonary dysfunction is common during a cytomegalovirus infection after renal transplantation even in asymptomatic patients. Possible relationship with complement activation. Am Rev Respir Dis 1987; 136:580–5.

[19] Quinnan Jr GV, Kirmani N, Rook AH, et al. Cytotoxic T cells in cytomegalovirus infection: HLA-restricted T-lymphocyte and non-T-lymphocyte cytotoxic responses correlate with recovery from cytomegalovirus infection in bone-marrow-transplant recipients. N Engl J Med 1982;307:7–13.

[20] Reusser P, Riddell SR, Meyers JD, et al. Cytotoxic T-lymphocyte response to cytomegalovirus after human allogeneic bone marrow transplantation: pattern of recovery and correlation with cytomegalovirus infection and disease. Blood 1991;78:1373–80.

[21] Li CR, Greenberg PD, Gilbert MJ, et al. Recovery of HLA-restricted cytomegalovirus (CMV)-specific T-cell responses after allogeneic bone marrow transplant: correlation with CMV disease and effect of ganciclovir prophylaxis. Blood 1994;83:1971–9.

[22] Meyers JD, Flournoy N, Thomas ED. Cytomegalovirus infection and specific cell-mediated immunity after marrow transplant. J Infect Dis 1986;153:478–88.

[23] Ljungman P, Griffiths P, Paya C. Definitions of cytomegalovirus infection and disease in transplant recipients. Clin Infect Dis 2002;34:1094–7.

[24] Leung AN, Gosselin MV, Napper CH, et al. Pulmonary infections after bone marrow transplantation: clinical and radiographic findings. Radiology 1999;210:699–710.

[25] Ljungman P. Cytomegalovirus pneumonia: presentation, diagnosis, and treatment. Semin Respir Infect 1995;10:209–15.

[26] Franquet T, Lee KS, Muller NL. Thin-section CT findings in 32 immunocompromised patients with cytomegalovirus pneumonia who do not have AIDS. AJR Am J Roentgenol 2003;181:1059–63.

[27] Tamm M, Traenkle P, Grilli B, et al. Pulmonary cytomegalovirus infection in immunocompromised patients. Chest 2001;119:838–43.

[28] Griffiths PD, Emery VC. Cytomegalovirus. In: Richman DD, Whitley RJ, Hayden FG, editors. Clinical virology. 2nd edition. Washington (DC): American Society of Microbiology Press; 2002.

[29] The TH, Andersen HK, Spencer ES, et al. Antibodies against cytomegalovirus-induced early antigens (CMV-EA) in immunosuppressed renal-allograft recipients. Clin Exp Immunol 1977;28:502–5.

[30] The TH, Grefte JM, van der Bij W, et al. CMV infection after organ transplantation: immunopathological and clinical aspects. Neth J Med 1994;45:309–18.

[31] Baldanti F, Revello MG, Percivalle E, et al. Use of the human cytomegalovirus (HCMV) antigenemia assay for diagnosis and monitoring of HCMV infections and detection of antiviral drug resistance in the immunocompromised. J Clin Virol 1998;11:51–60.

[32] Egan JJ, Barber L, Lomax J, et al. Detection of human cytomegalovirus antigenaemia: a rapid diagnostic technique for predicting cytomegalovirus infection/pneumonitis in lung and heart transplant recipients [see comments]. Thorax 1995;50:9–13.

[33] Michaelides A, Liolios L, Glare EM, et al. Increased human cytomegalovirus (HCMV) DNA load in peripheral blood leukocytes after lung transplantation correlates with HCMV pneumonitis. Transplantation 2001;72:141–7.

[34] Guiver M, Fox AJ, Mutton K, et al. Evaluation of CMV viral load using TaqMan CMV quantitative PCR and comparison with CMV antigenemia in heart and lung transplant recipients. Transplantation 2001;71:1609–15.

[35] Caliendo AM, Schuurman R, Yen-Lieberman B, et al. Comparison of quantitative and qualitative PCR assays for cytomegalovirus DNA in plasma. J Clin Microbiol 2001;39:1334–8.

[36] Caliendo AM, Yen-Lieberman B, Baptista J, et al. Comparison of molecular tests for detection and quantification of cell-associated cytomegalovirus DNA. J Clin Microbiol 2003;41:3509–13.

[37] Middeldorf J, Sillekens P, Lunenberg J. Diagnosis of active HCMV infection: the mRNA approach. Organ and Tissues 2000;2:99–107.

[38] Seehofer D, Meisel H, Rayes N, et al. Prospective evaluation of the clinical utility of different methods for the detection of human cytomegalovirus disease after liver transplantation. Am J Transplant 2004; 4:1331–7.

[39] Weill D, Zamora MR. Comparison of the efficacy and cost-effectiveness of pre-emptive therapy as directed

by CMV antigenemia and prophylaxis with ganciclovir in lung transplant recipients. J Heart Lung Transplant 2000;19:815–6.

[40] Kelly J, Hurley D, Raghu G. Comparison of the efficacy and cost effectiveness of pre-emptive therapy as directed by CMV antigenemia and prophylaxis with ganciclovir in lung transplant recipients. J Heart Lung Transplant 2000;19:355–9.

[41] Sanchez JL, Kruger RM, Paranjothi S, et al. Relationship of cytomegalovirus viral load in blood to pneumonitis in lung transplant recipients. Transplantation 2001;72:733–5.

[42] Westall GP, Michaelides A, Williams TJ, et al. Human cytomegalovirus load in plasma and bronchoalveolar lavage fluid: a longitudinal study of lung transplant recipients. J Infect Dis 2004;190:1076–83.

[43] Taplitz RA, Jordan MC. Pneumonia caused by herpesviruses in recipients of hematopoietic cell transplants. Semin Respir Infect 2002;17:121–9.

[44] Boeckh M, Leisenring W, Riddell SR, et al. Late cytomegalovirus disease and mortality in recipients of allogeneic hematopoietic stem cell transplants: importance of viral load and T-cell immunity. Blood 2003;101:407–14.

[45] Enright H, Haake R, Weisdorf D, et al. Cytomegalovirus pneumonia after bone marrow transplantation. Risk factors and response to therapy. Transplantation 1993;55:1339–46.

[46] Nagler A, Elishoov H, Kapelushnik Y, et al. Cytomegalovirus pneumonia prior to engraftment following T-cell depleted bone marrow transplantation. Med Oncol 1994;11:127–32.

[47] Grob JP, Grundy JE, Prentice HG, et al. Immune donors can protect marrow-transplant recipients from severe cytomegalovirus infections. Lancet 1987;1:774–6.

[48] Olding LB, Jensen FC, Oldstone MB. Pathogenesis of of cytomegalovirus infection. I. Activation of virus from bone marrow-derived lymphocytes by in vitro allogenic reaction. J Exp Med 1975;141:561–72.

[49] Reusser P. Cytomegalovirus infection and disease after bone marrow transplantation: epidemiology, prevention, and treatment. Bone Marrow Transplant 1991;7(Suppl 3):52–6.

[50] Gentile G, Donati PP, Capobianchi A, et al. Evaluation of a score system for the severity and outcome of cytomegalovirus interstitial pneumonia in allogeneic bone marrow recipients. J Infect 1997;35:117–23.

[51] Wingard JR, Chen DY, Burns WH, et al. Cytomegalovirus infection after autologous bone marrow transplantation with comparison to infection after allogeneic bone marrow transplantation. Blood 1988;71:1432–7.

[52] Reusser P, Fisher LD, Buckner CD, et al. Cytomegalovirus infection after autologous bone marrow transplantation: occurrence of cytomegalovirus disease and effect on engraftment. Blood 1990;75:1888–94.

[53] Konoplev S, Champlin RE, Giralt S, et al. Cytomegalovirus pneumonia in adult autologous blood and marrow transplant recipients. Bone Marrow Transplant 2001;27:877–81.

[54] Holmberg LA, Boeckh M, Hooper H, et al. Increased incidence of cytomegalovirus disease after autologous CD34-selected peripheral blood stem cell transplantation. Blood 1999;94:4029–35.

[55] Bailey TC, Trulock EP, Ettinger NA, et al. Failure of prophylactic ganciclovir to prevent cytomegalovirus disease in recipients of lung transplants. J Infect Dis 1992;165:548–52.

[56] Duncan SR, Paradis IL, Dauber JH, et al. Ganciclovir prophylaxis for cytomegalovirus infections in pulmonary allograft recipients. Am Rev Respir Dis 1992;146:1213–5.

[57] Ettinger NA, Bailey TC, Trulock EP, et al. Cytomegalovirus infection and pneumonitis. Impact after isolated lung transplantation. Washington University Lung Transplant Group. Am Rev Respir Dis 1993;147:1017–23.

[58] Soghikian MV, Valentine VG, Berry GJ, et al. Impact of ganciclovir prophylaxis on heart-lung and lung transplant recipients. J Heart Lung Transplant 1996;15:881–7.

[59] Trulock EP, Ettinger NA, Brunt EM, et al. The role of transbronchial lung biopsy in the treatment of lung transplant recipients. An analysis of 200 consecutive procedures. Chest 1992;102:1049–54.

[60] Cerrina J, Le Roy Ladurie F, et al. Role of CMV pneumonia in the development of obliterative bronchiolitis in heart-lung and double-lung transplant recipients. Transpl Int 1992;5(Suppl 1):S242–5.

[61] Sharples LD, McNeil K, Stewart S, et al. Risk factors for bronchiolitis obliterans: a systematic review of recent publications. J Heart Lung Transplant 2002;21:271–81.

[62] Paradis IL, Williams P. Infection after lung transplantation. Semin Respir Infect 1993;8:207–15.

[63] Dummer JS, Montero CG, Griffith BP, et al. Infections in heart-lung transplant recipients. Transplantation 1986;41:725–9.

[64] Smyth RL, Scott JP, Borysiewicz LK, et al. Cytomegalovirus infection in heart-lung transplant recipients: risk factors, clinical associations, and response to treatment. J Infect Dis 1991;164:1045–50.

[65] Fend F, Prior C, Margreiter R, et al. Cytomegalovirus pneumonitis in heart-lung transplant recipients: histopathology and clinicopathologic considerations. Hum Pathol 1990;21:918–26.

[66] Heurlin N, Brattstrom C, Tyden G, et al. Cytomegalovirus the predominant cause of pneumonia in renal transplant patients. A two-year study of pneumonia in renal transplant recipients with evaluation of fiberoptic bronchoscopy. Scand J Infect Dis 1989;21:245–53.

[67] Reichenberger F, Dickenmann M, Binet I, et al. Diagnostic yield of bronchoalveolar lavage following renal transplantation. Transpl Infect Dis 2001;3:2–7.

[68] Gane E, Saliba F, Valdecasas GJ, et al. Randomized trial of efficacy and safety of oral ganciclovir in the prevention of cytomegalovirus disease in liver-transplant recipients. Lancet 1997;350:1729–33.

[69] Falagas ME, Snydman DR, George MJ, et al. Incidence and predictors of cytomegalovirus pneumonia in orthotopic liver transplant recipients. Boston Center for Liver Transplantation CMVIG Study Group. Transplantation 1996;61:1716–20.

[70] Pescovitz MD, Rabkin J, Merion RM, et al. Valganciclovir results in improved oral absorption of ganciclovir in liver transplant recipients. Antimicrob Agents Chemother 2000;44:2811–5.

[71] John GT, Manivannan J, Chandy S, et al. Leflunomide therapy for cytomegalovirus disease in renal allograft recipients. Transplantation 2004;77:1460–1.

[72] Waldman WJ, Knight DA, Blinder L, et al. Inhibition of cytomegalovirus in vitro and in vivo by the experimental immunosuppressive agent leflunomide. Intervirology 1999;42:412–8.

[73] Waldman WJ, Knight DA, Lurain NS, et al. Novel mechanism of inhibition of cytomegalovirus by the experimental immunosuppressive agent leflunomide. Transplantation 1999;68:814–25.

[74] Avery RK, Bolwell BJ, Yen-Lieberman B, et al. Use of leflunomide in an allogeneic bone marrow transplant recipient with refractory cytomegalovirus infection. Bone Marrow Transplant 2004;34:1071–5.

[75] Bowden RA. Transfusion-transmitted cytomegalovirus infection. Hematol Oncol Clin North Am 1995;9:155–66.

[76] Bowden RA, Slichter SJ, Sayers M, et al. A comparison of filtered leukocyte-reduced and cytomegalovirus (CMV) seronegative blood products for the prevention of transfusion-associated CMV infection after marrow transplant. Blood 1995;86:3598–603.

[77] Nichols WG, Price TH, Gooley T, et al. Transfusion-transmitted cytomegalovirus infection after receipt of leukoreduced blood products. Blood 2003;101:4195–200.

[78] Snydman DR, Werner BG, Dougherty NN, et al. Cytomegalovirus immune globulin prophylaxis in liver transplantation. A randomized, double-blind, placebo-controlled trial. The Boston Center for Liver Transplantation CMVIG Study Group. Ann Intern Med 1993;119:984–91.

[79] Snydman DR, Werner BG, Heinze-Lacey B, et al. Use of cytomegalovirus immune globulin to prevent cytomegalovirus disease in renal-transplant recipients. N Engl J Med 1987;317:1049–54.

[80] Kruger RM, Paranjothi S, Storch GA, et al. Impact of prophylaxis with cytogam alone on the incidence of CMV viremia in CMV-seropositive lung transplant recipients. J Heart Lung Transplant 2003;22:754–63.

[81] Messori A, Rampazzo R, Scroccaro G, et al. Efficacy of hyperimmune anti-cytomegalovirus immunoglobulins for the prevention of cytomegalovirus infection in recipients of allogeneic bone marrow transplantation: a meta-analysis. Bone Marrow Transplant 1994;13:163–7.

[82] Maurer JR, Tullis DE, Scavuzzo M, et al. Cytomegalovirus infection in isolated lung transplantations. J Heart Lung Transplant 1991;10:647–9.

[83] Zaia JA. Prevention and treatment of cytomegalovirus pneumonia in transplant recipients. Clin Infect Dis 1993;17(Suppl 2):S392–9.

[84] Ljungman P, de La Camara R, Milpied N, et al. Randomized study of valacyclovir as prophylaxis against cytomegalovirus reactivation in recipients of allogeneic bone marrow transplants. Blood 2002;99:3050–6.

[85] Schmidt GM, Horak DA, Niland JC, et al. A randomized, controlled trial of prophylactic ganciclovir for cytomegalovirus pulmonary infection in recipients of allogeneic bone marrow transplants; The City of Hope-Stanford-Syntex CMV Study Group [see comments]. N Engl J Med 1991;324:1005–11.

[86] Winston DJ, Ho WG, Bartoni K, et al. Ganciclovir prophylaxis of cytomegalovirus infection and disease in allogeneic bone marrow transplant recipients. Results of a placebo-controlled, double-blind trial. Ann Intern Med 1993;118:179–84.

[87] Goodrich JM, Bowden RA, Fisher L, et al. Ganciclovir prophylaxis to prevent cytomegalovirus disease after allogeneic marrow transplant. Ann Intern Med 1993;118:173–8.

[88] Atkinson K, Nivison-Smith I, Dodds A, et al. A comparison of the pattern of interstitial pneumonitis following allogeneic bone marrow transplantation before and after the introduction of prophylactic ganciclovir therapy in 1989. Bone Marrow Transplant 1998;21:691–5.

[89] Lowance D, Neumayer HH, Legendre CM, et al. Valacyclovir for the prevention of cytomegalovirus disease after renal transplantation. International Valacyclovir Cytomegalovirus Prophylaxis Transplantation Study Group [see comments]. N Engl J Med 1999;340:1462–70.

[90] Singh N. Preemptive therapy versus universal prophylaxis with ganciclovir for cytomegalovirus in solid organ transplant recipients. Clin Infect Dis 2001;32:742–51.

[91] Couchoud C, Cucherat M, Haugh M, et al. Cytomegalovirus prophylaxis with antiviral agents in solid organ transplantation: a meta-analysis. Transplantation 1998;65:641–7.

[92] Duncan SR, Grgurich WF, Iacono AT, et al. A comparison of ganciclovir and acyclovir to prevent cytomegalovirus after lung transplantation. Am J Respir Crit Care Med 1994;150:146–52.

[93] Duncan SR, Paradis IL, Yousem SA, et al. Sequelae of cytomegalovirus pulmonary infections in lung allograft recipients. Am Rev Respir Dis 1992;146:1419–25.

[94] Speich R, Thurnheer R, Gaspert A, et al. Efficacy and cost effectiveness of oral ganciclovir in the

prevention of cytomegalovirus disease after lung transplantation. Transplantation 1999;67:315–20.

[95] Paya C, Humar A, Dominguez E, et al. Efficacy and safety of valganciclovir vs. oral ganciclovir for prevention of cytomegalovirus disease in solid organ transplant recipients. Am J Transplant 2004; 4:611–20.

[96] Boivin G, Goyette N, Gilbert C, et al. Absence of cytomegalovirus-resistance mutations after valganciclovir prophylaxis, in a prospective multicenter study of solid-organ transplant recipients. J Infect Dis 2004;189:1615–8.

[97] Valantine HA, Luikart H, Doyle R, et al. Impact of cytomegalovirus hyperimmune globulin on outcome after cardiothoracic transplantation: a comparative study of combined prophylaxis with CMV hyperimmune globulin plus ganciclovir versus ganciclovir alone. Transplantation 2001;72:1647–52.

[98] Zamora MR. Controversies in lung transplantation: management of cytomegalovirus infections. J Heart Lung Transplant 2002;21(8):841–9.

[99] Crumpacker CS. Ganciclovir. N Engl J Med 1996; 335:721–9.

[100] Shepp DH, Dandliker PS, de Miranda P, et al. Activity of 9-[2-hydroxy-1-(hydroxymethyl)ethoxymethyl] guanine in the treatment of cytomegalovirus pneumonia. Ann Intern Med 1985;103:368–73.

[101] Blacklock HA, Griffiths P, Stirk P, et al. Specific hyperimmune globulin for cytomegalovirus pneumonitis. Lancet 1985;2:152–3.

[102] Reed EC, Bowden RA, Dandliker PS, et al. Efficacy of cytomegalovirus immunoglobulin in marrow transplant recipients with cytomegalovirus pneumonia. J Infect Dis 1987;156:641–5.

[103] Bacigalupo A, Bregante S, Tedone E, et al. Combined foscarnet-ganciclovir treatment for cytomegalovirus infections after allogeneic hemopoietic stem cell transplantation (HSCT). Bone Marrow Transplant 1996;18(Suppl 2):110–4.

[104] Watson FS, O'Connell JB, Amber IJ, et al. Treatment of cytomegalovirus pneumonia in heart transplant recipients with 9(1,3-dihydroxy-2-proproxymethyl)-guanine (DHPG). J Heart Transplant 1988;7:102–5.

[105] Cerrina J, Bavoux E, Le Roy Ladurie F, et al. Ganciclovir treatment of cytomegalovirus infection in heart-lung and double-lung transplant recipients. Transplant Proc 1991;23:1174–5.

[106] Steinhoff G, Behrend M, Wagner TO, et al. Early diagnosis and effective treatment of pulmonary CMV infection after lung transplantation. J Heart Lung Transplant 1991;10:9–14.

[107] Hecht DW, Snydman DR, Crumpacker CS, et al. Ganciclovir for treatment of renal transplant-associated primary cytomegalovirus pneumonia. J Infect Dis 1988;157:187–90.

[108] Snydman DR. Historical overview of the use of cytomegalovirus hyperimmune globulin in organ transplantation. Transpl Infect Dis 2001;3(Suppl 2):6–13.

[109] Limaye AP, Raghu G, Koelle DM, et al. High incidence of ganciclovir-resistant cytomegalovirus infection among lung transplant recipients receiving preemptive therapy. J Infect Dis 2002;185:20–7.

[110] Chou SW. Cytomegalovirus drug resistance and clinical implications. Transpl Infect Dis 2001;3(Suppl 2): 20–4.

[111] Drew WL, Paya CV, Emery V. Cytomegalovirus (CMV) resistance to antivirals. Am J Transplant 2001;1:307–12.

[112] Chou S, Marousek G, Parenti DM, et al. Mutation in region III of the DNA polymerase gene conferring foscarnet resistance in cytomegalovirus isolates from 3 subjects receiving prolonged antiviral therapy. J Infect Dis 1998;178:526–30.

[113] Chou S, Miner RC, Drew WL. A deletion mutation in region V of the cytomegalovirus DNA polymerase sequence confers multidrug resistance. J Infect Dis 2000;182:1765–8.

[114] Manion DJ, Vibhagool A, Chou TC, et al. Susceptibility of human cytomegalovirus to two-drug combinations in vitro. Antivir Ther 1996;1:237–45.

[115] Mylonakis E, Kallas WM, Fishman JA. Combination antiviral therapy for ganciclovir-resistant cytomegalovirus infection in solid-organ transplant recipients. Clin Infect Dis 2002;34:1337–41.

[116] Weiss RL, Snow GW, Schumann GB, et al. Diagnosis of cytomegalovirus pneumonitis on bronchoalveolar lavage fluid. Comparison of cytology, immunofluorescence, and in situ hybridization with viral isolation. Diagn Cytopathol 1991;7:243–7.

[117] Bewig B, Haacke TC, Tiroke A, et al. Detection of CMV pneumonitis after lung transplantation using PCR of DNA from bronchoalveolar lavage cells. Respiration (Herrlisheim) 2000;67:166–72.

[118] Sakamaki H, Yuasa K, Goto H, et al. Comparison of cytomegalovirus (CMV) antigenemia and CMV in bronchoalveolar lavage fluid for diagnosis of CMV pulmonary infection after bone marrow transplantation. Bone Marrow Transplant 1997;20:143–7.

Clin Chest Med 26 (2005) 707 – 720

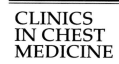

Viral Pneumonias Other Than Cytomegalovirus in Transplant Recipients

Todd D. Barton, MD[a,b],*, Emily A. Blumberg, MD[a]

[a]Division of Infectious Diseases, Hospital of the University of Pennsylvania, Silverstein Building Suite E,
34th and Spruce Streets, Philadelphia, PA 19104, USA
[b]Internal Medicine Residency Program, Hospital of the University of Pennsylvania, 34th and Spruce Streets,
Philadelphia, PA 19104, USA

Community-acquired respiratory viruses (CARVs) are frequent causes of upper respiratory infection (URI) in adult and pediatric populations, usually occurring in seasonal outbreaks. In healthy outpatients, the morbidity caused by these infections is minimal, because progression to lower respiratory tract infection (LRTI) is rare, and most infections are self-limited in duration.

Although case reports of viral pneumonia complicating hematopoietic stem cell transplantation (HSCT) or solid organ transplantation (SOT) have been described for decades, it is only in recent years that larger case series and therapeutic trials have been conducted and reported, providing greater insight into the impact of CARV on these immunosuppressed hosts. After some general observations about CARV infections, this article focuses on this important recent literature and specifically on the four most common pathogens, respiratory syncytial virus (RSV), influenza virus, parainfluenza virus (PIV), and adenovirus. It concludes by briefly touching on several less commonly reported causes of viral pneumonia, including some potentially important emerging pathogens.

General observations

Epidemiology

Although dozens of published studies have described the epidemiology of some or all of the CARVs, their findings are often widely disparate. This differences in part result from the nature of the diseases, because both their seasonality and relative frequencies may vary depending on the climate of the reporting institutions. Similarly, studies that track only a single year's incidence of the CARVs may over- or underestimate the general relative frequency of the pathogens based on a particularly widespread epidemic of a single viral pathogen, as might be seen in a year with an especially widespread influenza epidemic. Table 1 reviews the relative frequencies of the CARVs in several recent reports. Depending on the center and the year, RSV, PIV, or influenza has been the most common pathogen, whereas adenovirus generally accounts for fewer than 10% of CARV infections [1–8]. Finally, studies that include children may report higher rates of CARV infections than those focusing on adult populations, probably reflecting in part the higher carriage of CARVs in children.

Most commonly, investigators have employed two major strategies to gain an understanding of the general epidemiology of respiratory virus infections. In the first, consecutive tranplant recipients have been screened at regular intervals, usually in the first 6 to 18 months after transplantation, regardless of symptomatology. Results of such studies have shown overall incidence rates of CARV infection in HSCT

---

* Corresponding author. Division of Infectious Diseases, Hospital of the University of Pennsylvania, 3rd Floor, Silverstein Building Suite E, 34th and Spruce Streets, Philadelphia, PA 19104.

E-mail address: todd.barton@uphs.upenn.edu
(T.D. Barton).

Table 1
Frequency of respiratory viruses in recent published case series

Reference	No. of patients	No. of culture-positive episodes	RSV[a] (%)	PIV[a] (%)	Flu[a] (%)	Adeno[a] (%)	Other[a] (%)
Ljungman [1]	545 HSCT	39	21	21	38	21	0
Raboni [2]	722 HSCT	62	48	11	37	3	0
Hassan [3]	626 HSCT	29	27	13	17	0	37 Rhino
							7 Entero
Machado [4]	179 HSCT	68	33	15	52	0	0
Chakrabarti [5]	89 HSCT	25	37	49	14	0	0
Roghmann [7]	62 HSCT	22	46	21	21	0	13
Lujan-Zilbermann [6]	281 HSCT	32	14	47	17	19	0
Khalifah [8]	259 lung transplant	21	38	33	19	10	0

Abbreviations: Adeno, adenovirus; Entero, enterovirus; Flu, influenza virus; HSCT, hematologic stem cell transplant; PIV, parainfluenza virus; Rhino, rhinovirus; RSV, respiratory syncytial virus.

[a] Percentages are percent of all isolates; may not add to 100 because of rounding.

recipients ranging from 11% to 65% [5–7,9]. In contrast, a recent prospective surveillance study in SOT recipients showed only a 4% incidence of CARV in adult liver transplant recipients during the first 12 weeks after transplantation, although interpretation of this study is limited by the investigators' use of throat swabs alone to detect CARV infection [10]. More frequently published are large retrospective case series of CARV infections. Because these series do not include patients who had asymptomatic infection, overall reported rates of CARV infection are predictably lower, ranging from 4% to 27% in HSCT recipients [1–3,11] to 8% to 21% in lung transplant recipients [8,12,13]. Although these larger reported series represent the best estimates of the CARV disease burden in the general transplant population, it is important to remember that the reports are biased by the seasonal occurrence of CARV in both nosocomial and community settings and the potentially devastating impact of these infections on HSCT and SOT patients [14].

Diagnosis

A major limiting factor in the understanding of CARV infection has been the limited sensitivity of what currently are the most widely used diagnostic tests. In three patient series involving more than 1500 episodes of symptomatic URI in HSCT recipients [2,4,11], fewer than half the patients had a virus isolated from clinical specimens. Most studies (and clinical centers) use a combination of direct (DFA) or indirect (IFA) fluorescent antibody testing and viral culture. Results of fluorescent antibody testing are typically available in about 24 hours, but viral culture may not be positive for 7 to 14 days. In

children, these tests are often performed on samples from nasopharyngeal lavage. In adults, swabs from the nasopharynx or throat often are substituted. Whereas the DFA or IFA tests may have a sensitivity of up to 90% for CARV infection in immunocompetent hosts, two studies comparing IFA and viral culture in HSCT recipients have shown a composite IFA sensitivity of 52% [2–4,11,15]. Palmer and colleagues [16] reported a DFA sensitivity of 20% in their series of lung tranplant recipients who had CARV infections. Both fluorescent antibody testing and viral culture probably have higher yields when the sample is obtained from the lower respiratory tract. In one recent study, two thirds of CARV diagnoses were made from bronchoalveolar lavage (BAL) samples [17]. Recently, two series have used real-time polymerase chain reaction (PCR) assays to test for CARV infections in HSCT recipients [9,15]. In one series of 72 adult HSCT recipients being monitored with routine nasal and throat swabs over a 6-month period, real-time PCR was positive in 33 patients, whereas viral culture was positive in only 11 [9]. Many of the additional positive tests were asymptomatic patients who had rhinovirus infection. Bredius and colleagues [15] tested 39 children with symptomatic respiratory tract infection; IFA was positive in 5; viral culture was positive in 10; and real-time PCR was positive in 13.

Viruses, perhaps especially PIV, are often copathogens with other bacterial or fungal infections [18,19]. Infection with both a CARV and cytomegalovirus, *Aspergillus* species, or *Pneumocystis jiroveci* have been described in up to 53% of CARV pneumonias [18,19]. Conversely, because providers may halt a diagnostic work-up after isolation of a single bacterial or fungal pathogen, it is not known how often infection with these more traditionally opportunistic pathogens is complicated by coinfection with a CARV.

Outcomes

The overall reported mortality from CARV infection has varied widely in published series. Probably no mortality is associated directly with CARV infection limited to the upper respiratory tract. In older case series of predominantly hospitalized HSCT or SOT recipients who had LRTI, mortality was frequently greater than 50% [1]. It can be difficult to compare some series based on varying definitions of LRTI: in some series, a positive chest radiograph is required to define LRTI or pneumonia, whereas in others series physical examination findings (eg, rales, hypoxia) consistent with lower tract disease have sufficed.

Most recent series in HSCT recipients have included more outpatients who have URI and have shown much lower mortality, ranging from 2% to 18% [4,6,11,20]. Raboni and colleagues [2] in Brazil reported 37% mortality from CARV infection in a cohort of patients. Many of these patients had received allogeneic bone marrow transplants within the previous year. Fewer case series exist in SOT recipients. Palmer and colleagues [16] reported 20% mortality in their series of CARV in lung transplant recipients , but case series in renal and liver transplant recipients showed no mortality from the infection [10,17].

Of particular recent interest has been the possible link between CARV infection and the development of chronic rejection in lung transplant recipients. This link is supported by a mouse model in which PIV infection aggravated chronic rejection of lung allografts [13]. Epidemiologically, the possibility that CARV infection contributes to chronic lung transplant rejection manifesting as bronchiolitis obliterans syndrome (BOS) has been supported by the observation that BOS may have a seasonal pattern of onset [17]. This observation has not been true in all studies, however [13]. Although BOS occurs in up to 60% to 80% of lung transplant recipients after 5 years [21], the overall incidence rates for each of the four most commonly reported CARVs generally have not exceeded 5% in lung transplant cohorts [8,13, 21–23]. As noted previously, this percentage may reflect a limitation in current diagnostics rather than a lower incidence of these infections.

CARV infection may produce wheezing and bronchospasm in immunocompetent adults, so it is not surprising that case series of CARV infections in lung transplant recipients report a decline in perfor-

mance on pulmonary function tests during the acute illness [22,24]. In two reports that have followed serial pulmonary function tests for several months after CARV infection, there have been no significant changes in the pulmonary function testing after a few months' follow-up [24,25], although one investigator reported impairment of pulmonary function persisting beyond 90 days in 21% of patients [25]. Three reports demonstrated marked variability in rates of acute rejection at the time of CARV infection. Vilchez and colleagues [23] reported allograft rejection in 18 (82%) of 22 patients who had PIV infection, whereas two other series reported acute rejection in 0 (0%) of 11 and 1 (7%) of 14 patients, respectively, at the time of CARV infection [24,25]. Further study is needed to clarify this important disparity.

Two larger series specifically designed to investigate the link between any CARV infection and BOS bear closer analysis. Khalifah and colleagues [8] followed 259 adult lung transplant recipients prospectively and identified 21 CARV infections. Nearly all were lower respiratory infections found on bronchoscopy performed either for surveillance or in response to a new clinical syndrome. Patients who had any history of CARV infection in this cohort were more likely to develop severe BOS (38% versus 14%), to die from BOS (29% versus 9%), or to die from any cause (43% versus 23%) than were patients who had no history of CARV infection [8]. Additionally, the authors note that of eight patients who had RSV infection, three who were treated with antiviral agents did not develop BOS, whereas four of five patients not treated with antiviral agents did develop BOX. Billings and colleagues [13] followed 219 adult lung transplant recipients and found 40 CARV infections in 33 patients over an 11-year follow-up period. Again, the majority of identified CARV infections in this series were LRTI, and many were identified from bronchoscopy specimens when bronchoscopy was performed for surveillance or follow-up of treatment for rejection. In this series, CARV LRTI was found to be predictive of severe (grade 3) BOS, but not of moderate (grade 2) BOS. The authors noted that BOS was clearly a risk factor for CARV [13]. It is possible that the chronic rejection facilitates colonization, infection, or progression to LRTI by CARVs. It is also probable; however, that patients who have BOS undergo more frequent bronchoscopy, making it more likely that CARV infection will be identified. Taken together, the reports from Khalifah [8] and Billings [13] strongly suggest an association between CARV infection and BOS. The significance and directionality of this association remain to be determined.

Respiratory syncytial virus

Epidemiology

RSV occurs annually in late autumn or winter outbreaks in the general population, with a low level of persistent year-round activity. These same seasonal patterns have been found in HSCT recipients [26,27]. Like most CARVs, RSV affects children more than adults, and this observation has been confirmed in single-center analyses where adult and pediatric HSCT programs coexist [28]. The epidemic nature of RSV infections must be stressed, because these outbreaks have been responsible for significant morbidity and mortality [14]. Several important factors may contribute to RSV outbreaks among HSCT or SOT recipients. On inpatient units, HSCT or SOT recipients tend to be housed on dedicated wards, thus exposing them to each other and also to a common group of hospital staff and care providers. In fall or winter seasons, 15% to 20% of these providers may shed RSV asymptomatically, and that number may increase to 50% during community outbreaks [29]. Additionally, HSCT or SOT recipients are more likely than immunocompetent patients to have prolonged shedding of RSV, thus introducing the potential for a single index case to infect many other patients [10,29,30]. Together, these factors may explain why multiple reported series of RSV infection note that more than 50% of cases were nosocomially acquired [27,30,31].

Among HSCT and SOT recipients, RSV is the most commonly reported CARV in most series (see Table 1). Large series of RSV infection have been reported in recipients of allogeneic HSCT [28, 32–34], autologous HSCT [28,31], liver transplants [12], and lung transplants [12,21], in addition to case reports or small series from nearly all other transplant types. It is difficult, however, to compare the incidences reported in these trials directly, because study designs include longitudinal studies, single-year surveys, and prospective surveillance data. McCarthy and colleagues [32] reported a cumulative RSV incidence of 6.3% in allogeneic HSCT recipients over a 5-year period. Small and colleagues [28] reviewed consecutive HSCT recipients over a 6-year period and demonstrated an incidence of 8.8% in allogeneic HSCT recipients as compared with 1.5% in autologous HSCT recipients. Other reports have confirmed this higher rate in allogeneic HSCT recipients, including a multicenter European study that showed a single-year incidence of symptomatic RSV of 3.5% in recipients of allogeneic HSCT and of 0.4% in autologous HSCT recipients [34]. Longitudinal stud-

ies of pediatric liver transplant recipients and adult lung transplant recipients showed incidence rates similar to the longitudinal studies, at 3.4% and 5% to 10%, respectively [12,21].

Clinical features and diagnosis

RSV infection begins in the upper respiratory tract, with cough present in 87% to 100% of immunocompromised patients [35]. Most patients also report rhinorrhea or sinus congestion, and nearly half report subjective wheezing [35]. Although fever may be present in most immunocompromised patients, the prevalence of fever in HSCT and SOT recipients has not been well clarified; in one series, only 35% of patients who had RSV LRTI were febrile [25].

Morbidity and mortality from RSV are directly attributable to progression of the infection to pneumonia. Although bacterial infection may occur coincidentally with other CARV infections, it is not seen frequently with RSV in HSCT or SOT recipients [36]. Many recent series have documented that about 50% of patients who have RSV infection develop pneumonia; some present with pneumonia, and others develop pneumonia after initial presentation with URI (Table 2). Nearly all patients who present with pneumonia give a history of several days of antecedent URI symptoms. Once the infection progresses to pneumonia, mortality rates are high. The results of several recent reports are presented in Table 2 and show that 66 (41%) of 161 HSCT recipients who had RSV pneumonia died [1,4–6,11,27,28,32,34,37,38].

Diagnosis of RSV infection at most centers is done primarily by fluorescent antibody testing because of the wide availability of the tests (IFA or DFA) and the rapid turnaround time. In immunocompetent hosts, DFA or IFA for RSV may be up to 90% sensitive, whereas culture is only 33% to 67% sensitive [35]. Englund and colleagues [39], however, reported concerning data in immunocompromised adults who had hematologic malignancies, in whom DFA testing on specimens from throat swabs and nasopharyngeal washing had a sensitivity of only 15%. When applied to specimens from BAL, the DFA was 70% to 90% sensitive [39]. These results parallel those reported by Billings and colleagues [17], in which 67% of RSV diagnoses were made from BAL samples. The poor yield of DFA on easily obtained samples highlights the need for newer diagnostic tests or strategies. Preliminary data suggest that real-time PCR may have a sensitivity of greater than 90% for RSV infection [35]. There are no large series employing this diagnostic modality, however.

Table 2
Outcomes of respiratory syncytial virus infection in case series of hematopoietic stem cell transplant recipients published from 1997 to 2003

Reference	No. of cases	No. LRTI (%)	No. of deaths in LRTI (% of LRTI)	Treatment?
Ljungman [34]	46	27 (59)	11 (41)	No
Abdallah [27]	8	4 (50)	2 (50)	No
McCarthy [32]	26	15 (58)	5 (33)	No
Bowden [37]	88	35 (40)	24 (69)	No
Machado [4]	18	10 (55)	1 (10)	Yes
Small [28]	58	25 (43)	3 (12)	Yes, in majority
Whimbey [11]	33	20 (61)	12 (60)	No
Lujan-Zilbermann [6]	5	0 (0)	0 (0)	No
Ljungman [1]	19	15 (79)	6 (40)	No
Chakrabarti [5]	13	6 (46)	0 (0)	Yes
Sparrelid [38]	6	4 (67)	2 (50)	Yes
Total not treated	**225**	**116 (52)**	**60 (52)**	**No**
Total treated	**95**	**45 (47)**	**6 (13)**	**Yes**
Total	**320**	**161 (50)**	**66 (41)**	**[Mixed]**

Abbreviation: LRTI, lower respiratory tract infection.

As with other PCR testing, there may be issues with false-positive tests (in this case, defined as a positive PCR for RSV when RSV is not the true cause of the patient's symptomatology), and the definition of an appropriate criterion standard test may prove difficult in future studies. One recent series used real-time PCR on all samples, and found four cases of RSV, three of which were missed by viral culture and were found only by real-time PCR [7]. Serology has a reported sensitivity of up to 80% but is not commercially available [35].

Treatment

Ribavirin, a synthetic guanosine analogue, is an antiviral agent with activity against RSV. Its exact role in the treatment of HSCT or SOT recipients who have RSV infection remains unclear, however. Dozens of studies using ribavirin in various forms—intravenous, oral, or aerosolized—and at different points in the illness now have been reported. Although generalization of so many studies is difficult, the preponderance of data suggests a benefit to ribavirin therapy, which may be augmented by the addition of nonspecific or RSV-specific intravenous immune globulin. This benefit has been demonstrated best in trials using aerosolized ribavirin, in contrast with decidedly mixed evidence for oral or intravenous ribavirin. This combination therapy is now endorsed in several sets of consensus guidelines [40,41], although most of the data on which this recommendation is made are from experience in treatment of HSCT recipients. The reader is referred to the excellent review by Englund and colleagues [36] for a detailed summary of 17 years of ribavirin trials for RSV infection through 1996.

Despite the recommendations in favor of ribavirin therapy for RSV, the patient population that might benefit most from the therapy has not been identified definitively. As noted previously, morbidity and mortality from RSV are linked to progression of infection to the lower respiratory tract. Several investigators, therefore, have sought to use ribavirin-based therapy for the treatment of documented RSV URI. Recent series by Ghosh and colleagues [42] and Small and colleagues [28] have demonstrated low rates of progression to pneumonia in HSCT recipients who had RSV URI and who received early therapy with ribavirin and intravenous immune globulin. Antiviral treatment of RSV URI is specifically not recommended by the American Society of Transplantation, however [40]. In the Ghosh [42] and Small [28] series, those patients progressing to pneumonia while receiving therapy also had low mortality rates in comparison with historical controls. Interestingly, the benefit of therapy for established pneumonia, which is recommended in the guidelines, has not been as clear in the literature [40]. Mortality rates in SOT or HSCT recipients who had respiratory failure caused by RSV pneumonia have been estimated at 90%, however [36], and at least one consensus group does not favor treatment at that late stage [41].

It is important to highlight the potential difficulties of administering aerosolized ribavirin, which requires a small-particle nebulizer machine that may not be present in all hospitals. In addition, ribavirin is teratogenic, so pregnant women may not enter the room of a patient receiving the therapy. Those who do enter the room (including the patient) may develop a number of bothersome side effects from exposure to the drug, including headache, rash, and conjunctivitis [41]. These potential barriers to drug delivery are best addressed in advance if a provider group wishes to ensure timely administration of the drug when a patient is identified.

Parainfluenza virus

Epidemiology

PIV and RSV are both members of the paramyxovirus family, but, unlike RSV, there are four major serotypes of PIV that cause disease in humans. PIV-1 and PIV-2 cause annual winter outbreaks in a pattern similar to RSV or influenza, whereas PIV-3 circulates in low levels year-round, with epidemic spread frequently seen in the spring or summer [19]. PIV-1 and PIV-2 are the classic causes of childhood croup, whereas PIV-3 is more associated with adult disease and with LRTI or pneumonia. The epidemiology of PIV-4 is not clearly defined, because it is the least commonly isolated serotype. As in the case of RSV, epidemics of PIV are frequently reported both in the community and in dedicated HSCT units and have been the cause of significant morbidity and mortality [14,43]. Data on factors contributing to epidemics in these settings are limited; one series reported PIV shedding for 4 months in two HSCT recipients [18].

PIV infections account for 10% to 50% of CARV infections in recent case series of HSCT and SOT recipients (see Table 1) [1–8]. Two excellent longitudinal surveys of PIV infection in HSCT recipients were published in 2001 [18,19]. Nichols and col-leagues [19] at the Fred Hutchinson Cancer Research Center reviewed 3577 HSCT recipients who received transplants between 1990 and 1999 and found 253 (7.1%) PIV infections. Of these, PIV-3 accounted for 90%, PIV-1 for 6%, and PIV-2 for 4%. Elizaga and colleagues [18] in London similarly reviewed 456 HSCT recipients from 1990 to 1996 and found 24 (5.3%) with PIV-3 infection. Unlike most reports of RSV in HSCT recipients, PIV was found with similar frequency in recipients of allogeneic (5.2%) and autologous (5.5%) HSCT [18]. Among SOT recipients, case series of PIV have been reported in renal transplant [17] and lung transplant recipients [21–23]. Between 1.6% and 11.9% of lung transplant recipients may develop PIV infection, although some may be asymptomatic infections detected during frequent bronchoscopies [22]. In lung transplant recipients, PIV-3 accounted for 63% of PIV isolates, PIV-1 for 29%, and PIV-2 for 8% [23].

Clinical features and diagnosis

Cough is the hallmark symptom of PIV infection, but other URI symptoms (eg, rhinorrhea) may be absent. Fever is uncommon: in lung transplant recipients who have PIV LRTI, only 17% to 35% are febrile [23,25].

The frequency of LRTI in recent series of PIV infection in HSCT recipients is reviewed in Table 3 [1,5,11,18–20,37,38,43]. Overall, LRTI (as either the presenting syndrome or as progression from URI) is reported in one third of patients, and half of those with LRTI die, but considerable variability exists among series. Of patients in series with at least 10 cases of PIV infection, rates of LRTI vary from 18% to 77%, and mortality among patients who have LRTI varies from 15% to 73%. Importantly, both large reviews of PIV infection in HSCT recipients demon-

Table 3
Outcomes of parainfluenza virus infection in case series of hematopoietic stem cell transplant recipients published from 1997 to 2003

Reference	No. of cases	No. LRTI (%)	No. of deaths in LRTI (% of LRTI)
Nichols [19]	253	56 (22)	41 (73)
Elizaga [18]	24	14 (58)	8 (57)
Chakrabarti [5]	17	13 (76)	2 (15)
Whimbey [11]	45	26 (58)	10 (38)
Ljungman [1]	13	10 (77)	2 (20)
Sparrelid [38]	3	3 (100)	0 (0)
Chakrabarti [20]	5	4 (80)	0 (0)
Hohenthal [43]	5	2 (40)	0 (0)
Bowden [37]	38	7 (18)	4 (57)
Total	403	135 (33)	67 (50)

Abbreviation: LRTI, lower respiratory tract infection.

strated a 50% rate of bacterial or fungal coinfection in patients who have PIV pneumonia, emphasizing the need for comprehensive diagnostic testing in this population [18,19].

The diagnosis of PIV infection usually is made with IFA or DFA testing of respiratory secretions, along with viral culture. It is notable that most widely available fluorescent antibody tests for PIV do not test for PIV-4, which may explain in part why there has been only one reported case in an HSCT recipient [44]. Although real-time PCR testing is being developed, there are not yet sufficient data to permit comment on its relative usefulness in comparison with conventional testing.

Treatment

Ribavirin has activity against PIV, and a number of smaller recent reports in which ribavirin was given to all HSCT recipients who had PIV have demonstrated LRTI and mortality rates lower than historical controls [5,20,25,38,43]. The two largest series, however, demonstrated no benefit of ribavirin given alone or in combination with intravenous immune globulin [18,19]. Furthermore, Nichols and colleagues [19] demonstrated a failure of ribavirin therapy to shorten duration of shedding time. A recent consensus statement from the Infectious Disease Community of Practice of the American Society of Transplantation recommends for PIV LRTI that providers "consider aerosolized ribavirin as no other options exist but experience to date provides little evidence for efficacy" [40].

Influenza virus

Epidemiology

Influenza, an orthomyxovirus, is one of the most common community-acquired respiratory viruses and is a significant cause of morbidity in transplant recipients. The actual incidence of influenza in transplant recipients is unknown; many cases are likely undiagnosed, and case reports of influenza illness probably overestimate the severity of illness in this population. Although most cases of influenza are acquired in community settings, nosocomial acquisition has been noted in both SOT and HSCT units. Because nosocomial acquisition often is associated with earlier acquisition after transplantation, these cases are more likely to result in worse outcomes.

Influenza occurs on a seasonal basis, with the vast majority of cases occurring during winter months.

Both influenza A and B have been described in transplant recipients; the distribution of these infections mirrors community patterns of infection. Influenza virus has been reported to be a significant pathogen in both HSCT and SOT recipients; among SOT recipients, lung transplant recipients may be at special risk for infection [45,46]. Transplant recipients have been documented to have persistent influenza viral shedding, serving as a potentially significant reservoir of virus that can spread to others in both community and institutional settings [47,48].

Clinical features and diagnosis

The timing of influenza infection with respect to transplantation significantly affects the outcome of infection, with more severe infection occurring in the earlier posttransplantation period. In most cases, upper respiratory tract symptoms predominate. Lower respiratory tract involvement is uncommon. Other complications of influenza include bacterial superinfection, central nervous system involvement, myocarditis, and transplant rejection [49,50]. Influenza mortality remains low.

Influenza should be suspected in any individual presenting with fever, rhinorrhea, coryza, myalgia, and headache during the winter months. Diagnosis of influenza typically relies on isolation of the virus, either by fluorescent antibody techniques (DFA or IFA) or by viral culture of nasal and oropharyngeal epithelial cell samples obtained by nasal lavage (in pediatric patients) or swab sampling [40,51]. Alternatively, BAL specimens can be assayed. Serologic diagnoses are retrospective and may be limited by impairment of humoral responses in recent HSCT recipients or SOT recipients, especially those receiving mycophenolate mofetil.

Treatment

There are several antiviral agents with demonstrated efficacy against influenza, most of which have been used to varying degrees in transplant recipients [46,52]. Amantadine and rimantadine have antiviral activity limited to influenza A; oseltamivir and zanamivir have activity against both influenza A and B. To date, no significant drug interactions have been reported with any of these medications and immunosuppressive therapies including calcineurin inhibitors. The recommended dosages and duration of treatment are the same as those for the normal host. Antiviral resistance has been reported rarely in transplant recipients [47], but there are currently no specific recommendations for altering antiviral therapy.

Adenovirus

Epidemiology

There are several fundamental differences between adenovirus infection and infection with the other common CARVs. Adenovirus may be acquired by person-to-person transmission as a primary respiratory tract infection, as is the norm for RSV or PIV. Most adenovirus disease in immunocompromised patients, however, is probably reactivation of latent infection. In addition, adenovirus infection can produce a wide variety of clinical syndromes—gastroenteritis, hepatitis, and hemorrhagic cystitis—in addition to respiratory tract illness. These patterns of illness may vary by host and by adenovirus serotypes [53].

Adenovirus infections account for 0% to 21% of CARV infections in recent large case series (see Table 1) [1–8]. In general, adenovirus is more common in children, in whom infection with a new serotype may be primary infection and more likely to produce true clinical disease. Although adenovirus may be the least commonly reported of the four main CARV infections in these series, it is important to recall that most of these series test patients who had symptomatic URI; the true incidence of adenovirus infection in these patient populations probably would be higher if other clinical manifestations were included.

Clinical features and diagnosis

In general, three patterns of adenovirus infection are described in HSCT and SOT recipients who have positive sputum testing for adenovirus infection: (1) asymptomatic; (2) symptomatic respiratory tract infection; and (3) disseminated disease, with or without respiratory tract involvement. Mortality from adenovirus clearly is tied to dissemination of the infection, but dissemination does not require progressive respiratory tract infection. Therefore, unlike RSV or PIV infections, many cases of fatal adenovirus infection are reported in patients who have adenovirus isolated from the upper respiratory tract only and without radiographic evidence of pneumonia or positive testing from lower respiratory tract samples [11,15].

Outcomes from adenovirus respiratory tract infection after HSCT have been poor. Four recent series describe mortality rates ranging from 38% to 100%, with a cumulative mortality of 56% (30 of 54 cases) [1,2,11,15]. Although mortality from adenovirus pneumonia is high, it is noteworthy that one third of these deaths occurred in patients who had adenovirus URI without evidence of pneumonia.

Fewer cases of adenovirus infection have been reported in SOT recipients, but details presented in some reports shed important light on the nature of the disease in this population. McGrath and colleagues [54] performed the largest review of adenovirus infection in adult liver transplant recipients and showed an overall incidence rate of 5.8%. Four (36%) of their 11 patients who had positive cultures were asymptomatic. Of the seven who had clinical disease, three had pneumonia, but all had evidence of disseminated disease, making it unclear if the pneumonia was a primary event or the result of dissemination of uncontrolled infection. Therefore, it is unclear if any patients in this series had a true, newly community-acquired respiratory tract infection with adenovirus.

Several papers have reviewed the potential significance of adenovirus infection in lung transplant recipients. Approximately 1% to 3% of lung transplant recipients may develop adenovirus infection in longitudinal studies [16,21,55,56]. In many of these patients, adenovirus has been tied closely to graft failure and to acute and chronic rejection, but the numbers of patients involved prevent rigorous statistical analysis or the ability to draw a firm conclusion. In the two largest recent series examining the potential link between BOS and CARV infection, for example, adenovirus accounted for only 2 of 61 isolates [8,13].

Adenovirus infection may be diagnosed using the widely available immunofluorescent antibody kits. This test is insensitive for adenovirus in sputum, however, with a reported sensitivity of perhaps 50% in immunocompetent hosts. Given that DFA and IFA are the most commonly used assays, this lack of sensitivity may explain, in part, the relative infrequency of adenovirus in some surveys of CARV infection. The virus can be cultured as well and is identified readily by characteristic smudge cells on histopathology. Because adenovirus frequently may be a reactivation disease, more sensitive assays, perhaps PCR based, may detect the infection more frequently. Further study is needed to determine whether patients who have more indolent adenovirus replication actually have clinical disease, or whether another pathogen is responsible for the clinical presentation.

Treatment

The widely reported high mortality rates from adenoviral infection, particularly in the early post-transplantation period, have prompted many clinicians to push for early and aggressive treatment of documented adenovirus infections in HSCT and SOT recipients. Unfortunately, there are limited data to support the efficacy of available therapeutics. Recently cidofivir has been shown to improve outcomes in small studies of children after HSCT and has had anecdotal reports of success in adults. Because of the significant risk of nephrotoxicity associated with cidofivir, this agent should be used with caution in transplant recipients who may be at increased risk for renal impairment. Although both have been tried in the past, neither ribavirin nor ganciclovir has demonstrated significant efficacy; consequently, neither agent is recommended [53].

Two recent articles have questioned the need for treatment in all patients who have documented adenovirus infections. Walls and colleagues [57] recently reported the results of retrospective testing for adenovirus in 26 consecutive pediatric HSCT recipients. In this series, 11 children had at least one positive test for adenovirus, but 7 of the 11 spontaneously cleared the infection without antiviral therapy. Two children died of disseminated disease, and each first tested positive in the first 2 weeks after HSCT. A recent prospective monitoring study by van Kraaij and colleagues [9] in HSCT recipients also demonstrated several cases of early but asymptomatic adenovirus infection.

Miscellaneous respiratory viruses

Rhinovirus

The rhinoviruses (comprised of more than 100 serotypes) are among the most common causes of the common cold in immunocompetent adults and children. Only a few studies have addressed their potential role as respiratory pathogens in SOT and HSCT recipients, but the available data suggest that rhinovirus infection may be underappreciated. Four studies of prospective active surveillance for CARV infection—one in adult lung transplant recipients [56], one in pediatric HSCT recipients [15], and two in adult HSCT recipients [7,9]—noted rhinovirus infection in their cohorts; in two studies, rhinovirus was the most common isolate. In these groups, most rhinovirus infections were asymptomatic, but, taken together, three other longitudinal studies of HSCT recipients who had symptomatic respiratory tract infection identified rhinovirus in a total of 42 (27%) of 157 isolates [3,37]. Of these 42 reported cases of symptomatic rhinovirus respiratory tract infection, 7 (17%) progressed to LRTI, and two (29% of LRTI)

deaths were attributed to rhinovirus pneumonia. Several of these series used real-time PCR for viral surveillance; as this newer diagnostic technology becomes more widely used, the true epidemiology and impact of rhinovirus infections in HSCT or SOT recipients will become clearer. At present, there is no specific antiviral therapy available for the treatment of rhinovirus infections.

Coronavirus

Coronaviruses, like rhinoviruses, are frequent causes of benign URI occurring in annual wintertime community outbreaks. Laboratory isolation of these agents is difficult, so no systematic study of their possible role in LRTI in HSCT or SOT recipients has been undertaken [11]. The recent experience with the newly identified causative agent of severe acute respiratory syndrome (SARS), SARS coronavirus, bears mention. Kumar and colleagues [58] in Toronto reported a liver transplant recipient who died from SARS. A study of tissue obtained at autopsy revealed that a dramatically higher concentration of the SARS coronavirus was present in this patient's tissues than in those of other case patients, suggesting both a reason for the fatal course and the possible role of immunosuppressed patients as 'super-spreaders' of the epidemic.

Herpes viruses

Nearly all viruses in the herpes virus family have been reported as occasional causes of pneumonia in HSCT and SOT recipients. Herpes simplex virus type 1 (HSV-1) will reactivate almost universally after HSCT or SOT in the 70% to 80% of adults with latent infection, and several reports have documented pneumonia, occasionally fatal, from this pathogen [56,59–61]. HSV-1 is suppressed effectively by agents used for cytomegalovirus prophylaxis, however, and reports of HSV-1 pneumonia have greatly decreased in the era of universal prophylaxis. At most centers, prophylactic acyclovir is given to suppress reactivation of herpes simplex disease even when the recipient and the donor are cytomegalovirus negative. Similarly, acyclovir and ganciclovir are active against varicella-zoster virus (VZV), which has been reported as a rare cause of pneumonia in SOT or HSCT recipients [56,59,61]. VZV may reactivate at any point in the posttransplantation course, and shingles is a common disease in all immunosuppressed populations. Because most cases of VZV pneumonia in HSCT or SOT recipients are preceded by the characteristic vesicular skin rash [61], and because

VZV pneumonia is rare, it is assumed that prompt antiviral therapy with acyclovir can abort the progression of reactivation disease to pneumonia. VZV pneumonia may be more of a concern in children or adult patients who have no innate immunity to VZV from either natural exposure or previous vaccination, because primary VZV infection is more likely to cause pneumonia.

Finally, the roles of human herpesvirus 6 and human herpesvirus 7 (HHV-7) as pulmonary pathogens remain poorly understood. Active replication with both viruses can be detected, probably as reactivation of latent infection, in 20% to 50% of HSCT or SOT recipients [62]. Several authors have reported isolation of human herpesvirus 6 from sputum or lung tissue in patients who have otherwise idiopathic pneumonia after HSCT [62–64]. The overall data, however, conflict as to whether a causative role can be established [62,65]. Ross and colleagues [66] have reported HHV-7 in seven (100%) of seven lung transplant recipients who had early bronchiolitis obliterans with organizing pneumonia and in three (75%) of four patients who had diffuse alveolar damage. In this series, HHV-7 was detected in 5 (19%) of 26 lung transplant recipients who had no pathology on biopsy and in 2 (14%) of 14 patients who had acute or chronic rejection (ie, BOS). These findings are thought-provoking and confirm the need for further research into the potential role of HHV-7 as a single or copathogen for certain patterns of pulmonary disease.

Prevention of community-acquired respiratory virus infection

Given that CARV infections in HSCT or SOT recipients occur frequently and are associated with poor outcomes, attention must be given to the prevention of CARV infection. Recommendations for a multifaceted approach to the prevention of morbidity and mortality from these infections are presented in Box 1.

Any approach to the prevention of CARV infection must start with appropriate hand hygiene. With the possible exception of influenza [67], which may be transmitted in part by aerosolized droplets, CARV infections are transmitted by larger droplet particles that are introduced to the host oropharynx from the hands. Regular hand washing with attention to hand washing before food preparation or meals significantly reduces the incidence of CARV infection. In the inpatient setting, the widespread availability of alcohol-based hand-washing products has reduced the transmission of most hospital-acquired infections.

Additional infection control measures are recommended to prevent the spread of CARV infections on inpatient units. The Centers for Disease Control and Prevention recommend contact isolation for all patients who have CARV infection [67]. In addition, droplet precautions should be taken in the rooms of patients who have adenovirus or influenza respiratory tract infections. Importantly, patients should be placed under special precautions when the infections are first suspected, not when they are first confirmed, to limit the exposure of other patients and staff to infectious droplets [67]. These measures have been used successfully on a number of occasions to limit nosocomial spread of CARV infections. One group reported an 81% reduction in RSV cases on a HSCT unit with institution of droplet precautions and with cohorting case patients [30]. Many authorities, including the Centers for Disease Control and Prevention, advocate strongly for restricting visitors during the winter months as well [29,67].

Infection with many CARVs produces a measurable, type-specific antibody response. This response is neither long lasting nor protective [17]. Unfortunately, trials of active vaccination for RSV or PIV have been disappointing, including trials of subunit vaccines and live attenuated viruses [36]. Cortez and colleagues [68] recently reported on the use of passive vaccination (pavilizumab) in 54 allogeneic bone marrow transplant recipients. Although titers of RSV-specific immune globulins were increased, no difference in the rates of RSV infection were observed.

Prevention of influenza in transplant recipients has been focused on vaccination, and transplant recipients are among the immunosuppressed hosts targeted for influenza vaccination [69]. The standard inactivated vaccine is composed of two influenza A and one influenza B strain. Vaccine composition varies annually based on predicted antigenic drifts and shifts in circulating virus; consequently, annual reimmunization is recommended for optimal protection. Live attenuated intranasal influenza vaccine is not recommended for immunosuppressed hosts, including transplant recipients, or for family or health care providers who are in close contact with the patients. Numerous studies over several decades have examined vaccine responses in transplant recipients and have demonstrated conflicting results. In general, both humoral and cellular vaccine responses seem to be suboptimal when compared with healthy controls and cannot be reliably predicted based on the level of

---

Box 1. Approaches to reducing morbidity and mortality from community-acquired respiratory virus infections in hematopoietic stem cell transplant or solid organ transplant recipients

Prevention of CARV infection

  Careful hand hygiene, especially during fall and winter months
  Vaccination of patients and close contacts (particularly for influenza)
  Avoidance of contact with patients who have symptomatic URI
  Patient education (eg, how CARV infection is spread, how to avoid sick contacts, how to perform appropriate hand hygiene)

Diagnosis of CARV infection

  Combination nasal/throat swab fluorescent antibody testing in early URI
  Consideration of bronchoscopy for BAL sample if symptoms progress or in any HSCT or SOT patient with an unexplained LRTI or pneumonia
  Routine testing for CARV infection in all SOT or HSCT recipients presenting with pneumonia, including those patients who have an already identified bacterial or fungal pathogen
  Expanded use of newer diagnostic tools (eg, real-time PCR)
  Awareness of seasonal patterns of CARV infection and of circulating viruses in the local community
  Patient education (eg, regarding need to contact a physician when URI symptoms occur)

Prevention of CARV LRTI

  Consideration of pre-emptive antiviral therapy for RSV or PIV URI in the early posttransplantation period
  Specific antiviral therapy for influenza

Treatment of established CARV LRTI or pneumonia

  Specific antiviral therapy for influenza
  Aerosolized ribavirin therapy for RSV, possibly in combination with intravenous immune globulin
  Appropriate therapy for bacterial or fungal coinfections

Prevention of CARV outbreaks

  Strict adherence to infection-control guidelines in hospitals, including attention to hand hygiene and contact, droplet, or aerosol isolation as dictated by accepted guidelines
  Consideration of cohorting patients on inpatient units
  Active surveillance or case finding by infection control personnel
  Careful monitoring of staff and visitors for symptoms of URI, particularly during times of heightened CARV prevalence in the community
  Separation of sick from healthy patients in outpatient waiting areas

---

immunosuppression [70–73]. Anecdotal reports have suggested a potential linkage between vaccination and organ rejection; however, this association has not been supported by the majority of studies examining the immunogenicity of vaccine in SOT recipients. Current recommendations support annual vaccination of all SOT recipients, although it is likely that those with more recent transplants may be less likely to respond to vaccine. HSCT recipients may be especially poor vaccine responders within the first 2 years after transplantation [46]. Prophylactic administration of licensed antiviral agents (including oseltamivir and zanamavir) may serve as an alternative preventive measure for individuals who are unable to receive influenza vaccination (eg, those with egg allergy) or who are anticipated to be especially unlikely to respond to vaccine [74]. Although not specifically studied in transplant recipients, these antiviral agents have been demonstrated to be effective in preventing the acquisition of influenza when administered to immunocompetent individuals during periods of peak influenza activity [69]. Because transplant recipients may be suboptimal vaccine responders and are at increased risk for adverse outcomes from influenza, consideration should be given to immunization of household contacts before the influenza season.

Summary

CARVs are frequent causes of both URI and LRTI in HSCT or SOT recipients. In most series, RSV and PIV are the most common CARVs. Significant morbidity and mortality are associated with these infections, particularly when they progress to LRTI. Outcomes are also poor with adenovirus, frequently reflecting disseminated infection. Efforts to prevent morbidity and mortality from CARV infection should focus on prevention, because treatment options are limited, with inconclusive data to support their efficacy.

References

[1] Ljungman P. Respiratory virus infections in bone marrow recipients: the European perspective. Am J Med 1997;102:44–7.

[2] Raboni SM, Nogueira MB, Tsuchiya LRV, et al. Respiratory tract viral infections in bone marrow transplant patients. Transplantation 2003;76:142–6.

[3] Hassan IA, Chopra R, Swindell R, et al. Respiratory viral infections after bone marrow / peripheral stem-cell transplantation: the Christie hospital experience. Bone Marrow Transplant 2003;32:73–7.

[4] Machado CM, Boas LSV, Mendes AVA, et al. Low mortality rates related to respiratory virus infections after bone marrow transplantation. Bone Marrow Transplant 2003;31:695–700.

[5] Chakrabarti S, Avivi I, Mackinnon S, et al. Respiratory virus infections in transplant recipients after reduced-intensity conditioning with Campath-1H: high incidence but low mortality. Br J Haematol 2002;119: 1125–32.

[6] Lujan-Zilbermann J, Benaim E, Tong X, et al. Respiratory virus infections in pediatric hematopoietic stem cell transplantation. Clin Infect Dis 2001;33: 962–8.

[7] Roghmann M, Ball K, Erdman D, et al. Active

surveillance for respiratory virus infections in adults who have undergone bone marrow and peripheral blood stem cell transplantation. Bone Marrow Transplant 2003;32:1085–8.

[8] Khalifah AP, Hachem RR, Chakinala MM, et al. Respiratory viral infections are a distinct risk for bronchiolitis obliterans syndrome and death. Am J Respir Crit Care Med 2004;170:181–7.

[9] van Kraaij MGJ, van Elden LJR, van Loon AM, et al. Frequent detection of respiratory viruses in adult recipients of stem cell transplants with the use of real-time polymerase chain reaction, compared with viral culture. Clin Infect Dis 2005;40:662–9.

[10] Singhal S, Muir DA, Ratcliffe DA, et al. Respiratory viruses in adult liver transplant patients. Transplantation 1999;68:981–4.

[11] Whimbey E, Englund JA, Couch RB. Community respiratory virus infections in immunocompromised patients with cancer. Am J Med 1997;102:10–8.

[12] Wendt CH. Community respiratory viruses: organ transplant recipients. Am J Med 1997;102:31–6.

[13] Billings JL, Hertz MI, Savik K, et al. Respiratory viruses and chronic rejection in lung transplant recipients. J Heart Lung Transplant 2002;21:559–66.

[14] McCann S, Byrne JL, Rovira M, et al. Outbreaks of infectious diseases in stem cell transplant units: a silent cause of death for patients and transplant programmes. Bone Marrow Transplant 2004;33:519–29.

[15] Bredius RGM, Templeton KE, Scheltinga SA, et al. Prospective study of respiratory viral infections in pediatric hemopoietic stem cell transplantation patients. Pediatr Infect Dis J 2004;23:518–22.

[16] Palmer SM, Henshaw NG, Howell DN, et al. Community respiratory viral infection in adult lung transplant recipients. Chest 1998;113:944–50.

[17] Billings JL, Hertz MI, Wendt CH. Community respiratory virus infections following lung transplantation. Transpl Infect Dis 2001;3:138–48.

[18] Elizaga J, Olavarria E, Apperley JF, et al. Parainfluenza virus 3 infection after stem cell transplant: relevance to outcome of rapid diagnosis and ribavirin treatment. Clin Infect Dis 2001;32:413–8.

[19] Nichols WG, Corey L, Gooley T, et al. Parainfluenza virus infections after hematopoietic stem cell transplantation: risk factors, response to antiviral therapy, and effect on transplant outcome. Blood 2001;98: 573–8.

[20] Chakrabarti S, Collingham KE, Holder K, et al. Parainfluenza virus type 3 infections in hematopoietic stem cell transplant recipients: response to ribavirin therapy. Clin Infect Dis 2000;31:1516–8.

[21] Vilchez RA, Dauber J, Kusne S. Infectious etiology of bronchiolitis obliterans: the respiratory viruses connection—myth or reality? Am J Transplant 2003;3:245–9.

[22] Vilchez RA, Dauber J, McCurry K, et al. Parainfluenza virus infection in adult lung transplant recipients: an emergent clinical syndrome with implications on allograft function. Am J Transplant 2003;3:116–20.

[23] Vilchez RA, McCurry K, Dauber J, et al. The

epidemiology of parainfluenza virus infection in lung transplant recipients. Clin Infect Dis 2001;33: 2004–8.

[24] Garbino J, Gerbase MW, Wunderli W, et al. Respiratory viruses and severe lower respiratory tract complications in hospitalized patients. Chest 2004;125: 1033–9.

[25] McCurdy LH, Milstone A, Dummer S. Clinical features and outcomes of paramyxoviral infection in lung transplant recipients treated with ribavirin. J Heart Lung Transplant 2003;22:745–53.

[26] Anaissie EJ, Mahfouz TH, Aslan T, et al. The natural history of respiratory syncytial virus infection in cancer and transplant patients: implications for management. Blood 2004;103:1611–7.

[27] Abdallah A, Rowland KE, Schepetiuk SK, et al. An outbreak of respiratory syncytial virus infection in a bone marrow transplant unit: effect on engraftment and outcome of pneumonia without specific antiviral treatment. Bone Marrow Transplant 2003;32:195–203.

[28] Small TN, Casson A, Malak SF, et al. Respiratory syncytial virus infection following hematopoietic stem cell transplantation. Bone Marrow Transplant 2002;29: 321–7.

[29] Hall CB. Nosocomial respiratory syncytial virus infections: the "cold war" has not ended. Clin Infect Dis 2000;31:590–6.

[30] Raad I, Abbas J, Whimbey E. Infection control of nosocomial respiratory viral disease in the immuno-compromised host. Am J Med 1997;102:48–52.

[31] Ghosh S, Champlin RE, Ueno NT, et al. Respiratory syncytial virus infections in autologous blood and marrow transplant recipients with breast cancer: combination therapy with aerosolized ribavirin and parenteral immunoglobulins. Bone Marrow Transplant 2001;28:271–5.

[32] McCarthy AJ, Kingman HM, Kelly C, et al. The outcome of 26 patients with respiratory syncytial virus infection following allogeneic stem cell transplantation. Bone Marrow Transplant 1999;24:1315–22.

[33] Khushalani NI, Bakri FG, Wentling D, et al. Respiratory syncytial virus infection in the late bone marrow transplant period: report of three cases and review. Bone Marrow Transplant 2001;27:1071–3.

[34] Ljungman P, Ward KN, Crooks BNA, et al. Respiratory virus infections after stem cell transplantation: a prospective study from the Infectious Diseases Working Party of the European Group for Blood and Marrow Transplantation. Bone Marrow Transplant 2001;28:479–84.

[35] Falsey AR, Walsh EE. Respiratory syncytial virus infection in adults. Clin Microbiol Rev 2000;13:371–84.

[36] Englund JA, Piedra PA, Whimbey E. Prevention and treatment of respiratory syncytial virus and parainfluenza viruses in immunocompromised patients. Am J Med 1997;102:61–70.

[37] Bowden RA. Respiratory virus infections after marrow transplant: the Fred Hutchinson Cancer Research Center experience. Am J Med 1997;102:27–30.

[38] Sparrelid E, Ljungman P, Ekelof-Andstrom E, et al. Ribavirin therapy in bone marrow transplant recipients with viral respiratory tract infections. Bone Marrow Transplant 1997;19:905–8.

[39] Englund JA, Piedra PA, Jewell A, et al. Rapid diagnosis of respiratory syncytial virus infections in immunocompromised patients. J Clin Microbiol 1996; 34:1649–53.

[40] Community-acquired respiratory viruses. Am J Transplant 2004;4:105–9.

[41] Swedish Consensus Group. Management of infections caused by respiratory syncytial virus. Scand J Infect Dis 2001;33:323–8.

[42] Ghosh S, Champlin RE, Englund JA, et al. Respiratory syncytial virus upper respiratory tract illnesses in adult blood and marrow transplant recipients: combination therapy with aerosolized ribavirin and intravenous immunoglobulin. Bone Marrow Transplant 2000;25: 751–5.

[43] Hohenthal U, Nikoskelainen J, Vainionpaa R, et al. Parainfluenza virus type 3 infections in a hematology unit. Bone Marrow Transplant 2001;27:295–300.

[44] Miall F, Rye A, Fraser M, et al. Human parainfluenza type 4 infection: a case report highlighting pathogenicity and difficulties in rapid diagnosis in the post-transplant setting. Bone Marrow Transplant 2002;29: 541–2.

[45] Vilchez RA, Fung J, Kusne S. The pathogenesis and management of influenza virus infection in organ transplant recipients. Transplant Infectious Diseases 2002;4:177–82.

[46] Hayden FG. Prevention and treatment of influenza in immunocompromised patients. Am J Med 1997;102: 55–60.

[47] Weinstock DM, Gubareva LV, Zuccotti G. Prolonged shedding of multidrug-resistant influenza A virus in an immunocompromised patient. N Engl J Med 2003; 348:867–8.

[48] Apalsh AM, Green M, Ledesma-Medina J, et al. Parainfluenza and influenza virus infection in pediatric organ transplant recipients. Clin Infect Dis 1994;20: 394–9.

[49] Vilchez RA, McCurry K, Dauber J, et al. Influenza virus infection in adult solid organ transplant recipients. Am J Transplant 2002;2:287–91.

[50] Mauch TJ, Bratton S, Myers T, et al. Influenza B virus infection in pediatric solid organ transplant recipients. Pediatrics 1994;94:225–9.

[51] Hopkins PM, Plit ML, Carter IW, et al. Indirect fluorescent antibody testing of nasopharyngeal swabs for influenza diagnosis in lung transplant recipients. J Heart Lung Transplant 2003;22:161–8.

[52] Machado CM, Boas LSV, Mendes AVA, et al. Use of oseltamivir to control influenza complications after bone marrow transplantation. Bone Marrow Transplant 2004;34:111–4.

[53] Adenovirus. Am J Transplant 2004;4:101–4.

[54] McGrath D, Falagas ME, Freeman R, et al. Adenovirus infection in adult orthotopic liver transplant recipi-

ents: incidence and clinical significance. J Infect Dis 1998;177:459–62.

[55] Ohori NP, Michaels MG, Jaffe R, et al. Adenovirus pneumonia in lung transplant recipients. Hum Pathol 1995;26:1073–9.

[56] Holt ND, Gould FK, Taylor CE, et al. Incidence and significance of noncytomegalovirus viral respiratory infection after adult lung transplantation. J Heart Lung Transplant 1997;16:416–9.

[57] Walls T, Hawrami K, Ushiro-Lumb I, et al. Adenovirus infection after pediatric bone marrow transplantation: is treatment always necessary? Clin Infect Dis 2005; 40:1244–9.

[58] Kumar D, Tellier R, Draker R, et al. Severe acute respiratory syndrome (SARS) in a liver transplant recipient and guidelines for donor SARS screening. Am J Transplant 2003;3:977–81.

[59] Anderson DJ, Jordan MC. Viral pneumonia in recipients of solid organ transplants. Semin Respir Infect 1990;5:38–49.

[60] Liebau P, Kuse E, Winkler M, et al. Management of herpes simplex virus type 1 pneumonia following liver transplantation. Infection 1996;24:130–5.

[61] Taplitz RA, Jordan MC. Pneumonia caused by herpesviruses in recipients of hematopoietic cell transplants. Semin Respir Infect 2002;17:121–9.

[62] Yoshikawa T. Human herpesvirus-6 and -7 infections in transplantation. Pediatr Transplant 2003;7:11–7.

[63] Cone RW, Hackman RC, Huang MLW, et al. Human herpesvirus 6 in lung tissue from patients with pneumonitis after bone marrow transplantation. N Engl J Med 1993;329:156–61.

[64] Buchbinder S, Elmaagacli AH, Schaefer UW, et al. Human herpesvirus 6 is an important pathogen in infectious lung disease after allogeneic bone marrow transplantation. Bone Marrow Transplant 2000;26: 639–44.

[65] Kadakia MP, Rybka WB, Stewart JA, et al. Human herpesvirus 6: infection and disease following autologous and allogeneic bone marrow transplantation. Blood 1996;87:5341–54.

[66] Ross DJ, Chan RCK, Kubak B, et al. Bronchiolitis obliterans with organizing pneumonia: possible association with human herpesvirus-7 infection after lung transplantation. Transplant Proc 2001;33:2603–6.

[67] Centers for Disease Control and Prevention. Guidelines for preventing health-care-associated pneumonia, 2003: recommendations of CDC and the Healthcare Infection Control Practices Advisory Committee. Morb Mortal Wkly Rep 2004;53:1–36.

[68] Cortez K, Murphy BR, Almeida KN, et al. Immuneglobulin prophylaxis of respiratory syncytial virus infection in patients undergoing stem-cell transplantation. J Infect Dis 2002;186:834–8.

[69] Harper SA, Fukuda K, Uyeki TM, et al. Prevention and control of influenza. Recommendations of the advisory committee on immunization practices (ACIP). Morb Mortal Wkly Rep 2004;53:1–40.

[70] Blumberg EA, Albano C, Pruett T, et al. The immunogenicity of influenza virus vaccine in solid organ transplant recipients. Clin Infect Dis 1996;22: 295–302.

[71] Duchini A, Hendry RM, Nyberg LM, et al. Immune response to influenza vaccine in adult liver transplant recipients. Liver Transpl 2001;7:311–3.

[72] Mazzone PJ, Mossad SB, Mawhorter SD, et al. The humoral immune response to influenza vaccination in lung transplant recipients. Eur Respir J 2001;18:971–6.

[73] Mazzone PJ, Mossad SB, Mawhorter SD, et al. Cellmediated immune response to influenza vaccination in lung transplant recipients. J Heart Lung Transplant 2004;23:1175–81.

[74] Chik KW, Li CK, Chan PKS. Oseltamivir prophylaxis during the influenza season in a paediatric cancer centre: prospective observational study. Hong Kong Med J 2004;10:103–6.

ELSEVIER
SAUNDERS

Clin Chest Med 26 (2005) 721–739

CLINICS
IN CHEST
MEDICINE

Cumulative Index 2005

Note: Page numbers of article titles are in **boldface** type.

A

ACE. See *Angiotensin-converting enzyme (ACE).*

Acinetobacter sp.
  A. baumannii, VAP due to, 89–90
  VAP due to, mechanisms of resistance of, 76–77

Acremonium sp., in transplant recipients, 676, 677

Acute high-altitude pulmonary illness, in sojourners, 396–397

Acute lung injury (ALI), **105–112**
  altered immunity during, 106–107
  bacterial superinfection in animals with, 105–106

Acute lung injury, after HSCT, **561–569.** See also *Hematopoietic stem cell transplantation (HSCT), acute lung injury after.*

Acute mountain sickness, features of, 397

Acute respiratory distress syndrome (ARDS), VAP during, clinical studies of, 140

Acute respiratory failure, after transplantation, 623–624

Adaptive immunity, pneumonia in SOT recipients and, 114

Adenovirus, in transplant recipients, 714–715

Aerobic fitness, in divers, 489

Aerobic gram-negative pneumonia, CAP due to, 50

Aerobic gram-positive cocci, VAP due to, 91–92

Aerosol(s), inhaled, in microgravity studies, 432

Aerospace exposures, pulmonary function effects of, 492–493

Age
  advanced, as factor in delayed resolution of pneumonia, 147
  as factor in tuberculosis, 186

Aging, effects on respiratory system, **469–483.**
  See also *Respiratory system, aging effects on.*

Air travel, pulmonary function effects of, 493–499

Airspace consolidation
  after transplantation, 546–551
  defined, 546

Airway(s)
  artificial, colonization of, in pneumonia, 41–42
  extra-thoracic, limitations of, respiratory response to exercise and, 446–448
  intra-thoracic, limitations of, respiratory system response to exercise and, 448–453
  limitations of, exercise and, 453–454
  lower, colonization of, in pneumonia, 41
  peripheral, age-associated changes in, 472
  upper, injury of, after HSCT, 561

Airway resistance and conductance, in older persons, 476

ALI. See *Acute lung injury (ALI).*

Allograft rejection, after lung transplantation, **599–612.** See also *Lung transplantation, allograft rejection after.*

Altitude
  high
    drive to breathe at, 406
    respiration at, limits of, **405–414.** See also *High-altitude environment.*
  pulmonary effects of, 491
  terrestrial, pulmonary function effects of, 499–503

Alveolar ventilation, EIAH and, 463

Aminoglycoside(s), for active tuberculosis, 277

Amphotericin B, for *Aspergillus* pulmonary infections in transplant recipients, 667

Amplification, phage, in pulmonary tuberculosis diagnosis, 261–262

Anaerobe(s), VAP due to, 93

Anaerobic bacterial pneumonia, CAP due to, 50

United States Postal Service
Statement of Ownership, Management, and Circulation

1. Publication Title	2. Publication Number	3. Filing Date
Clinics in Chest Medicine	0 2 7 2 - 5 2 3 1	9/15/05

4. Issue Frequency	5. Number of Issues Published Annually	6. Annual Subscription Price
Mar, Jun, Sep, Dec	4	$185.00

7. Complete Mailing Address of Known Office of Publication (*Not printer*) (*Street, city, county, state, and ZIP+4*)

Elsevier Inc.
6277 Sea Harbor Drive
Orlando, FL 32887-4800

Contact Person
Gwen C. Campbell

Telephone
215-239-3685

8. Complete Mailing Address of Headquarters or General Business Office of Publisher (*Not printer*)

Elsevier Inc., 360 Park Avenue South, New York, NY 10010-1710

9. Full Names and Complete Mailing Addresses of Publisher, Editor, and Managing Editor (*Do not leave blank*)

Publisher (*Name and complete mailing address*)

Tim Griswold, Elsevier Inc., 1600 John F. Kennedy Blvd. Suite 1800, Philadelphia, PA 19103-2899

Editor (*Name and complete mailing address*)

Sarah Barth, Elsevier Inc., 1600 John F. Kennedy Blvd. Suite 1800, Philadelphia, PA 19103-2899

Managing Editor (*Name and complete mailing address*)

Heather Cullen, Elsevier Inc., 1600 John F. Kennedy Blvd. Suite 1800, Philadelphia, PA 19103-2899

10. Owner (*Do not leave blank. If the publication is owned by a corporation, give the name and address of the corporation immediately followed by the names and addresses of all stockholders owning or holding 1 percent or more of the total amount of stock. If not owned by a corporation, give the names and addresses of the individual owners. If owned by a partnership or other unincorporated firm, give its name and address as well as those of each individual owner. If the publication is published by a nonprofit organization, give its name and address.*)

Full Name	Complete Mailing Address
Wholly owned subsidiary of	4520 East-West Highway
Reed/Elsevier Inc., US holdings	Bethesda, MD 20814

11. Known Bondholders, Mortgagees, and Other Security Holders Owning or Holding 1 Percent or More of Total Amount of Bonds, Mortgages, or Other Securities. If none, check box ► ☐ None

Full Name	Complete Mailing Address
N/A	

12. Tax Status (*For completion by nonprofit organizations authorized to mail at nonprofit rates*) (*Check one*)
The purpose, function, and nonprofit status of this organization and the exempt status for federal income tax purposes:
☐ Has Not Changed During Preceding 12 Months
☐ Has Changed During Preceding 12 Months (*Publisher must submit explanation of change with this statement*)

(*See Instructions on Reverse*)

PS Form 3526, October 1999

---

13. Publication Title	14. Issue Date for Circulation Data Below
Clinics in Chest Medicine	June 2005

15. Extent and Nature of Circulation		Average No. Copies Each Issue During Preceding 12 Months	No. Copies of Single Issue Published Nearest to Filing Date
a. Total Number of Copies (*Net press run*)		5075	4900
b. Paid and/or Requested Circulation	(1) Paid/Requested Outside-County Mail Subscriptions Stated on Form 3541. (*Include advertiser's proof and exchange copies*)	2795	2746
	(2) Paid In-County Subscriptions Stated on Form 3541 (*Include advertiser's proof and exchange copies*)		
	(3) Sales Through Dealers and Carriers, Street Vendors, Counter Sales, and Other Non-USPS Paid Distribution	902	1001
	(4) Other Classes Mailed Through the USPS		
c. Total Paid and/or Requested Circulation [*Sum of 15b (1), (2), (3), and (4)*] ►		3697	3747
d. Free Distribution by Mail (*Samples, complimentary, and other free*)	(1) Outside-County as Stated on Form 3541	77	76
	(2) In-County as Stated on Form 3541		
	(3) Other Classes Mailed Through the USPS		
e. Free Distribution Outside the Mail (*Carriers or other means*)			
f. Total Free Distribution (*Sum of 15d. and 15e.*) ►		77	76
g. Total Distribution (*Sum of 15c. and 15f.*) ►		3774	3823
h. Copies not Distributed		1301	1077
i. Total (*Sum of 15g. and h.*) ►		5075	4900
j. Percent Paid and/or Requested Circulation (*15c. divided by 15g. times 100*)		98%	98%

16. Publication of Statement of Ownership
☐ Publication required. Will be printed in the **December 2005** issue of this publication. ☐ Publication not required

17. Signature and Title of Editor, Publisher, Business Manager, or Owner

[signature] Date 9/15/05

Jason Donatin - Executive Director of Subscription Services

I certify that all information furnished on this form is true and complete. I understand that anyone who furnishes false or misleading information on this form or who omits material or information requested on the form may be subject to criminal sanctions (including fines and imprisonment) and/or civil sanctions (including civil penalties).

Instructions to Publishers

1. Complete and file one copy of this form with your postmaster annually on or before October 1. Keep a copy of the completed form for your records.
2. In cases where the stockholder or security holder is a trustee, include in items 10 and 11 the name of the person or corporation for whom the trustee is acting. Also include the names and addresses of individuals who are stockholders who own or hold 1 percent or more of the total amount of bonds, mortgages, or other securities of the publishing corporation. In item 11, if none, check the box. Use blank sheets if more space is required.
3. Be sure to furnish all circulation information called for in item 15. Free circulation must be shown in items 15d, e, and f.
4. Item 15h, Copies not Distributed, must include (1) newsstand copies originally stated on Form 3541, and returned to the publisher, (2) estimated returns from news agents, and (3), copies for office use, leftovers, spoiled, and all other copies not distributed.
5. If the publication had Periodicals authorization as a general or requester publication, this Statement of Ownership, Management, and Circulation must be published; it must be printed in any issue in October or, if the publication is not published during October, the first issue printed after October.
6. In item 16, indicate the date of the issue in which this Statement of Ownership will be published.
7. Item 17 must be signed.
Failure to file or publish a statement of ownership may lead to suspension of Periodicals authorization.

PS Form 3526, October 1999 (Reverse)

Changing Your Address?

Make sure your subscription changes too! When you notify us of your new address, you can help make our job easier by including an exact copy of your Clinics label number with your old address (see illustration below.) This number identifies you to our computer system and will speed the processing of your address change. Please be sure this label number accompanies your old address and your corrected address—you can send an old Clinics label with your number on it or just copy it exactly and send it to the address listed below.

We appreciate your help in our attempt to give you continuous coverage. Thank you.

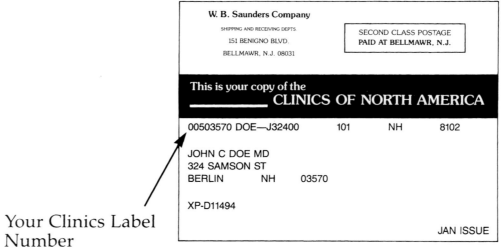

Your Clinics Label Number
Copy it exactly or send your label along with your address to:
W.B. Saunders Company, Customer Service
Orlando, FL 32887-4800
Call Toll Free 1-800-654-2452

Please allow four to six weeks for delivery of new subscriptions and for processing address changes.